616. 028076 HAL

Accession no.
01054756

£31.50

WITHDRAWN

PRINCIPLES OF
CRITICAL CARE

PreTest® Self-Assessment and Re...

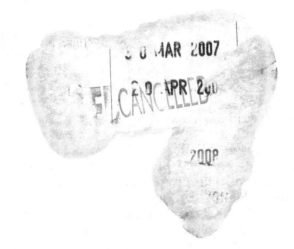

30 MAR 2007

CANCELLED APR 2

2008

NOTICE

Medicine is an ever-changing science. As new research and clinical experience broaden our knowledge, changes in treatment and drug therapy are required. The editors and the publisher of this work have checked with sources believed to be reliable in their efforts to provide information that is complete and generally in accord with the standards accepted at the time of publication. However, in view of the possibility of human error or changes in medical sciences, neither the editors nor the publisher nor any other party who has been involved in the preparation or publication of this work warrants that the information contained herein is in every respect accurate or complete, and they are not responsible for any errors or omissions or for the results obtained from use of such information. Readers are encouraged to confirm the information contained herein with other sources. For example and in particular, readers are advised to check the product information sheet included in the package of each drug they plan to administer to be certain that the information contained in this book is accurate and that changes have not been made in the recommended dose or in the contraindications for administration. This recommendation is of particular importance in connection with new or infrequently used drugs.

PRINCIPLES OF CRITICAL CARE

PreTest® Self-Assessment and Review

SECOND EDITION

Edited by

Jesse B. Hall, M.D.
Director of Critical Care Services
Professor of Anesthesiology & Critical Care and of Medicine
The University of Chicago, Chicago, Illinois

Gregory A. Schmidt, M.D.
Director of Academic Programs
Associate Professor of Anesthesiology & Critical Care and of Medicine
The University of Chicago, Chicago, Illinois

Lawrence D.H. Wood, M.D., Ph.D.
Faculty Dean of Medical Education,
Pritzker School of Medicine
Professor of Anesthesiology & Critical Care and of Medicine
The University of Chicago, Chicago, Illinois

McGRAW-HILL
Health Professions Division

PreTest® Series

New York   St. Louis   San Francisco   Auckland   Bogotá   Caracas   Lisbon   London
Madrid   Mexico City   Milan   Montreal   New Delhi   San Juan   Singapore   Sydney   Tokyo   Toronto

McGraw-Hill
A Division of The McGraw·Hill Companies

Principles of Critical Care, 2/e:
PreTest® Self-Assessment and Review

Copyright © 1998, 1991 by The McGraw Hill Companies, Inc. All rights reserved. Printed in the United States of America. Except as permitted under the United States Copyright Act of 1976, no part of this publication may be reproduced or distributed in any form or by any means, or stored in a data base or retrieval system without the prior written permission of the publisher.

1 2 3 4 5 6 7 8 9 0   MALMAL   9 9 8 7

ISBN 0-07-052294-4

This book was set in Times Roman by V&M Graphics, Inc.
The editors were Martin J. Wonsiewicz and Peter J. Boyle.
The production supervisor was Richard C. Ruzycka.
Malloy Lithographers, Inc., was printer and binder.

Cataloging-in-publication data is on file for this book at the Library of Congress.

CONTENTS

CONTRIBUTORS

Jeffrey Christenson, MD
Fellow, Section of Pulmonary
* and Critical Care Medicine*
University of Chicago Medical Center
Chicago, Illinois

John Kress, MD
Fellow, Section of Pulmonary
* and Critical Care Medicine*
University of Chicago Medical Center
Chicago, Illinois

Thomas Corbridge, MD
Northwestern University Medical Center
Department of Pulmonary Medicine
Chicago, Illinois

Steven Koenig, MD
University of Virginia Health Sciences Center
Division of Pulmonary and Critical Care
Charlottesville, Virginia

Theodore Lewis, MD
Northern Arizona Medical Specialist
Flagstaff, Arizona

Avi Nahum, MD
Assistant Professor of Medicine
Staff Physician
Department of Pulmonary and Critical Care
St. Paul-Ramsey Medical Center
St. Paul, Minnesota

Kenneth W. Presberg, MD
Assistant Professor of Medicine
Pulmonary and Critical Care
Medical College of Wisconsin
Milwaukee, Wisconsin

Mary Strek, MD
Assistant Professor of Medicine
Pulmonary and Critical Care Medicine
University of Chicago Medical Center
Chicago, Illinois

PREFACE

The Critical Care Program at the University of Chicago is based on our belief that learning is fundamental to the delivery of quality care. Physicians learn by reading, teaching, engaging in research, and treating patients. In this text we try to assist the learning physician by providing a tool for self-assessment. Of course it is impossible to recreate in a text the complex decision making that occurs at the bedside. Nevertheless, a substantial science of medicine underlies the art: Here we aim to facilitate the building of a solid database. Factual information is only a part of critical care, but it is an essential part. In addition, we offer a unified pathophysiologic approach that makes mastery of the broad scope of critical illness more possible. Following review of this book, we ask that students of critical care return to the bedside to integrate their knowledge with the more challenging and exciting reality of the critically ill patient. The remaining ingredients of empathy, judgment, technical expertise, and experience can best be found there.

We wish to thank our contributors—Thomas Corbridge, Steven Koenig, Theodore Lewis, Avi Nahum, Kenneth Presberg, and Mary Strek—who carefully and thoughtfully created most of the questions for the first edition. We especially thank Jeff Christenson and John Kress who updated, revised, or added about 150 new questions and reorganized this second edition in accord with the revised content of the second edition of *Principles of Critical Care*, to which we refer the reader for further explication of the answers. These gifted physicians have succeeded in distilling their own knowledge and experience into relevant and challenging scenarios. We consider ourselves fortunate to have known physicians who are so excited by critical care.

We are grateful to the medical students at the Pritzker School of Medicine and the residents from Medicine, Surgery, and Anesthesiology who have learned with us over the years. Our skillful editors at McGraw-Hill, deserve credit for guiding us to this finished text. Most importantly, we owe a great debt to our editorial assistant, Cora Taylor, who organized, motivated, corrected, prodded, and aided us. Without her expertise and guidance this task would never have been completed.

INTRODUCTION

Principles of Critical Care: PreTest Self-Assessment and Review, 2/e, was written to assist physicians in evaluating their mastery of topics related to the care of the critically ill. This comprehensive and up-to-date text should be especially useful to clinicians and fellows planning to take Critical Care Board examinations sponsored by the American Board of Internal Medicine, the American Board of Surgery, and the American Board of Anesthesiology. However, the questions are intended to be relevant to the experienced critical care practitioner who wishes to identify areas for further study. In addition, the questions and cases are of sufficient interest that this text can stand alone as a tool for sharpening any physician's case analysis and decision-making skills. Finally, resident physicians and medical students will find the pathophysiologic underpinning of the questions a useful guide as they begin to discover the principles of critical care. This review book should aid the reader to: (1) learn the principles of organization and complications of critical care; (2) discover gaps in current knowledge of specific critical illnesses; and (3) become familiar with areas of new knowledge, controversy, and research in critical care.

This book contains 733 multiple-choice questions that correspond to the topics in *Principles of Critical Care,* 2/e (Hall JB, Schmidt GA, Wood LDH; McGraw-Hill, 1998). These questions have been organized into chapters that parallel those in the companion text, and this book may be used profitably a chapter at a time. By allowing no more than two and a half minutes to answer each question, you can simulate the time constraints of the actual board examinations. Answers and explanations are given at the end of each chapter. Furthermore, each answer is followed by a parenthetical reference to the chapter in *Principles of Critical Care* in which a full discussion of the topic and additional references can be found. We recommend that the reader keep a list of incorrect answers from which to select topics that may benefit from further study.

Although this book is organized to complement the larger text, it can be profitably used alone or in conjunction with other books in the literature.

The editors have invested substantial effort in the creation and selection of questions relevant to the daily practice of care in the ICU. This book should provide a means to assay, update, and round out your knowledge base in critical care. Interpretive skills, diagnostic acumen, and clinical problem solving can be honed by careful study of the answers. Most importantly, we hope that you find this text, like real medicine, to be challenging and stimulating.

PRINCIPLES OF CRITICAL CARE

PreTest® Self-Assessment and Review

ORGANIZATION AND COMPLICATIONS OF CRITICAL CARE

QUESTIONS

DIRECTIONS: Each question below contains four or five suggested responses. Select the **one best** response to each question.

1. ICU psychosis is correctly characterized by which of the following statements?

   (A) It is not life-threatening
   (B) It is usually worse in the early morning hours
   (C) It is best treated with haloperidol
   (D) It occurs in 10 percent of patients admitted to the ICU
   (E) It typically occurs after 5 to 7 days in the ICU

2. A 23-year-old man with right middle lobe pneumonia was intubated for progressive hypoxemia. After intubation, the peak pressure alarm sounded and breath sounds were not heard over the left hemithorax. The first response should be to

   (A) order a chest x-ray to evaluate the situation further as long as the patient remains stable
   (B) insert a needle into the left chest to rule out a pneumothorax
   (C) pull back the endotracheal tube slightly
   (D) add positive end-expiratory pressure (PEEP) in increments of 3 to 5 cm H_2O to treat left lung atelectasis, a common finding in mechanically ventilated patients
   (E) decrease tidal volume to lower peak airway pressure

3. A 69-year-old man with ARDS developed upper gastro-intestinal hemorrhage after 3 days of mechanical ventilation. The most likely cause of this patient's bleeding is ulceration

   (A) superficial to the muscularis mucosa in the gastric antrum
   (B) superficial to the muscularis mucosa in the gastric fundus
   (C) deep to the muscularis mucosa in the gastric fundus
   (D) deep to the muscularis mucosa in the gastric antrum
   (E) superficial to the muscularis mucosa in the duodenum

4. All the following are major metabolic complications of hyperalimentation EXCEPT

   (A) hypercapnia
   (B) hyperglycemia
   (C) hyperchloremia
   (D) hyperphosphatemia
   (E) hyperlipidemia

5. All the following complications are associated with the placement of a pulmonary artery catheter EXCEPT

   (A) left bundle branch block (LBBB)
   (B) ventricular tachycardia
   (C) atrial tachyarrhythmias
   (D) pericardial tamponade
   (E) phrenic nerve injury

6. A 37-year-old woman with histiocytosis-X needs mechanical ventilation for a spontaneous right-sided pneumothorax that requires tube thoracostomy. After 24 hours of mechanical ventilation, peak airway pressure suddenly increases to 80 cm H_2O with a resistive pressure drop of 60 cm H_2O. Breath sounds are markedly decreased bilaterally but are heard better on the left. Which of the following responses is correct?

   (A) Increase F_{IO_2} to 1.0 and obtain a stat chest x-ray
   (B) Insert a needle into the right hemithorax anteriorly to rule out tension pneumothorax
   (C) Disconnect the patient from the ventilator, manually bag the patient with F_{IO_2} of 1.0, and call for a new ventilator as soon as possible
   (D) Manually bag the patient with oxygen and pass a suction catheter down the airway to assess airway patency
   (E) Pull back the endotracheal tube slightly while listening carefully for the return of breath sounds

7. All the following statements regarding nosocomial pneumonia are true EXCEPT

(A) it usually results from aspiration of oropharyngeal or gastric contents colonized by pathogens
(B) gram-negative bacilli represent over half the organisms responsible for infection
(C) it occurs in 20 percent of mechanically ventilated patients in a medical ICU and as many as 68 percent of patients with ARDS
(D) most infections result from exogenous sources, such as respiratory therapy equipment and medical personnel
(E) oropharyngeal colonization occurs rapidly, often within the first 2 to 3 days in the ICU

8. Which of the following statements regarding nosocomial pneumonia is true?

(A) It can be diagnosed most of the time by clinical criteria (fever, white blood cell count, chest x-ray)
(B) Patients receiving appropriate antibiotics have higher survival rates
(C) The prior use of antibiotics increases the rate of infections by *Pseudomonas, Acinetobacter,* and *Staphylococcus*
(D) Specimens obtained by bronchoalveolar lavage have not been shown to be helpful in making the diagnosis
(E) Specimens obtained by a protected brush have not been shown to be helpful in making the diagnosis

---

9. A 49-year-old man was found by paramedics to be unresponsive and was intubated for airway protection. A left subclavian central venous catheter was placed for venous access. This subsequent portable chest radiograph is most consistent with

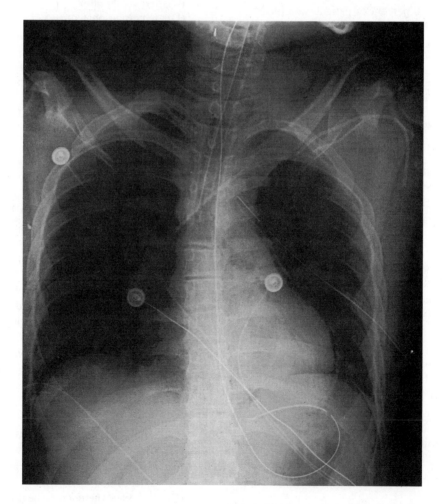

(A) left pneumothorax
(B) pneumopericardium
(C) left tension pneumothorax
(D) pneumomediastinum
(E) rotational artifact

10. The complication most feared in a transbronchial biopsy in a patient who is being mechanically ventilated is

(A) refractory hypoxemia
(B) severe dysrhythmias
(C) tension pneumothorax
(D) uncontrollable hemorrhage
(E) myocardial infarction

11. In all the following situations, transfer from a community hospital to a tertiary care hospital is considered safe EXCEPT

(A) acute myocardial infarction after thrombolytic therapy
(B) acute head injury
(C) acute cervical spine injury
(D) status asthmaticus after intubation
(E) premature labor with active contractions and fetal crowning

12. A 55-year-old man is intubated for hypotension and hypoxemia. Arterial blood gas measurements while the patient was being ventilated with $F_{I_{O_2}}$ at 0.70 on PEEP at 10 cm H_2O showed pH 7.36, Pa_{CO_2} 34 mm Hg, and Pa_{O_2} 65 mm Hg. A right subclavian introducer sheath is inserted, through which a pulmonary artery catheter is passed, but a wedge tracing cannot be obtained. The chest radiograph below is obtained. A blood sample is withdrawn from the distal port of the pulmonary artery catheter and sent for blood gas analysis. Of the following possible results, the one predicted by the chest radiograph is

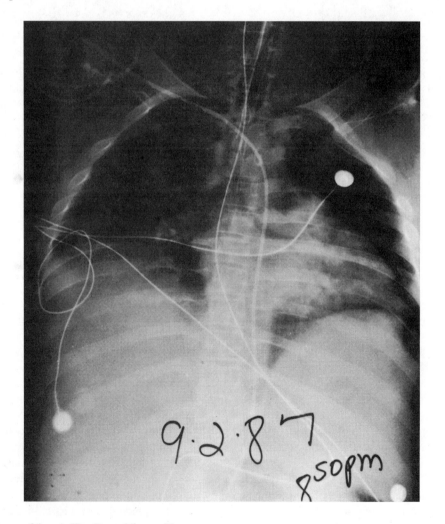

(A) pH 7.36, Pa_{CO_2} 34 mm Hg, Pa_{O_2} 35 mm Hg
(B) pH 7.33, Pa_{CO_2} 41 mm Hg, Pa_{O_2} 35 mm Hg
(C) pH 7.22, Pa_{CO_2} 66 mm Hg, Pa_{O_2} 35 mm Hg
(D) pH 7.36, Pa_{CO_2} 34 mm Hg, Pa_{O_2} 65 mm Hg
(E) pH 7.33, Pa_{CO_2} 41 mm Hg, Pa_{O_2} 65 mm Hg

13.   A 65-year-old woman is recovering in the first few hours after coronary artery bypass grafting and mitral valve replacement with a porcine heterograft. She suddenly becomes hypotensive to a blood pressure of 75/55, with a heart rate of 115. The chest radiograph below is obtained. Based on the findings of the film, the most likely cause of her hypotension is

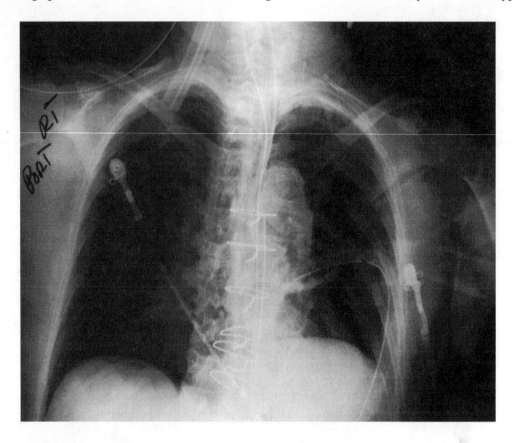

(A) cardiac tamponade
(B) acute hemorrhage
(C) valve dehiscence
(D) occlusion of the bypass graft
(E) tension pneumothorax

---

14.   A 45-year-old woman requires tube thoracostomy for drainage of an empyema. One hour after insertion she complains of dizziness. On examination, she is pale and afebrile with a pulse of 120 beats per minute and a blood pressure of 95/70 mm Hg. Which of the following could have occurred during tube thoracostomy to account for the clinical picture described?

(A) Sepsis from the introduction of bacteria
(B) Perforation of the thoracic duct with subsequent chylothorax
(C) Hemorrhage from laceration of an intercostal or internal mammary artery
(D) Bronchopleural fistula from perforation of the lung
(E) Incomplete reexpansion of the lung

15.   A 62-year-old man presented with pneumonia that proceeded to the adult respiratory distress syndrome (ARDS). He has had a pulmonary artery catheter in for 4 days, and his hemodynamics, which originally were consistent with septic shock, are now normalizing. Which of the following is true regarding proper management of the pulmonary artery catheter and the risk of line infection?

(A) This line can be continued with no additional risk for up to 7 days
(B) Changing this line over a guidewire and culturing a subcutaneous catheter segment are acceptable
(C) The appearance of the cutaneous insertion site is not predictive of possible infection
(D) The catheter should be changed and a new insertion site should be attempted in almost all cases
(E) An increased incidence of bacteremia is suggested if a catheter segment culture grows more than 10 colony-forming units. Treatment of the organism is generally recommended in this setting

16. A 25-year-old woman underwent liver transplantation 8 months ago for chronic active hepatitis. Her postoperative course was complicated by lower gastrointestinal hemorrhage attributed to cytomegalovirus colitis, for which a left hemicolectomy was performed. She now has a right-upper-quadrant colostomy. She recovered and was doing well as an outpatient on chronic immunosuppression until 5 days before admission, when she noted extreme weakness. On the day of admission she developed shortness of breath, which progressed rapidly to extreme dyspnea and then hypoxemic respiratory failure, which necessitated intubation and mechanical ventilation. One hour ago the Pa_{O_2} was 65 mm Hg and the Pa_{CO_2} was 52 mm Hg on assist control at a rate of 30, tidal volume of 450 mL, FI_{O_2} of 1.0, and PEEP of 15 cm H_2O. The peak airway pressure was 60 cm H_2O, and the static pressure was 53 cm H_2O. Now the pressure alarm (set at 75 cm H_2O) is sounding with each breath, and the ventilator is delivering only 325 mL per breath. A repeat arterial blood gas reveals pH 7.24, Pa_{CO_2} 60 mm Hg, and Pa_{O_2} 56 mm Hg. The chest radiograph is shown below. The most appropriate next step is to

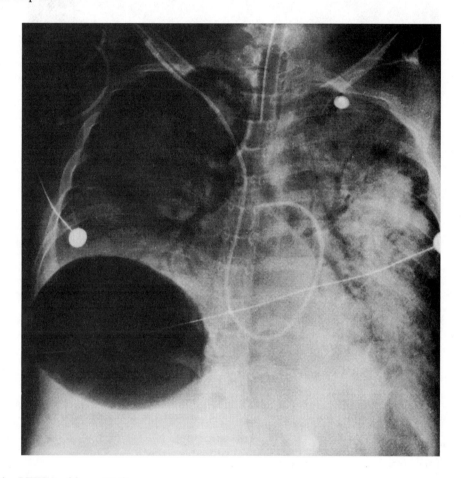

(A) increase the PEEP to 20 cm H_2O

(B) change the endotracheal tube

(C) insert a chest tube

(D) increase the tidal volume to 700 mL

(E) raise the pressure limit to 90 cm H_2O

17. An 84-year-old woman with fulminant hepatic failure developed hypotension (BP 90/40 mm Hg) and oliguria despite fluid administration. A chest x-ray 1 hour ago revealed only a well-positioned endotracheal tube and mild cardiomegaly. A right subclavian introducer sheath was inserted, and a pulmonary artery catheter was passed to a wedge position. The pulmonary capillary wedge pressure (PCWP) was 19 cm H_2O, and the cardiac output was 6.9 L/min. While you are waiting for the postprocedure chest x-ray, the blood pressure falls further to 82/52 mm Hg, while the cardiac output falls to 4.8 L/min and the PCWP to 15 cm H_2O. Based on the chest x-ray below and the clinical course, the best explanation for the right pleural fluid is

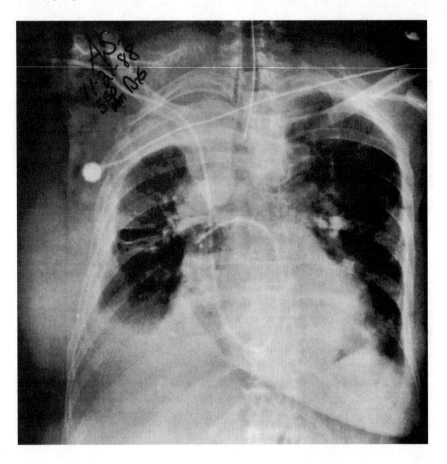

(A) hemothorax as a result of subclavian vein puncture in the setting of severe coagulopathy
(B) congestive heart failure
(C) ascitic fluid that has traversed the diaphragm
(D) malposition of the catheter into the pleural space
(E) erosion of the endotracheal tube into the innominate artery

18. Regarding ICU management in the United States, the following statements are true EXCEPT

(A) it is estimated that the ratio of daily ICU bed costs to general acute care bed costs is 5:1
(B) physicians' fees represent only 20 percent of health care costs, and up to 80 percent of expenditures for services are prescribed by physicians
(C) educational programs administered by mail are not as effective as programs communicated personally
(D) over 90 percent of all U.S. acute care hospitals have at least one ICU

19. Appropriate responsibilities for an intensive care unit fellow (as determined by current training guidelines) include all the following EXCEPT

(A) delegating responsibility to the junior staff
(B) having the final say in critical management decisions
(C) educating residents, nurses, and students
(D) documenting patient status and treatment plans
(E) participating in ICU quality assurance

DIRECTIONS: Each question below contains four suggested responses of which **one or more** is correct. Select

A	if	**1, 2, and 3**	are correct
B	if	**1 and 3**	are correct
C	if	**2 and 4**	are correct
D	if	**4**	is correct
E	if	**1, 2, 3, and 4**	are correct

20. A 41-year-old woman with sepsis and multisystem organ failure is noted by her physicians on morning rounds to be comatose. Thirty minutes earlier, her nurse reported spontaneous movement of the right lower extremity and withdrawal of the right upper extremity to painful stimuli. Explanations for this change in neurologic status include

(1) subarachnoid hemorrhage
(2) recent sedation or paralysis
(3) status epilepticus
(4) embolic stroke

21. Manifestations of ventilator-induced barotrauma include

(1) cardiovascular collapse
(2) air embolization
(3) pneumomediastinum
(4) hemothorax

22. A 64-year-old female is admitted to the ICU for an upper gastrointestinal hemorrhage and type IV respiratory failure, for which she is intubated. A pulmonary artery catheter is placed through the right internal jugular vein to guide volume replacement in the setting of ongoing hemorrhage. After the procedure, a chest x-ray is obtained which shows the pulmonary artery catheter in the proximal right pulmonary artery. There is a small right apical pneumothorax. True statements include which of the following?

(1) She may be extubated only after her blood loss is replaced
(2) She should receive a daily chest x-ray as long as she is intubated
(3) She should be observed and a chest tube should be placed if the pneumothorax appears to be increasing in size
(4) A chest tube should be placed now

23. Pneumoperitoneum caused by barotrauma usually

(1) is associated with other forms of barotrauma, such as pneumomediastinum and pneumothorax
(2) may be a harbinger for subsequent air embolism
(3) requires no specific therapy
(4) results from microscopic disruption of the diaphragm

24. The frequency of stress ulceration may be decreased by

(1) antacids and H_2 blockers
(2) enteral nutrition
(3) sucralfate
(4) correction of hypoperfusion and acidosis

25. Positive end-expiratory pressure (PEEP) may

(1) widen the difference between arterial and venous oxygen content
(2) increase West's zone I conditions
(3) increase intrapulmonary shunt in patients with pneumonic consolidation
(4) decrease lung water

26. Nephrotoxic drugs used in critical illness include

(1) cyclosporine
(2) methotrexate
(3) adriamycin
(4) heparin

Questions 27–28.

27. A 54-year-old alcoholic aspirated gastric contents and developed four-quadrant alveolar infiltrates. Arterial blood gases on 100% oxygen delivered by face mask were pH 7.29, Pa_{CO_2} 32 mm Hg, and Pa_{O_2} 45 mm Hg. Correct statements concerning this patient include

   (1) the alveolar-arterial oxygen gradient $[(A-a)PO_2]$ can be calculated as 628 mm Hg, assuming atmospheric pressure is 760 mm Hg, RQ is 0.8, and water vapor pressure is 47 mm Hg
   (2) PEEP probably will improve $(A-a)PO_2$
   (3) corticosteroids probably will improve $(A-a)PO_2$
   (4) decreasing the pulmonary capillary wedge pressure (PCWP) may improve $(A-a) PO_2$

28. After 2 weeks of mechanical ventilation, the patient in the previous question has a "honeycomb" appearance on chest x-ray. The following changes in arterial blood gases between morning and early afternoon rounds are noted (without a change in ventilator settings: FI_{O_2} 0.6, tidal volume 550 mL, respiratory rate 28, PEEP 10 cm H_2O):

	Morning	**Afternoon**
BP (mm Hg)	115/60	90/55
Pa_{O_2} (mm Hg)	64	49
Pa_{CO_2} (mm Hg)	36	45
pH	7.43	7.35

The intern makes the following changes in ventilator settings: FI_{O_2} 1.0, tidal volume 700, RR 28, PEEP 12.5 cm H_2O. The following measurements are now obtained: BP 86/50 mm Hg, pH 7.27, Pa_{CO_2} 51 mm Hg, and Pa_{O_2} 53 mm Hg. What should you do next?

   (1) Increase tidal volume
   (2) Consider gastrointestinal hemorrhage
   (3) Increase respiratory rate
   (4) Perform fluid challenge

29. A 22-year-old woman is undergoing a craniotomy and resection of a glioblastoma. The procedure is done in the sitting position. During the procedure, the patient is noted to become hypotensive and tachycardic. Which of the following procedures would be useful intraoperatively?

   (1) Transesophageal echocardiography
   (2) End-tidal nitrogen
   (3) Capnography
   (4) Airway pressure monitoring

30. In the ICU, bronchoscopy with bronchoalveolar lavage would be contraindicated in a patient

   (1) with an acute myocardial infarction 5 weeks ago
   (2) with a stabilized fracture of the cervical spine
   (3) suspected of having epiglottitis
   (4) with chronic renal failure and a BUN of 75 mg/dL

31. Correct statements regarding pulmonary infarction resulting from the placement of a Swan-Ganz catheter include

   (1) it occurs from persistent wedging and thrombosis
   (2) it appears as a focal, pleural-based density
   (3) infiltrates usually resolve in 7 to 14 days
   (4) it is more likely to occur in patients with pulmonary venous hypertension

32. Complications of central venous cannulation include

   (1) thrombosis
   (2) brachial plexus injury
   (3) pneumothorax
   (4) airway obstruction

33. In planning a new intensive care unit, it is best to

   (1) limit the number of beds to less than 16
   (2) provide eight electrical outlets per bed
   (3) locate the sink next to the door in each room
   (4) carpet patient rooms to decrease noise

34. True statements regarding legally effective consent include

   (1) consent must be voluntary
   (2) consent must be adequately informed
   (3) persons giving consent must have adequate mental capacity
   (4) consent must be written

35. Correct statements regarding decisions to limit treatment include

   (1) minors are legally incapable of ever making their own medical decisions to limit treatment
   (2) a properly informed capable patient always has the right to limit treatment that could prolong life
   (3) a living will document requesting maximum medical intervention requires physicians to provide maximum treatment even if it is futile
   (4) in a patient kept alive in a persistent vegetative state, feeding and hydration may be withheld if there is clear documentation that this was the wish of the patient while the patient was competent

36. True statements regarding intrahospital transport of a critically ill patient include

(1) deterioration in status during transport is uncommon
(2) a portable model ventilator is superior to manual ventilation during transport
(3) if personnel are limited, a qualified medical student can be given transport responsibility for an ICU patient
(4) some ventilator models can be used in an MRI scanner

37. Air transport of critically ill patients may result in

(1) increased supplemental oxygen requirements
(2) expansion of gas within the gastrointestinal cavity
(3) extrusion of the globe contents of the eye
(4) acute pulmonary edema

38. Disaster management requires

(1) a prearranged disaster plan
(2) regularly scheduled drills
(3) dedicated phone lines and radio backup communications
(4) a preprinted schedule of assigned shifts for the staff

DIRECTIONS: Each group of questions below consists of four lettered headings followed by a set of numbered items. For each numbered item select

A	if the item is associated with	(A) **only**
B	if the item is associated with	(B) **only**
C	if the item is associated with	**both** (A) and (B)
D	if the item is associated with	**neither** (A) nor (B)

Each lettered heading may be used **once, more than once, or not at all.**

Questions 39–40.

   (A) Hypercapnia
   (B) Hypoxemia
   (C) Both
   (D) Neither

39. May result from high levels of PEEP

40. May increase pulmonary vascular resistance

Questions 41–42.

   (A) Nasotracheal intubation
   (B) Orotracheal intubation
   (C) Both
   (D) Neither

41. May be complicated by bacterial sinusitis

42. May be safely performed in most awake, spontaneously breathing patients

Questions 43–45.

   (A) Peripheral venous cannulation
   (B) Central venous cannulation
   (C) Both
   (D) Neither

43. Can be used for nutritional support

44. Can deliver large volumes of fluid to the venous circulation

45. Can be complicated by air embolism

ORGANIZATION AND COMPLICATIONS OF CRITICAL CARE

ANSWERS

1. **The answer is E.** *(Chapter 57)* ICU psychosis should be considered only after other causes of altered mental status have been rigorously considered. The diagnosis is strengthened if typical features are present, such as emergence 5 to 7 days after admission and deterioration in the evening. It may occur to some degree in up to 70 percent of patients and is life-threatening when it results in self-extubation or the pulling of arterial or venous catheters. Treatment includes improving sleep quality and duration, communication, and orientation and interrupting the monotony of ICU life with radio, television, and reading to the patient. There is little place for major tranquilizers.

2. **The answer is C.** *(Chapter 11)* High airway pressures and decreased or absent breath sounds on the left suggest intubation of the right main stem bronchus, which occurs in 7 to 9 percent of intubations. The appropriate first step is to pull back the endotracheal tube gradually until airway pressures fall or breath sounds are heard bilaterally. Waiting for a chest x-ray places the patient at risk for ventilator-induced barotrauma.

3. **The answer is B.** *(Chapter 79)* Stress ulcerations are erosions superficial to the muscularis mucosa that involve the gastric fundus with sparing of the antrum. They result in critically ill patients when gastric defense mechanisms fail. Other than in stress ulcers associated with disorders of the CNS, increased gastric acid and increased pepsin usually are not found. Risk factors include major trauma, shock, sepsis, renal failure, jaundice, and acute respiratory failure.

4. **The answer is D.** *(Chapter 15)* In addition to the listed metabolic complications, the complications of hyperalimentation include complications related to line placement, infection, fatty liver, cholestasis, and triaditis. Hypercapnia may arise from increases in V_{CO_2} and the respiratory quotient during nutritional support. Hyperglycemia is common given the relative insulin resistance of critical illness, and hyperlipidemia may result from infusion of fat emulsion. Hyperchloremia is common and requires appropriate adjustment of the electrolyte composition of nutritional and other fluids.

5. **The answer is A.** *(Chapter 14)* Complications of the insertion of a pulmonary artery catheter include pneumothorax, air embolism, phrenic nerve injury, arterial injury, cardiac perforation, hemothorax, and arrhythmias. Common arrhythmias include atrial and ventricular tachyarrhythmias and right bundle branch block (RBBB). Left bundle branch block (LBBB) usually is not associated with right heart catheterization.

6. **The answer is D.** *(Chapters 12, 15)* When peak airway pressure is high, an inspiratory hold maneuver should be performed to determine whether it is static or resistive pressure that is high. High resistive pressure suggests airflow obstruction from kinking or plugging of the endotracheal tube or airflow obstruction below the endotracheal tube, which most often means bronchospasm. In this case, F_{IO_2} should be increased to 1.0, the endotracheal tube should be inspected, and a suction catheter should be passed to assess airway patency. An obstructed endotracheal tube that cannot be cleared quickly with instillation of saline, manual bagging, and suctioning should be replaced emergently.

7. **The answer is D.** *(Chapters 38, 47)* Nosocomial pneumonia usually results from aspiration of oropharyngeal or gastric contents colonized by pathogens, not from exogenous

sources. It is common in mechanically ventilated patients, particularly patients with ARDS, and is caused by gram-negative bacilli in over half the cases.

8. **The answer is C.** *(Chapters 38, 47)* Nosocomial pneumonia usually cannot be diagnosed on clinical grounds. Quantitative cultures from specimens obtained from protected brush catheters or bronchoalveolar lavage have been shown to be useful in making this diagnosis when more than 10^3 cfu/mL is found. Antibiotics have not been shown to increase survival, and prior use of antibiotics may increase the rate of serious gram-negative and gram-positive infections.

9. **The answer is B.** *(Chapter 15)* The patient has pneumopericardium that probably is related to the central line placement. The left pneumothorax has been evacuated with a chest tube. With positive-pressure ventilation, the pleural air can track up the bronchus into the mediastinum and rupture into the pericardial sac. With evacuation of the pneumothorax, the pneumopericardium probably will resolve spontaneously, though vigilance for possible cardiac compromise should be maintained.

10. **The answer is C.** *(Chapter 15)* In mechanically ventilated patients, it is probably best to avoid transbronchial biopsy if there is a good alternative. It is preferable to take these patients to the operating room for open-lung biopsy, since improved control over bleeding and pneumothorax in the operating room greatly lessens the risk of a catastrophic complication.

11. **The answer is E.** *(Chapter 9)* Critically ill patients can be safely transported, provided that the transport is carefully planned and trained transport personnel accompany the patient. Several series have shown successful transport of patients with an acute myocardial infarction who have just received thrombolytic therapy. Patients with an acute head injury or cervical spine injury require adequate restraint if they are combative and the cervical spine must be stabilized. Patients who are intubated can be transported safely as long as close attention is paid to endotracheal tube position and ventilation. Transport of pregnant patients who will deliver imminently should be avoided, since it is difficult to care for two critically ill patients in the transport environment. Examination of the pelvic station and cervical dilation should be performed before deciding on the safety of transport.

12. **The answer is D.** *(Chapter 15)* The chest radiograph shows that the catheter is malpositioned and is crossing the diaphragm into an abdominal vessel. After the catheter passes the medial aspect of the right clavicle, it turns caudad as it is projected over the aortic knob. As it is traced inferiorly toward the abdomen, the catheter is seen to the left of the midline, confirming its position in the aorta rather than the vena cava. Therefore, the introducer sheath has been placed into the right subclavian artery. The expected blood gas finding from the tip of the catheter should be identical to the arterial blood gas result obtained from the radial artery: Pa_{O_2} 65 mm Hg, Pa_{CO_2} 34 mm Hg.

13. **The answer is E.** *(Chapters 15, 20)* There are numerous etiologies for acute hypotension after open-heart surgery. In addition to those listed, acute myocardial infarction, right ventricular infarction, valve dysfunction, rhythm disturbance, and drug effect should be considered. The lucency of the right hemithorax should prompt the physician to examine the patient carefully for a pneumothorax. In this case, it is extremely difficult to see a pleural line laterally. However, the costophrenic sulcus on the right side is abnormally deep, narrow, and sharply defined (the "deep sulcus sign"), which confirms the suspicion of pneumothorax.

14. **The answer is C.** *(Chapter 15)* The incidence of complications of tube thoracostomy is 5 to 25 percent. While infection of the pleural space and perforation of the thoracic duct are considered iatrogenic complications of tube thoracostomy, they would not account for the clinical picture presented here. The patient's tachycardia and narrow pulse pressure and hypotension suggest bleeding, which could occur after laceration of an intercostal or internal mammary artery by the tube. Incomplete reexpansion of the underlying lung would not be expected to cause hypotension.

15. **The answer is B.** *(Chapter 46)*   It is generally recommended, as supported by studies, that these lines should be changed within 4 days. This can be done once over a guide-wire. The subcutaneous catheter segment should be cultured and the line should be dis-continued if the colony count is greater than or equal to 15 colony-forming units.

16. **The answer is C.** *(Chapter 15)*   The chest x-ray shows a diffuse lung lesion consistent with ARDS. In addition, there is an unusual air collection over the right lower lung field. While one possible explanation for this shadow is the right-upper-quadrant colostomy bag, the fact that the x-ray finding is delimited by the chest wall laterally and the mediastinum medially clearly points to this being a loculated subpulmonic pneumothorax. The lower edge of the air collection is the inverted hemidiaphragm, establishing that the pneumotho-rax is under pressure. The subpulmonic space is one of the most common sites for occult, or loculated, pneumothoraces in critically ill patients. Changing an endotracheal tube in a patient like this is an extremely delicate maneuver and is highly likely to lead to the demise of the patient. It should be attempted only when the endotracheal tube is clearly the source of the problem. Increasing the PEEP, tidal volume, or pressure limit on the ventilator will not correct the underlying problem and probably will exacerbate the barotrauma.

17. **The answer is A.** *(Chapter 15)*   The change in hemodynamics suggests an acute loss of volume from the vascular space, consistent with hemorrhage. After placement of a subclavian line in the setting of fulminant hepatic failure, the volume loss most likely represents hemorrhage from the subclavian vein into the pleural space. Because the sub-clavian vein is not compressible, it is not the preferred choice for central access in this setting. Erosion of an artificial airway into the innominate artery typically presents with hemoptysis and in any case is much less common than iatrogenic hemothorax.

18. **The answer is A.** *(Chapter 3)*   In both Canada and the United States the estimated ratio of ICU bed costs to general acute care bed costs is 3:1. Educational programs appear to have the greatest potential when professional role models effect change in physicians' professional environments. It has been shown that when information from such sources is transmitted by mail, it is less effective than it is when communicated personally.

19. **The answer is B.** *(Chapters 2, 4)*   An intensive care unit fellow has numerous respon-sibilities and is a critical member of the intensive care unit team. The fellow must mon-itor and manage critically ill patients; educate residents, nurses, and students; document patient status and treatment plans in the patient's chart; and participate in unit quality assurance programs. Because these responsibilities are time-consuming, a fellow must be able to appropriately delegate responsibility to junior members of the team. The ultimate responsibility for management decisions in critically ill patients should rest with the intensive care unit attending physician, who should be readily available for consultation.

20. **The answer is E (all).** *(Chapters 57, 58, 59)*   Status epilepticus should be considered in patients with a profound reduction in the level of consciousness or neurologic exami-nations that vary significantly over short periods of time or between observers. Tonic-clonic or focal motor activity need not be present. A review of recent medications is indicated in all patients with a decline in neurologic status, along with a detailed exami-nation to identify focal abnormalities.

21. **The answer is A (1, 2, 3).** *(Chapter 12)*   Pulmonary barotrauma is defined as the presence of extraalveolar air in areas not normally found in mechanically ventilated patients. Manifestations include pulmonary interstitial emphysema, pneumothorax, sub-cutaneous emphysema, pneumomediastinum, pneumoperitoneum, and air embolization. Hypotension is a manifestation of tension pneumothorax. Central nervous system depres-sion is a manifestation of air embolization. Hemothorax is not usually a complication of mechanical ventilation.

22. **The answer is C (2, 4).** *(Chapters 15, 30, 79)*   This patient has been intubated for hemorrhagic shock and should remain intubated until the bleeding is controlled and her blood loss is replaced. If blood loss is replaced but there is ongoing bleeding, she should

not be extubated. Her pneumothorax probably is iatrogenic from pulmonary artery catheter placement, and since she requires positive-pressure ventilation, it should be evacuated with a chest tube. Observation carries the risk of progression to tension pneumothorax while the patient receives positive-pressure ventilation. A daily chest x-ray while she is intubated to follow the pneumothorax after chest tube placement is indicated.

23. **The answer is A (1, 2, 3).** *(Chapters 12, 98)*   Pneumoperitoneum may result from a perforated viscus or from barotrauma. When it is the result of barotrauma, it usually is associated with thoracic manifestations and generally does not cause abdominal signs or symptoms. Peritoneal gas results when gas leaving a ruptured alveolus travels through the mediastinum, from which it escapes retroperitoneally into the abdomen. Retroperitoneal air may dissect into the venous circulation (inferior vena cava and tributaries), leading to a venous air embolism. Evacuation with a tube is necessary only if a large amount of air results in abdominal distention and difficulty in ventilation.

24. **The answer is E (all).** *(Chapter 79)*   All the listed treatments may be protective in stress ulceration; however, prophylaxis has not decreased mortality. Severe hemorrhage tends to occur in very critically ill patients in whom bleeding may be another manifestation of multisystem organ failure; thus, mortality may be unresponsive to prophylaxis.

25. **The answer is A (1, 2, 3).** *(Chapters 12, 33)*   By decreasing venous return to the right atrium, PEEP can lower cardiac output and Pv_{O_2} and can widen the difference between arterial and venous oxygen content. In patients with focal lung lesions such as lobar pneumonia, PEEP may increase alveolar pressure more in "normal" areas, thus diverting blood flow from normal areas to diseased areas and increasing shunt. PEEP does not decrease (and may in fact increase) lung water; instead, it redistributes edema and lowers shunt.

26. **The answer is A (1, 2, 3).** *(Chapter 70)*   Many immunosuppressive drugs—including cyclosporine, methotrexate, adriamycin, cisplatin, methyl-CCNU, and mitomycin-C— are nephrotoxic. Their use requires frequent monitoring of renal function. Use of serum drug levels when available is helpful in critically ill patients with complex pharmacokinetics.

27. **The answer is C (2, 4).** *(Chapter 33)*   Patients with respiratory distress who are receiving nasal cannula or mask oxygen have an unknown FI_{O_2} because these patients entrain room air gas during breathing. FI_{O_2} is known only when patients are breathing room air or are intubated with a tightly fitting endotracheal tube. FI_{O_2} must be known to determine $(A-a)P_{O_2}$. The correct $(A-a)P_{O_2}$ is 628 mm Hg if the FI_{O_2} is 1.0. PEEP lowers $(A-a)P_{O_2}$ in many patients with diffuse alveolar infiltrates by redistributing edema. Lowering PCWP also may improve gas exchange by decreasing the hydrostatic gradient that favors edema formation. Steroids have not been shown to be useful in treating patients with ARDS.

28. **The answer is C (2, 4).** *(Chapter 33)*   In patients with proliferative-phase ARDS, the dead-space fraction increases. Ventilatory maneuvers that increase alveolar pressure, such as high tidal volume and high respiratory rate, contribute to total dead space and may increase Pa_{CO_2}. PEEP and hypovolemia are frequent contributors to this process. In this patient, Pa_{CO_2} increased when tidal volume was increased. When this happens, minute ventilation should not be continually increased to try to lower Pa_{CO_2}; instead, strategies to lower dead space should be considered, such as ensuring an adequate circulating volume (and excluding reasons for hypovolemia) and lowering tidal volume, respiratory rate, or PEEP.

29. **The answer is A (1, 2, 3).** *(Chapter 26)*   The patient in the question probably is suffering from venous air emboli. Significant venous air embolization may cause hemodynamic collapse. The diagnosis may be made directly by aspiration of air from central veins or by visualization of air within the right ventricle with echocardiography. Transesophageal echocardiography is currently the most sensitive means of detecting a venous air embolism. End-tidal CO_2 is a slightly less sensitive means of detecting a venous air embolism. The drop in the end-tidal carbon dioxide tension is caused by the dilution of

expired carbon dioxide by alveolar gas from nonperfused lung units. End-tidal nitrogen as measured by mass spectrometry can detect the nitrogen from air bubbles not normally found in the blood. It appears to be even more sensitive than is capnography. Venous air embolism also is suggested by hypercapnia in a patient with relatively fixed carbon dioxide production and minute ventilation, suggesting a sudden increase in dead space (caused by occlusion of pulmonary capillaries by bubbles). Changes in airway pressures are not typically noted with venous air embolism.

30. **The answer is B (1, 3).** *(Chapter 15)* There are a number of contraindications to bronchoscopy in the ICU, including unstable cervical neck fractures, a problem with severe posterior nosebleeds, epiglottitis, unstable angina, an acute myocardial infarction within the past 6 weeks, dangerous dysrhythmias such as ventricular tachycardia, hemoglobin saturation less than 90 percent on supplemental oxygen, and hypotension. However, a patient with a cervical fracture may undergo fiber-optic bronchoscopy if the fracture is well stabilized. Patients with recent active posterior nosebleeds can have bronchoscopy done via the transoral route. If bronchial brushing or biopsy is contemplated, the patient should have adequate PT/PTT, a BUN less than 60 mg/dL, and a platelet count greater than 50,000 per cubic millimeter of blood. However, if only inspection and bronchoalveolar lavage are performed, normal clotting function is not absolutely required.

31. **The answer is E (all).** *(Chapter 14)* The most commonly seen complications of placement of a Swan-Ganz catheter are the formation of a loop within the heart and an excessively distal location. Ideally, the catheter tip should be in the area of the central pulmonary vessels, such as a proximal lobar branch. Pulmonary infarction can result from a persistently wedged catheter or from catheter-induced thrombosis. Infarction usually results in a focal, pleural-based infiltrate that resolves in 7 to 14 days. Pulmonary venous hypertension is a risk factor for catheter-induced infarction.

32. **The answer is E (all).** *(Chapter 15)* Central venous cannulation frequently is required in hospitalized patients for the administration of fluids, blood products, medications, or nutrition. Pneumothorax and central vein thrombosis are well-recognized complications of central venous line placement. Brachial plexus injury may occasionally be seen, usually in patients with landmarks in the neck that are difficult to locate. Acute airway closure is a rare complication of carotid artery puncture secondary to hematoma formation in the neck.

33. **The answer is B (1, 3).** *(Chapter 2)* Critical care beds are best clustered into units of 6 to 16 to optimize quality care and economic efficiency. A minimum of 12 to 18 electrical outlets is advised. Sinks are ideally located near the door of each patient room to encourage hand washing on entering and leaving the room. Although carpets may decrease noise and have not proved to be an infectious problem, they tend to develop odors with time and are best avoided.

34. **The answer is A (1, 2, 3).** *(Chapter 6)* Legally effective consent is a process of communication that must have three parts: it must be voluntary, adequately informed, and given by persons with adequate mental capacity. A written consent form is not the equivalent of legally effective informed consent and only provides evidence that the communication process occurred.

35. **The answer is D (4).** *(Chapter 6)* Minors (usually defined as those younger than age 18) who are granted "mature" status are legally capable of decision making. A properly informed capable patient has the right to make medical decisions to limit life-prolonging treatment, except when the welfare of a third party (such as a child) is jeopardized. Physicians are not required to provide futile interventions even in the face of previous patient wishes or family insistence. In the case of Nancy Cruzan, the United States Supreme Court ruled that a state may require "clear and convincing" evidence of treatment preference before incompetence before withdrawing life-prolonging therapy, including artificial feeding and hydration.

36. **The answer is C (2, 4).** *(Chapter 9)* Portable ventilators have been associated with better control of gas exchange during the transport of patients who require mechanical ventilation. Special models free of ferrous metals can be used in MRI scanners.

37. **The answer is A (1, 2, 3).** *(Chapter 9)* Air transport of critically ill patients in unpressurized helicopters or small pressurized aircraft may result in patients flying at an "effective altitude" of up to 8000 feet. Barometric pressure at this altitude is 565 mm Hg with a Pa_{O_2} of 55 mm Hg in healthy persons. Thus, supplemental oxygen requirements will be increased greatly in critically ill patients who require oxygen. Barometric pressure changes also will result in an increase in gas volume—30 percent at 8000 feet in all air-containing cavities, including the gastrointestinal tract. In addition, depressurization can lead to extrusion of the globe contents of the eye. Acute pulmonary edema occurs after prolonged exposure to very high altitude and would not occur as a direct result of air transport.

38. **The answer is E (all).** *(Chapters 2, 4)* The ability to cope with a disaster that necessitates the involvement of an intensive care unit requires a prearranged disaster plan; regularly scheduled drills; dedicated phone lines and radio backup communications systems between police, fire personnel, other hospitals, and the disaster scene; and an arrangement by which intensive care unit staff members have preassigned shifts to work during the disaster. Preparation and rehearsal for situations of mass casualties have been found to be the most beneficial factors in patient salvage.

39–40. **The answers are 39-C, 40-C.** *(Chapters 30, 33)* When alveolar pressure is high or intravascular pressure is low, large regions of physiologic dead space may occur (which will increase Pa_{CO_2} for a constant level of minute ventilation). Additionally, high alveolar pressure increases right atrial pressure, thus lowering venous return to the right atrium and reducing cardiac output and Pv_{O_2}. Perfusion of lung units with low V/Q and a low Pv_{O_2}, contributes to hypoxemia. Both hypercapnia and hypoxemia increase pulmonary vascular resistance, hypoxemia to a greater degree.

41–42. **The answers are 41-C, 42-A.** *(Chapter 11)* Endotracheal intubation is associated with bacterial sinusitis regardless of whether the endotracheal tube is placed orotracheally or nasotracheally. Although there is a higher incidence of sinusitis with nasotracheal intubation, prolonged periods in the supine position appear to cause pooling of secretions in the sinuses, with colonization leading to acute infection. Awake nasotracheal intubation can be performed safely in the absence of coagulopathy or basilar skull fracture. Orotracheal intubation with direct laryngoscopy is difficult to perform in most awake, spontaneously breathing patients. Sedation is usually required, and many patients require neuromuscular blockade to facilitate the procedure.

43–45. **The answers are 43-C, 44-C, 45-C.** *(Chapter 15)* Indications for venous catheterization include the administration of fluids, medications, or blood products. Both peripheral and central venous catheters can deliver large volumes of fluid as long as large-gauge catheters are used. Both can be used for alimentation, although fewer calories can be delivered peripherally, since high concentrations of glucose or amino acids will result in thrombosis of smaller veins. Both routes of catheterization can be complicated by air embolism.

MULTIPLE SYSTEM ORGAN FAILURE

QUESTIONS

DIRECTIONS: Each question below contains four or five suggested responses. Select the **one best** response to each question.

46. Multiple system organ failure (MSOF) develops in what percentage of patients who require admission to the ICU?

(A) 5 percent
(B) 15 percent
(C) 30 percent
(D) 40 percent

47. The most common cause of MSOF is

(A) trauma
(B) iatrogenic complications
(C) liver failure
(D) sepsis

48. Failure of which of the following organs or organ systems confers the highest risk of mortality?

(A) Central nervous system
(B) Respiratory system
(C) Liver
(D) Renal system

49. When used to predict individual ICU mortality in patients with MSOF, APACHE II may incorrectly classify what percentage of patients?

(A) < 5 percent
(B) 10 to 15 percent
(C) 25 to 35 percent
(D) 35 to 45 percent

50. Regarding MSOF, which of the following statements is true?

(A) Contributions of individual organ system failures to MSOF are equal
(B) Microbial infection is equivalent to sepsis
(C) Sepsis and the systemic inflammatory response syndrome (SIRS) are equivalent
(D) Progression of the initial infection or injury to MSOF does not depend on persistently elevated plasma levels of tumor necrosis factor-α (TNF-α)

51. A 40-year-old trauma victim opens his eyes to pain, withdraws his extremities to pain, and makes incomprehensible sounds. His Glasgow coma score is

(A) 7
(B) 9
(C) 11
(D) 13

52. The highest incidence of the adult respiratory distress syndrome (ARDS) is seen in patients suffering from

(A) neutropenic fevers
(B) sepsis syndrome
(C) CNS catastrophes
(D) multiple trauma
(E) drug overdose

53. The physiologic definition of MSOF is failure of

(A) at least three organs
(B) at least two organs on admission to the ICU
(C) at least two organs lasting at least 24 to 48 hours
(D) at least two organs lasting longer than 48 hours

54. Positive end-expiratory pressure (PEEP) often is used in therapy for the adult respiratory distress syndrome (ARDS). While PEEP often is useful in reducing shunt and allowing the use of a less toxic oxygen concentration, it also may have deleterious effects. The potential deleterious effects of PEEP include all the following EXCEPT

(A) reduction of venous return in hypovolemic patients
(B) hyperinflation of nonflooded alveoli with the risk of barotrauma
(C) increased left ventricular afterload
(D) increased right ventricular afterload
(E) increased dead space in patients with hypovolemia

55. The hematologic effects of sepsis include all the following EXCEPT

(A) leukocytosis resulting from catecholamine-induced PMN demargination

(B) leukocytosis caused by cytokine-induced release of immature PMNs from bone marrow

(C) erythrocytosis resulting from elevated levels of erythropoietin

(D) thrombocythemia caused by an acute-phase reaction to infection

(E) thrombocytosis caused by platelet consumption

56. Initial therapy for patients with the sepsis syndrome complicating gram-negative infection might include all the following EXCEPT

(A) restoration of intravascular volume

(B) identification of potential sources of sepsis

(C) improvement of tissue perfusion with vasoactive medications

(D) diuretic therapy

(E) eradication of infection

57. Findings compatible with the proliferative phase of the adult respiratory distress syndrome (ARDS) include all the following EXCEPT

(A) increased cellularity of the lung parenchyma

(B) improved efficiency of gas exchange

(C) diminished pulmonary compliance

(D) diminished pulmonary capillary leak

(E) radiographic appearance of pulmonary fibrosis

58. The hypermetabolic state of MSOF is characterized by

(A) decreased carbon dioxide production

(B) a requirement for excess glucose calories

(C) decreased hepatic glucose release

(D) increased total body protein catabolism

(E) decreased total body protein synthesis

DIRECTIONS: Each question below contains four suggested responses of which **one or more** is correct. Select

A	if	**1, 2, and 3**	are correct
B	if	**1 and 3**	are correct
C	if	**2 and 4**	are correct
D	if	**4**	is correct
E	if	**1, 2, 3, and 4**	are correct

59. Factors that promote bacterial translocation through the gut wall include

(1) systemic trauma
(2) total parenteral nutrition
(3) intestinal obstruction
(4) thermal injury

60. Noninfectious causes of multisystem dysfunction that simulate sepsis-induced MSOF include

(1) acute pancreatitis
(2) systemic lupus erythematosus
(3) trauma
(4) thrombotic thrombocytopenic purpura

61. In patients with intraabdominal sepsis, the risk of death increases with

(1) shock
(2) malnutrition
(3) history of alcoholism
(4) bowel infarction

62. Major risk factors for the development of MSOF are

(1) an episode of hypotension during hospitalization
(2) age > 65 years
(3) acute respiratory failure
(4) a diagnosis of sepsis or infection at ICU admission

63. Which of the following can be identified as a primary mediator in the host inflammatory response to lipopolysaccharide A (endotoxin)?

(1) Tumor necrosis factor-α
(2) Eosinophilic major basic protein
(3) Interleukin-1
(4) Interferon-α

64. Criteria used to diagnose the adult respiratory distress syndrome (ARDS) include

(1) diffuse alveolar damage on lung biopsy
(2) static compliance less than 40 mL per cm H_2O
(3) the presence of intrinsic positive end-expiratory pressure (PEEP)
(4) infiltrates in three of four quadrants on chest x-ray

65. In patients with the adult respiratory distress syndrome (ARDS), the interplay between lung injury and infection is complex. True statements regarding this association include which of the following?

(1) Sepsis may initiate the development of ARDS
(2) Mortality in patients with ARDS is more often associated with superimposed infection than with hypoxemia
(3) In patients with ARDS who develop MSOF, there is frequently clinical evidence of sepsis
(4) Parenteral antibiotics have been shown to reduce the mortality caused by nosocomial pneumonia in patients with ARDS

66. The hypoalbuminemia noted in patients with the sepsis syndrome is due to

(1) increased capillary permeability to albumin caused by platelet activating factor
(2) decreased hepatic synthesis caused by the actions of interleukin-1
(3) dilution of albumin caused by aggressive volume resuscitation
(4) urinary loss caused by the unappreciated high incidence of renal vein thrombosis

Questions 67–68.

A 74-year-old man with a history of chronic lympho-cytic leukemia presents with fatigue and dyspnea. On physical examination, his temperature is 39°C (102.2°F), blood pressure is 85/40 mm Hg, heart rate is 124 beats per minute and regular, and respiratory rate is 38 breaths per minute and labored with the use of accessory muscles. Lung examination reveals diffuse crackles. Pulses are bounding. Laboratory data are notable for a white blood cell count of 19,000 mm^3 with 28 band forms, hematocrit 25, an anion gap metabolic acidosis, lactate 9, and an arterial blood gas showing pH 7.10, Pa_{CO_2} 24 mm Hg, Pa_{O_2} 40 mm Hg. Chest x-ray appearance is consistent with pulmonary edema. A pulmonary artery catheter demonstrates a cardiac output of 11.0, a pulmonary capillary wedge pressure of 8 cm H_2O, and an arterial-venous oxygen content difference of 2.0 mL O_2/dL. Blood cultures eventually grow *Klebsiella pneumoniae.*

67. Potentially useful interventions which may decrease oxygen consumption in this patient include

 (1) administration of acetaminophen
 (2) administration of ampicillin and gentamicin
 (3) mechanical ventilation with sedation and muscle paralysis
 (4) use of a cooling blanket

68. Interventions that might increase oxygen delivery in this patient include

 (1) transfusion of packed red blood cells
 (2) infusion of normal saline
 (3) administration of positive end-expiratory pressure (PEEP)
 (4) administration of nitroprusside

69. True statements regarding hepatic dysfunction in patients with the sepsis syndrome include

 (1) fulminant hepatic failure as manifested by jaundice, lactic acidosis, bleeding, and hypo-glycemia may develop and is uniformly associated with a poor outcome
 (2) anoxic liver injury manifested by marked but transient increases in blood transaminase levels is associated with significant functional impairment in patients with the sepsis syndrome
 (3) focal hepatic necrosis resulting in elevations in liver enzymes and bilirubin is a common finding
 (4) elevations in serum bilirubin and alkaline phosphatase are indicative of the increased incidence of gallstones seen in the sepsis syndrome

70. Organs involved in the syndrome of MSOF include

 (1) respiratory system
 (2) gastrointestinal tract
 (3) liver
 (4) skeletal muscle

71. Excess glucose calories given to patients with MSOF have which of the following effects?

 (1) Decreased carbon dioxide production and oxygen consumption
 (2) Increased lactate production
 (3) Decreased catecholamine release
 (4) Failure to suppress gluconeogenesis

72. Which of the following conditions may be associated with pathologic supply dependence of oxygen delivery?

 (1) Adult respiratory distress syndrome (ARDS)
 (2) Chronic states of low oxygen delivery
 (3) Sepsis
 (4) Chronic renal failure

73. Enriched inspired O_2 can worsen the lung toxicity of

 (1) cyclosporine
 (2) inhaled nitric oxide
 (3) phenytoin
 (4) bleomycin

DIRECTIONS: Each group of questions below consists of lettered headings followed by a set of numbered items. For each numbered item select the **one** lettered heading with which it is **most** closely associated. Each lettered heading may be used **once, more than once, or not at all.**

Questions 74–77.

Match each oxidant with the best defense mechanism

(A) Superoxide dismutase (SOD)
(B) Catalase
(C) Ferritin
(D) Vitamin E

74. Lipid peroxides

75. O_2^-

76. H_2O_2

77. OH•

DIRECTIONS: Each group of questions below consists of four lettered headings followed by a set of numbered items. For each numbered item select

A	if the item is associated with	(A) **only**
B	if the item is associated with	(B) **only**
C	if the item is associated with	**both** (A) and (B)
D	if the item is associated with	**neither** (A) nor (B)

Each lettered heading may be used **once, more than once, or not at all.**

Questions 78–79.

   (A) Tissue hypoxia resulting from decreased oxygen delivery

   (B) Tissue hypoxia resulting from decreased oxygen extraction

   (C) Both

   (D) Neither

78. Septic shock

79. Cardiogenic shock

MULTIPLE SYSTEM ORGAN FAILURE

ANSWERS

46. The answer is B. *(Chapter 17)* MSOF, as defined by at least two organ failures for a minimum of 24 to 48 hours, develops in 15 percent of patients requiring ICU admission. As medical and surgical therapies become more extensive and supportive care becomes more successful in averting early demise, it may become a more commonly encountered condition. The roles of hypermetabolism, infection, and host response in producing this syndrome are under investigation.

47. The answer is D. *(Chapter 17)* All the listed conditions can lead to MSOF, but sepsis is the most common cause. Liver failure may carry particular weight as a poor prognostic indicator in MSOF. To the extent that iatrogenic complications include or lead to infection or hypermetabolism, they may increase the likelihood of MSOF.

48. The answer is A. *(Chapter 17)* In the large, multicenter APACHE II study, CNS failure conferred the highest risk of mortality, with an approximate 10 percent incremental risk (overall risk, 40 percent) of hospital death compared with other single-organ-system failures.

49. The answer is B. *(Chapter 17)* The APACHE II severity of illness scoring system is a useful tool in predicting mortality in large populations. It was not intended for mortality prediction in individual patients and thus is associated with relatively substantial error.

50. The answer is D. *(Chapter 17)* Despite the fact that the definition of MSOF treats all organ systems equally, the mortality risks associated with dysfunction of different organ systems are very different. In prediction algorithms for mortality risk, various organ systems are given different weights. For instance, in APACHE II the highest weight is given to the CNS. Microbial infection is not equivalent to sepsis. Infection is a microbial phenomenon, while sepsis represents the sum total of host-derived immune and inflammatory responses over time that produce tissue injury, cardiovascular derangements, hypermetabolism, and the clinical syndrome of MSOF. Sepsis and the systemic inflammatory response syndrome (SIRS) should be distinguished to promote an understanding that the clinical expression of MSOF reflects generalized activation of humoral and cellular elements of the immune system and circulatory changes that escape normal host regulation. In fulminant liver failure, for instance, patients can present with SIRS without having sepsis.

51. The answer is B. *(Chapter 17)* The Glasgow coma score is the sum of the best eye opening, motor, and verbal responses. The scores for eye opening are as follows: eye opens spontaneously (4), to verbal command (3), to pain (2), no response (1). Motor scores are as follows: obedience to verbal command (6), response to painful stimuli (5), flexion-withdrawal (4), decorticate rigidity (3), decerebrate rigidity (2), no response (1). Verbal scores are as follows: oriented (5), disoriented but converses (4), inappropriate words (3), incomprehensible sounds (2), no response (1).

52. **The answer is B.** *(Chapter 17)* The highest incidence of ARDS, roughly one-third of all patients, occurs among patients with the sepsis syndrome. Patients with multiple trauma, drug overdose, and CNS catastrophes may develop pulmonary edema, which meets the physiologic criteria for the diagnosis of ARDS. Patients who are neutropenic are not protected from ARDS, although the syndrome frequently develops in patients with neutropenic fevers whose marrow function returns.

53. **The answer is C.** *(Chapter 17)* MSOF is defined as failure of at least two organs lasting at least 24 to 48 hours.

54. **The answer is C.** *(Chapter 17)* PEEP increases intrathoracic pressure (and consequently right atrial pressure) and thus decreases the pressure gradient for venous return. It may hyperinflate normal alveoli and increase the risk of rupture and barotrauma. This hyperinflation also may compress alveolar vessels and thus cause increased right ventricular afterload and create areas of West's zone I lung, thus increasing dead space. The addition of PEEP actually reduces the left ventricular transmural pressure necessary to eject into the extrathoracic aorta; thus, PEEP reduces left ventricular afterload. This is usually a salutary effect.

55. **The answer is C.** *(Chapter 17)* The hematologic effects of sepsis are many and varied. Leukocytosis may be seen as a result of both endogenous catecholamine-induced demargination of polymorphonuclear leukocytes (PMNs) and cytokine-induced release of immature PMNs from bone marrow. Platelets are a well-known acute-phase reactant and thus may be elevated in patients with sepsis. The consumption of platelets leading to thrombocytopenia is associated with more severe sepsis and may culminate in DIC. Increased production of erythropoietin is not associated with sepsis.

56. **The answer is D.** *(Chapter 17)* The initial therapy for the sepsis syndrome should be directed at the identification and treatment of the infectious source. Hypovolemia is usually profound because of the marked vasodilation and capillary leakage and requires aggressive volume repletion. The use of diuretics may aggravate this problem. Vasoactive medications should be considered in an effort to improve tissue perfusion.

57. **The answer is B.** *(Chapter 17)* The proliferative phase of ARDS is characterized by an increase in lung cellularity with a decrease in pulmonary capillary leak. Proliferation of type II alveolar cells within alveolar septae and fibroblasts and of myofibroblasts within the alveolar wall leads to abnormal collagen deposition and may result in extensive pulmonary fibrosis. The fibrotic changes associated with the proliferative phase of ARDS are clearly demonstrable on chest radiography. These changes are manifested clinically by a decrease in lung compliance and an increase in the dead space fraction necessitating high minute ventilation. Decreased efficiency of gas exchange is the rule.

58. **The answer is D.** *(Chapter 17)* Hypermetabolism is thought to be a phase of MSOF that deteriorates into metabolic dysregulation manifested by organ failure. An increase in oxygen consumption with increased carbon dioxide production is thought to be the primary event in the hypermetabolic state. Total body protein catabolism and protein synthesis are both increased. Hepatic glucose release is increased. Excess supplemental glucose calories have been shown to have detrimental effects on metabolism.

59. **The answer is E (all).** *(Chapter 17)* All the listed factors are associated with bacterial translocation. In general, conditions that decrease intestinal perfusion are associated with bacterial translocation. Other factors are disruption of the ecologic balance of normal indigenous flora, deficient T-cell-mediated immunity, endotoxemia, hemorrhagic shock, and intraabdominal abscess.

60. The answer is E (all). *(Chapter 17)* Numerous noninfectious conditions may result in multiple system organ failure that is indistinguishable from sepsis-induced MSOF. Tissue hypoperfusion and ischemia, microthrombosis, trauma, and systemic inflammatory conditions have all been implicated as triggers that initiate the pathophysiologic pathways that culminate in MSOF.

61. The answer is E (all). *(Chapter 17)* In a prospective study that included 106 patients found at operation to have intraabdominal sepsis, an increased risk of death was found in patients with shock, age > 65 years, a history of alcoholism, bowel infarction, or malnutrition. Thus, both preexisting chronic health status and severity of hypoperfusion are likely to determine the prognosis.

62. The answer is C (2, 4). *(Chapter 17)* Clinical risk factors for the development or lethal progression of MSOF include severity of disease (APACHE II score), sepsis or infection at ICU admission, age > 65 years, systemic inflammation, persistent deficit in O_2 delivery after resuscitation from circulatory shock, focus of devitalized or injured tissue, severe trauma or major operations, and preexisting end-stage liver failure.

63. The answer is B (1, 3). *(Chapter 17)* The importance of tumor necrosis factor-α (TNF-α, or cachectin) in the pathogenesis of the inflammatory response has been well demonstrated. Mice exposed to endotoxin that are genetically unable to make TNF-α are protected against the development of shock. Similarly, interleukin-1 has been shown to have direct physiologic effects as well as to play a key role in the amplification of the host immune response to endotoxin. Major basic protein of the eosinophil may play an important role in the inflammation associated with asthma and parasitic diseases but generally is not associated with sepsis. Interferon-γ may play a role in activating macrophages and stimulating antibody production in sepsis. No such role has been identified for interferon-α.

64. The answer is C (2, 4). *(Chapter 17)* The diagnosis of ARDS is a clinical one that relies largely on physiologic criteria because of a lack of other reliable markers. These criteria include low compliance, increased alveolar-to-arterial gradient or ratio, and exclusion of hydrostatic pulmonary edema. Chest radiographic evidence of diffuse involvement is also required. Pathologic material obtained in the early stage of ARDS frequently demonstrates diffuse alveolar damage but is not necessary to make, nor does it confirm, the diagnosis of ARDS. Intrinsic PEEP occurs most often in patients with airflow obstruction, particularly if delivered minute ventilation is high.

65. The answer is A (1, 2, 3). *(Chapter 17)* Infection probably plays a role in the development and propagation of lung injury and MSOF. Whether these effects reflect a direct action of bacteremia or a nonspecific inflammatory cascade initiated by local infection is not known, though the latter is more likely. Unfortunately, antibiotics have not been shown to reduce mortality in nosocomial pneumonia in patients with ARDS.

66. The answer is A (1, 2, 3). *(Chapter 17)* The hypoalbuminemia of sepsis is multifactorial in its origin. There is decreased synthesis of albumin as a result of the effects of interleukin-1 on the liver, which shifts protein synthesis toward acute-phase reactants. There is leakage of albumin into the extravascular space because of the effects of platelet-activating factor and other cytokines as well as the effect of complement activation. During the resuscitation of patients in septic shock, large amounts of volume may be necessary to maintain adequate oxygen delivery. If this volume is administered as crystalloid alone, dilutional hypoalbuminemia may result. There are no data suggesting that renal vein thrombosis plays an important role in the urinary loss of protein during sepsis.

67. The answer is A (1, 2, 3). *(Chapter 17)* Critically ill patients have increased oxygen consumption secondary to fever, work of breathing, sepsis, and the associated metabolic response to trauma. Acetaminophen could correct this patient's elevated temperature. Cooling blankets without concomitant muscle paralysis are ineffective and do more harm than good by stimulating shivering. In patients with respiratory distress, the diaphragm may receive 20 percent of the cardiac output. In this situation, sedation, muscle paralysis, and mechanical ventilation would dramatically decrease oxygen consumption. Antibiotics, by treating sepsis, could decrease oxygen demand.

68. The answer is E (all). *(Chapter 17)* Oxygen delivery (Q_{O_2}) is a function of oxygen saturation (Sa_{O_2}), hemoglobin concentration (Hgb), the partial pressure of oxygen in arterial blood (Pa_{O_2}), and the cardiac output (Q_t), expressed by the following relationship: $Q_{O_2} = Q_t [(Sa_{O_2} \times j \times Hgb) + (k \times Pa_{O_2})]$, where j and k are constants (j = 1.39 mL O_2 per gram Hgb, k = 0.003 mL O_2 per mm Hg per milliliter of plasma). Packed red blood cells, by increasing hemoglobin concentration, and PEEP, by increasing Pa_{O_2} and Sa_{O_2}, could increase oxygen delivery. Normal saline, by increasing preload, and nitroprusside, by decreasing afterload, could increase cardiac output and thus oxygen delivery.

69. The answer is B (1, 3). *(Chapter 17)* Liver function abnormalities are seen commonly in patients with the sepsis syndrome. Focal hepatic necrosis manifested by increased serum bilirubin and transaminase levels is seen commonly in patients with the sepsis syndrome. Fulminant hepatic failure is seen in cases of more severe and prolonged sepsis and is associated with high mortality. Anoxic liver injury is a relatively common hepatic abnormality seen in patients with the sepsis syndrome. Although significant elevations of transaminase levels are attained, these elevations are usually transient and are not associated with substantial functional impairment. Hyperbilirubinemia regularly occurs in the sepsis syndrome. It often is associated with focal hepatic necrosis and cholestasis of an unknown etiology. The incidence of gallstones has not been shown to be increased in this population.

70. The answer is E (all). *(Chapter 17)* MSOF occurs after trauma, major surgery, or sepsis, with a mortality between 90 and 95 percent when three or more organ systems become severely impaired. The respiratory system is involved early, followed by involvement of the kidneys, gastrointestinal tract, and liver. Because this is a hypermetabolic state with total body protein catabolism, there is a rapid loss of skeletal muscle mass and failure of the skeletal muscle to perform some of its metabolic functions.

71. The answer is C (2, 4). *(Chapter 17)* Excess total calories and excess glucose calories have both been shown to have adverse effects on metabolism and organ structure and function when given to patients with MSOF. These effects include increased lactic acid production, failure to suppress gluconeogenesis, fatty liver syndrome, and hyperosmolar states. Also noted are an increase in carbon dioxide and oxygen consumption and stimulation of catecholamine release.

72. The answer is A (1, 2, 3). *(Chapter 17)* Almost two decades ago, it was first reported that patients with ARDS exhibited a dependence of oxygen uptake on oxygen delivery despite normal or high levels of oxygen delivery. Similar findings were found in patients with sepsis. Because of the prevalence of both sepsis and peripheral oxygen extraction defects in patients with ARDS, it is possible that sepsis, rather than simple ARDS, accounts for the abnormalities. Patients with chronic states of low oxygen delivery, such as those which occur with chronic congestive heart failure and anemia, also show the same peripheral oxygen extraction defect.

73. **The answer is C (2, 4).** *(Chapter 17)* The lung toxicities of both bleomycin and inhaled nitric oxide (iNO) are worsened with O_2 therapy. ARDS has been reported to develop in patients after bleomycin therapy when they were exposed to $Fi_{O_2} > 0.30$. This synergy between bleomycin and O_2 can occur months after therapy with bleomycin. The production of toxic nitrogen oxides (NOx) varies directly with the concentration and duration of mixing of nitric oxide with oxygen. Cyclosporine is not associated with lung toxicity. Phenytoin is associated with hilar adenopathy as well as interstitial infiltrates and pneumonitis.

74–77. **The answers are 74-D, 75-A, 76-B, 77-C.** *(Chapter 17)* SOD converts O_{2^-} to H_2O_2 and O_2; catalase reduces H_2O_2 to H_2O. Ferritin is an iron-carrying protein that binds iron and effectively removes it from plasma so that it cannot catalyze Fenton-type reactions and form OH•. Vitamin E is a lipid that terminates lipid peroxidation in the membranes.

78–79. **The answers are 78-C, 79-A.** *(Chapter 17)* Tissue hypoxia may result from a number of pathologic conditions, including decreased oxygen supply, increased oxygen demand, and decreased oxygen extraction ratio. In septic shock, both oxygen delivery and oxygen extraction contribute to tissue hypoxemia. Oxygen demand often is increased by a variety of factors, including fever, work of breathing, and other associated metabolic responses to sepsis. Oxygen supply may be limited by inadequate cardiac output, anemia, and intrinsic pulmonary complications of sepsis such as ARDS. The extraction ratio of oxygen is diminished in septic shock in part as a result of functional arteriovenous shunting, microembolization, and impaired autoregulatory matching of oxygen delivery to tissue demands. In cardiogenic shock, tissue hypoxia is primarily the result of diminished oxygen supply rather than the extraction ratio. Diminished cardiac output, increased afterload, and the potential for gas exchange impairment resulting from pulmonary edema all contribute to diminished oxygen delivery. An increase in the oxygen extraction ratio is often seen in patients with this condition.

NUTRITION

QUESTIONS

DIRECTIONS: Each question below contains four or five suggested responses. Select the **one best** response to each question.

80. Which of the following statements about the nutritional requirements of critically ill patients is true?

   (A) Energy expenditure in malnourished patients may approach 150 percent of normal
   (B) Energy expenditure in severe burn victims may approach 200 percent of normal
   (C) Energy expenditure is diminished in patients who sustain head trauma
   (D) Decreased nitrogen excretion in critically ill patients is a protective mechanism aimed at preventing depletion of nitrogen stores
   (E) Chronically malnourished patients are unable to utilize administered calories and nutrients

81. Nitrogen loss in critically ill patients occurs in all the following organs EXCEPT

   (A) heart
   (B) skeletal muscle
   (C) liver
   (D) brain
   (E) kidney

82. Initial daily caloric requirements for a critically ill patient with respiratory failure would most likely be

   (A) 500 kcal
   (B) 1500 kcal
   (C) 2500 kcal
   (D) 3500 kcal
   (E) 4500 kcal

DIRECTIONS: Each question below contains four suggested responses of which **one or more** is correct. Select

A	if	**1, 2, and 3**	are correct
B	if	**1 and 3**	are correct
C	if	**2 and 4**	are correct
D	if	**4**	is correct
E	if	**1, 2, 3, and 4**	are correct

83.   The hyperglycemia of critical illness is due to

  (1)   insulin resistance resulting from catecholamine secretion
  (2)   decreased glucose utilization by the brain
  (3)   increased gluconeogenesis in muscle
  (4)   increased glycogenolysis and intestinal uptake of carbohydrate

84.   True statements regarding enteral versus parenteral nutrition include

  (1)   enteral feeding is more effective than parenteral nutrition in maintaining and restoring the nutritional state
  (2)   enteral nutrition is less expensive and involves fewer complications than parenteral feeding
  (3)   parenteral nutrition should be employed in all critically ill patients who develop gastrointestinal dysmotility
  (4)   enteral feeds help prevent intestinal mucosal atrophy and may diminish gastric stress ulcer formation

85.   True statements concerning lipid supplementation include

  (1)   it can be given enterally and intravenously
  (2)   medium-chain triglycerides are recommended for patients with hepatic dysfunction
  (3)   lipid administration has been associated with an increase in prostaglandin production and an increase in shunt in the lung
  (4)   pancreatic function is not a factor for consideration with the administration of intravenous preparations

86.   A 60-year-old woman with COPD is intubated and mechanically ventilated for acute-on-chronic ventilatory failure. Parenteral nutritional support with intravenous 25% dextrose and 4.25% amino acids at 50 mL/h (1200 cal/day) is started after 2 days of ventilatory support. Over the next 24 hours greater minute ventilation is required to achieve a Pa_{CO_2} of 50 mm Hg. Nutritional strategies that could lower minute ventilatory requirements include

  (1)   changing to a peripheral formula of 5% dextrose plus 3% amino acids and adding 500 mL/day Intralipid (a fat emulsion)
  (2)   adding 500 mL/day Intralipid to the current solution
  (3)   decreasing total caloric intake to 1000 kcal/day
  (4)   changing to 20% dextrose with 4.25% amino acids at 75 mL/h and adding 500 mL/day Intralipid

87.   A 45-year-old woman with diabetic gastroparesis is intubated for ventilatory failure from Guillain-Barré syndrome. After 3 weeks, no neurologic recovery has occurred. Reasonable ways of providing nutrition include

  (1)   nasoduodenal feeding tube
  (2)   peripheral parenteral nutrition
  (3)   jejunostomy tube
  (4)   gastrostomy tube

Questions 88–90.

An 80-kg man with a 60-pack-year smoking history sustained a 50 percent full-thickness body surface area burn in an industrial accident. He was intubated for airway protection and ventilated to facilitate early cardiopulmonary and burn management. Bronchoscopy excluded an airway burn. The initial fluid management included daily parenteral nutrition with a standard balanced amino acid solution containing 100 g protein and 3900 nonprotein calories given as glucose (3 L 25% glucose) and fat (1 L 10% Intralipid). One week later, the patient was initiating 30 breaths per minute from a ventilator set to deliver a tidal volume of 800 mL at an FI_{O_2} of 0.4. The arterial blood gases were pH 7.35, Pa_{CO_2} 48 mm Hg, and Pa_{O_2} 85 mm Hg. Concurrent indirect calorimetry revealed a mixed expired fraction of CO_2 (FE_{CO_2}) of 0.03 and a mixed expired fraction of O_2 (FE_{O_2}) of 0.38.

88. True statements include which of the following?

(1) The large ventilatory requirement is due entirely to the excess CO_2 production
(2) The patient's ratio of dead space to tidal volume (V_D/V_T) is abnormally high
(3) The normal respiratory quotient (V_{CO_2}/V_{O_2}) measured in this patient excludes excess carbohydrate administration as a cause of high CO_2 production
(4) This patient's O_2 consumption is greater than 5 mL/kg because of the extensive burn

89. In this patient, enrichment of the standard balanced amino acid solution with branched-chain amino acids (BCAA) will

(1) double the concentration of valine, leucine, and isoleucine to about 45 percent of the amino acids infused
(2) increase the rate of hepatic protein synthesis
(3) increase the absolute lymphocyte count
(4) decrease the negative nitrogen balance

90. In this patient, the 24-h urine urea nitrogen loss was 20 g, which indicates protein catabolism of about 136 g/day. Appropriate adjustment of nutritional therapy includes

(1) increasing the protein intake to 120 g/day
(2) increasing the fat calories to 2 L of 10% Intralipid
(3) reducing the daily carbohydrate calories to 2 L of 25% glucose
(4) reducing the daily carbohydrate calories to 3 L of 10% glucose

DIRECTIONS: The group of questions below consists of lettered headings followed by a set of numbered items. For each numbered item select the **one** lettered heading with which it is **most** closely associated. Each lettered heading may be used **once, more than once, or not at all.**

Questions 91–94.

Match each metabolic process with the respiratory quotient (RQ).

(A) 0.7
(B) 0.8
(C) 1.0
(D) 1.2
(E) 8.0

91. Conversion of carbohydrate to fat

92. Oxidation of fat

93. Oxidation of protein

94. Oxidation of carbohydrate

NUTRITION

80. The answer is B. *(Chapter 16)* Patients with severe burn injuries have markedly increased requirements for protein and calories. Burn patients may require up to 50 kcal/kg per day, roughly twice the normal daily requirement. Other critically ill patients, such as those with sepsis or trauma, have elevated energy expenditures, although their nutritional requirements are generally less than those of burn patients. Malnourished patients, by contrast, demonstrate diminished energy expenditures compared with normal individuals. These patients are more receptive to nutritional support than are normal individuals and often attain a markedly positive nitrogen balance. Finally, nitrogen excretion is elevated in all types of injuries that cause critical illness. Protein malnutrition is a common complication of critical illness that requires prompt attention and aggressive therapy.

81. The answer is D. *(Chapter 16)* Nitrogen loss occurs in all tissues except the brain and nervous system, which appear to be spared. The majority of nitrogen loss arises from skeletal muscle proteins.

82. The answer is C. *(Chapter 16)* Before measurement or in patients in whom energy expenditure is not measurable, 2500 kcal has been reported to be sufficient for 85 percent of patients.

83. The answer is B (1, 3). *(Chapter 16)* Patients who are stressed by sepsis or trauma demonstrate increased levels of insulin as well as glucose. They are therefore resistant to the hypoglycemic effects of insulin. This effect is probably mediated in part by catecholamines and steroids released in response to the stress. In addition to insulin resistance, there is increased breakdown of muscle protein to form glucose. While total body utilization of glucose is increased, this increase is offset by increased production, leading to an overall reduction in the proportion of energy derived from glucose. The brain continues to require glucose for energy, as appreciable ketogenesis does not occur even in starvation during critical illness. Finally, hyperglycemia does not result from increased carbohydrate uptake or from glycogenolysis, both of which are reduced during critical illness.

84. The answer is C (2, 4). *(Chapter 16)* The decision to initiate enteral versus parenteral feeding should be based on the patient's medical illness and the risks inherent in the placement of catheters and feeding tubes. Enteral feeding is less expensive to perform, is associated with fewer complications, and helps prevent intestinal mucosal atrophy. Both routes of delivery effectively maintain and restore nutritional states. While parenteral nutrition is preferred in conditions involving structural or functional obstruction distal to the source of enteral feeding, enteral nutrition may be used in many circumstances involving gastrointestinal motility disorders that do not involve complete obstruction.

85. **The answer is A (1, 2, 3).** *(Chapter 16)* Pancreatic function should be considered carefully during parenteral administration of lipids, and triglyceride levels should be followed during intravenous lipid infusion to minimize the potential for inducing pancreatitis. Intravenous fat emulsions have been associated with an increase in shunt and PGI_2 production in the lung. Enteral medium-chain triglycerides are absorbed and directly oxidized by the liver without the need for carnitine. These may be preferable forms of supplementation in patients with hepatic dysfunction.

86. **The answer is B (1,3).** *(Chapter 16)* Decreasing carbohydrate and caloric intake decreases CO_2 production, which lowers Pa_{CO_2} for a given minute ventilation and volume of dead space. Changing to a peripheral formula of 5% dextrose plus 3% amino acids (300 cal/L) with 500 mL/day Intralipid (1 cal/mL) decreases both carbohydrate load and total caloric intake.

87. **The answer is B (1, 3).** *(Chapter 16)* The patient is probably facing months of mechanical ventilation. Nutrition will be important to prevent protein catabolism and muscle wasting. Enteral alimentation is preferred over TPN, as it is easier to perform and cheaper, has fewer complications, may increase gastric pH and thus serve as prophylaxis against gastrointestinal bleeding, and prevents intestinal mucosal atrophy, thus decreasing the risk of bacterial translocation. Enteral alimentation may be given by mouth; through a nasogastric, duodenal, or jejunal tube; or via a gastrostomy or jejunostomy. This patient's gastroparesis is a contraindication to nasogastric or gastrostomy tube feedings, as the risk of aspiration will be increased. Nasoduodenal feeding tubes and jejunostomy tubes are reasonable alternatives. TPN via a long-term central vein catheter is less desirable, as it does not have the advantages of enteral feeding mentioned above. Peripheral parenteral nutrition is even less desirable as adequate calories could not be delivered and venous access would soon become limited.

88. **The answer is C (2, 4).** *(Chapter 16)* The CO_2 production is more than twice normal ($V_{CO_2} = 24$ lpm $\times$ $F_{E_{CO_2}}$, or about 700 mL/min), and so part of the increased ventilatory requirement is explained. However, the V_D / V_T is also abnormally increased [$V_D / V_T = (Pa_{CO_2} - P_{E_{CO_2}}) / Pa_{CO_2} = (48 - 21) / 48 = > 0.5$], perhaps owing to prior smoking-induced obstructive lung disease. Oxygen consumption is also increased ($V_{O_2} = 24$ lpm $\times$ [$F_{I_{O_2}} - F_{E_{O_2}}$] = 480 mL/min). Accordingly, the RQ (700 / 480) is much greater than 1.0, a finding compatible with the lipogenesis associated with excess carbohydrate administration.

89. **The answer is A (1, 2, 3).** *(Chapter 16)* Negative nitrogen balance is not reduced by BCAA in most controlled series.

90. **The answer is A (1, 2, 3).** *(Chapter 16)* This hypermetabolic, catabolic patient is in moderate negative nitrogen balance (136 − 100, or 36 g/day), which can be minimized by increasing protein intake and providing sufficient nonprotein calories (about 30 kcal per gram of protein). Although he was receiving 3900 kcal as carbohydrate (CHO = 3000 kcal) and fat (lipid = 900 kcal), providing the same calories with only 50% carbohydrate will reduce RQ and CO_2 production, which will decrease the ventilation required to maintain eucapnia. Reducing total calories by reducing carbohydrate intake will fail to meet the metabolic needs and will cause wasting and weakness of the respiratory muscles.

91–94. **The answers are 91-E, 92-A, 93-B, 94-C.** *(Chapter 16)* Values for RQ are well known for different metabolic processes. An RQ near 1 indicates that the main nutrient utilized is glucose. When it is close to 0.7, the main nutrient is fat. Oxidation of carbohydrate results in an RQ of 1.0, while metabolism of an average diet of mixed (predominantly carbohydrate) caloric sources results in 0.8. Conversion of carbohydrate to fat (lipogenesis) results in an RQ of 8.0. Since RQ is V_{CO_2} / V_{O_2}, lipogenesis greatly increases V_{CO_2} and the consequent need for alveolar ventilation. For this reason, over-feeding critically ill patients may impede their liberation from mechanical ventilation.

CARDIOVASCULAR DISORDERS IN THE CRITICALLY ILL

QUESTIONS

DIRECTIONS: Each question below contains four or five suggested responses. Select the **one best** response to each question.

95. A 30-year-old man in shock is given nitroprusside, to which he initially responds well. However, attempts to switch to oral medications are unsuccessful. He remains on nitroprusside at doses of 10 to 12 μg/kg per minute. On the fourth hospital day he requires increasingly large doses of nitroprusside to control his blood pressure. He becomes less oriented and develops a metabolic acidosis. The cause of this patient's symptoms is

(A) depressed cardiac output because of increased afterload
(B) depressed cardiac output because of depressed systolic function
(C) altered distribution of blood flow by nitroprusside, which causes shunting of blood past hypoxic capillary beds
(D) impaired release of oxygen from hemoglobin because of the toxic effect of nitroprusside
(E) altered ability of cells to utilize oxygen because of the toxic effect of nitroprusside

96. Which of the following statements best describes therapy for an acute myocardial infarction?

(A) Aspirin has been shown to decrease both mortality and the incidence of reinfarction
(B) The addition of warfarin to aspirin improves the outcome in patients with an acute MI
(C) Cost-benefit analysis clearly favors the use of heparin with aspirin over aspirin alone
(D) Intravenous heparin has been shown to provide distinct clinical benefit over high-dose subcutaneous heparin administration
(E) Aspirin confers little benefit to patients with an acute MI who present more than 48 hours after the onset of symptoms

97. The best noninvasive test for determining the presence and degree of pulmonary hypertension is

(A) hilar-to-thoracic ratio and diameter of the right descending pulmonary artery on posteroanterior chest x-ray
(B) electrocardiogram
(C) physical examination
(D) Doppler-aided echocardiography
(E) chest CT

Questions 98–99.

A 32-year-old man with a history of hypertension and mild renal insufficiency presents with altered mental status. Physical examination reveals the following: pulse 112, blood pressure 244/165 mm Hg, respirations 32, and temperature 37.2°C (99°F). His funduscopic exam reveals papilledema. Chest auscultation revealed crackles to the lower one-third of the lung fields. Cardiac examination reveals a jugular venous pulsation to the angle of the jaw, normal S_1 and S_2, a II/VI holosystolic murmur at the left base that radiates to the apex, and a I/IV decrescendo diastolic murmur. Abdominal examination is unremarkable. Extremities are cool with poor capillary refill. Neurologically, the patient is oriented only to his name. He follows some simple commands but no complex ones. There is no focality to the motor or sensory examinations. Laboratory data reveals a hemoglobin of 15.2 g/dL, normal sodium and potassium, a bicarbonate of 12 mEq/L, a blood urea nitrogen of 56 mg/dL, and a creatinine of 6.2 mg/dL; an arterial blood gas on oxygen revealed a pH of 7.20, a Pa_{CO_2} of 32 mm Hg, and a Pa_{O_2} of 110 mm Hg. Chest x-ray reveals pulmonary edema and a globular heart.

98. Evidence supporting a shock state in this case includes all the following EXCEPT

(A) a metabolic acidosis
(B) altered mental status
(C) pulmonary edema
(D) renal dysfunction
(E) cool extremities with poor capillary refill

99. An echocardiogram was obtained because of concern about the globular heart on chest x-ray. It revealed massive four-chamber enlargement and globally depressed left ventricular function. Given this information, the appropriate therapy should include

(A) dobutamine started at 5 μg/kg per minute
(B) nitroglycerin started at 5 μg per minute
(C) furosemide in a 40-mg intravenous bolus
(D) nitroprusside at 0.5 μg/kg per minute
(E) dialysis

100. A 68-year-old man with an anterior wall myocardial infarction has a pulmonary capillary wedge pressure (PCWP) of 16 mm Hg and a low cardiac output. He is started on dobutamine, and his blood pressure falls from 93/70 to 87/55 mm Hg. What is the best response?

(A) Stop dobutamine and start dopamine
(B) Continue dobutamine and add dopamine
(C) Give a bolus of 500 mL normal saline
(D) Start norepinephrine (Levophed)
(E) Consider an intraaortic balloon pump

101. Ventilation-perfusion scans can be difficult to interpret in critically ill patients. However, there are some instances in which they can be extremely useful. All the following ventilation-perfusion results are useful EXCEPT

(A) a normal perfusion scan in a 50-year-old man with chest pain
(B) multiple matched subsegmental ventilation and perfusion defects in a 65-year-old woman with COPD
(C) complete lack of perfusion to one lung in a 32-year-old neurosurgical patient with shock
(D) a single matched ventilation and perfusion defect in a patient with fever, leukocytosis, purulent sputum, and an infiltrate on chest x-ray in the same region as the ventilation and perfusion defects
(E) a segmental, unmatched ventilation-perfusion defect in a patient with a clear chest x-ray who has developed new-onset atrial fibrillation and hypoxemia after hip replacement

102. Common causes of cardiac arrhythmias in critically ill patients include all the following EXCEPT

(A) electrolyte abnormalities
(B) catecholamine excess
(C) myocardial ischemia
(D) infiltrative cardiomyopathies
(E) drug intoxication

103. All the following are risk factors for thromboembolic events in the perioperative period EXCEPT

(A) morbid obesity
(B) adenocarcinoma
(C) lupus anticoagulant
(D) nephrotic syndrome
(E) chronic renal failure

104. Heparin prophylaxis against venous thrombosis is indicated for patients in all the following situations EXCEPT

(A) recent repair of an abdominal aortic aneurysm
(B) status post myocardial infarction
(C) intrauterine pregnancy at 14 weeks with exacerbation of asthma
(D) status post subarachnoid hemorrhage
(E) septic shock

105. The following statements about digoxin therapy for congestive heart failure (CHF) are true EXCEPT

(A) the use of digoxin increases the likelihood of developing atrial tachyarrhythmias
(B) the use of digoxin increases the likelihood of developing ventricular tachyarrhythmias
(C) the use of digoxin increases the likelihood of developing advanced atrioventricular block
(D) digoxin therapy has been shown to decrease overall mortality in patients with CHF who receive diuretics and ACE inhibitors
(E) digoxin therapy has been shown to reduce the overall number of hospitalizations for worsening heart failure in patients with CHF who receive diuretics and ACE inhibitors

106. Causes of aortic insufficiency include all the following EXCEPT

(A) Marfan's syndrome
(B) syphilis
(C) rheumatoid arthritis
(D) scleroderma
(E) bicuspid aortic valve

107. A 48-year-old renal dialysis patient is brought to the emergency room with severe shortness of breath and hypotension. She requires immediate intubation, after which the pulse is 148 and the blood pressure is 90/65 mm Hg. The chest radiograph and electrocardiogram below are obtained. These studies indicate that the cause of the patient's deterioration is likely to be

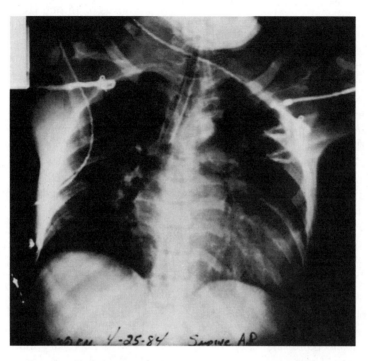

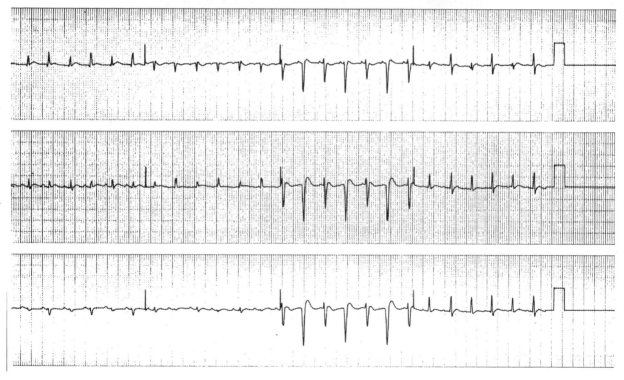

(A) anteroseptal myocardial infarction
(B) myocardial infarction and acute mitral regurgitation
(C) hypertrophic cardiomyopathy
(D) cardiac tamponade
(E) myocarditis

108. In patients who present with malignant hypertension,

(A) those who present with papilledema have a worse prognosis than do patients with hemorrhages or exudates seen on funduscopic examination
(B) prognosis does not depend on serum creatinine
(C) cerebral autoregulation is intact
(D) there is necrotizing arteriolitis in the later stages

109. A 48-year-old housewife with an unremarkable past medical history presented with a 2-day history of blurred vision in her left eye. Blood pressure was 210/120 with a regular heart rate of 82. On funduscopic examination, the physiologic cup of the optic disc was obscured. This blurring extended to diverging vessels, and the veins were distended and pulseless. Except for the funduscopic examination and a II/VI systolic ejection murmur, the remainder of her physical examination was normal. Laboratory data were notable for a creatinine of 2.1 and a normal urinalysis. Optimal management of this patient would consist of

(A) reduction of diastolic blood pressure to 90 to 100 mm Hg over several days
(B) reduction of diastolic blood pressure to 90 to 100 mm Hg over several hours
(C) reduction of mean arterial pressure to approximately 135 mm Hg in the first hour, followed by gradual reduction to a diastolic blood pressure of 100 to 110 mm Hg over several hours
(D) reduction of mean arterial pressure to approximately 120 mm Hg over several hours, followed by eventual reduction to a diastolic pressure of 90 to 100 mm Hg

110. Which of the following statements regarding aortic dissection is true?

(A) Medical therapy should target blood pressure reduction without decreasing cardiac contractility
(B) CT is more sensitive than aortography or echocardiography
(C) Transthoracic echocardiography is less accurate than transesophageal echocardiography in the diagnosis of aortic dissections
(D) In type A aortic dissections chest radiography reveals a widened mediastinum in 90 percent of cases

111. A 65-year-old man with widely metastatic bronchogenic carcinoma presents with complaints of dyspnea. On examination, his pulse is 110 beats per minute and his blood pressure is 90/65 mm Hg with a pulsus paradoxus of 15 mm Hg. His lungs are clear on examination, but cardiac auscultation reveals muffled heart sounds. ECG reveals low voltage with electrical alternans. Echocardiography might reveal

(A) diminished left ventricular systolic performance
(B) acute papillary muscle rupture
(C) right ventricular dilation and poor systolic function
(D) left ventricular hypertrophy with systolic anterior motion of the mitral valve
(E) diastolic collapse of the right atrium and right ventricle

112. Which of the following patients is at the greatest risk of death during cardiac catheterization?

(A) A 64-year-old man with New York Heart Association (NYHA) class IV congestive heart failure
(B) A 61-year-old man with significant three-vessel coronary artery disease
(C) A 60-year-old man with significant aortic stenosis and a right bundle branch block (RBBB)
(D) A 64-year-old man with severe peripheral vascular disease and an allergy to radiographic contrast dye

113. All the following statements regarding acute pericardial tamponade from penetrating chest trauma are true EXCEPT

(A) tamponade can occur with as little as 200 mL of fluid
(B) a normal cardiac silhouette is present in 15 percent of cases
(C) jugular venous distention may be absent
(D) hypotension is absent in close to 40 percent of these patients
(E) pericardiocentesis is an unreliable diagnostic procedure

114. Which of the following patients would be LEAST likely to benefit from coronary angioplasty?

(A) A 54-year-old man with the onset of severe substernal chest pain 1.5 hours ago who has just received tissue plasminogen activator (TPA)

(B) A 48-year-old man with a history of inferior myocardial infarction 3 weeks ago who presents with recurrence of chest pain and whose cardiac catheterization shows total occlusion of the right coronary artery

(C) A 50-year-old man with the onset of severe substernal chest pain 30 hours ago who is in cardiogenic shock secondary to severe mitral regurgitation

(D) A 56-year-old man with coronary artery bypass surgery 3 years ago and restenosis of two of his saphenous vein grafts

115. A patient with chronic pericardial tamponade develops worsening shortness of breath 3 hours after the performance of a subxiphoid pericardial window. The most likely cause of this patient's deterioration is

(A) pulmonary embolus

(B) noncardiogenic pulmonary edema

(C) cardiogenic pulmonary edema

(D) recurrent pericardial tamponade

(E) aspiration pneumonia

116. The use of an intraaortic balloon pump may be indicated in all the following EXCEPT

(A) a patient with a new infarct and cardiogenic shock who has a known history of moderate to severe aortic insufficiency

(B) a patient with continued angina and evidence of ischemia after other therapies have failed

(C) acute ventricular septal defect with shock

(D) acute mitral regurgitation with hypoperfusion

(E) as a bridge to cardiac transplantation

117. Direct-current cardioversion is typically useful for the treatment of

(A) sinus tachycardia

(B) multifocal atrial tachycardia

(C) torsade de pointes

(D) nonparoxysmal junctional tachycardia

(E) none of the above

118. A 70-year-old woman is being monitored after an acute inferior myocardial infarction. While talking with her nurse, she abruptly loses consciousness, and ventricular fibrillation is noted on the bedside monitor. The nurse calls for help, charges the defibrillator to 200 joule, and administers an asynchronous shock to the chest. The rhythm remains unchanged, and the shock is repeated. When ventricular fibrillation persists, she increases the charge to 360 joule and immediately repeats the attempt. The physician arrives on the scene and notes that the patient is still in ventricular fibrillation. All the following factors may negate the effects of electrical defibrillation EXCEPT

(A) hypomagnesemia

(B) digitalis intoxication

(C) pneumothorax

(D) encainide

(E) reversal of the polarity of the paddles

119. The following rhythm tracing is obtained in a patient with a temporary pacemaker in place, set at a rate of 68. This tracing demonstrates

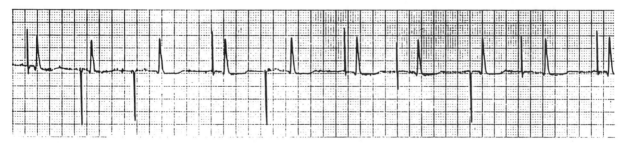

(A) electrical artifact

(B) failure to capture

(C) retrograde conduction

(D) pacemaker-induced tachycardia

(E) normal AV sequential pacing

120. The following is a rhythm tracing from a patient with a temporary pacemaker in place, set at a rate of 67. This tracing demonstrates

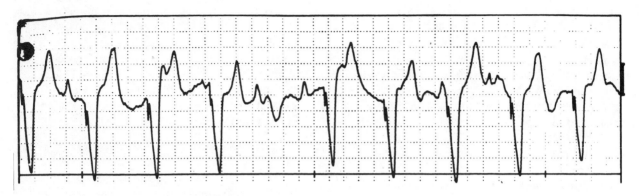

(A) electrical artifact
(B) normal pacemaker function
(C) failure to capture
(D) oversensing
(E) retrograde conduction

121. A 58-year-old male stockbroker presents with an acute anteroseptal myocardial infarction complicated by cardiogenic shock and pulmonary edema. To optimally manage this patient's hemodynamics, a pulmonary artery catheter is placed. To assure adequate delivery of oxygen to peripheral tissue beds, the mixed venous Pa_{O_2} should be kept above what threshold value?

(A) 40 mm Hg
(B) 35 mm Hg
(C) 25 mm Hg
(D) 20 mm Hg

DIRECTIONS: Each question below contains four suggested responses of which **one or more** is correct. Select

A	if	**1, 2, and 3**	are correct
B	if	**1 and 3**	are correct
C	if	**2 and 4**	are correct
D	if	**4**	is correct
E	if	**1, 2, 3, and 4**	are correct

122. In patients with shock, end-organ damage can accrue quickly and result in multiple system organ failure. Measures to prevent the development of this disastrous consequence include

(1) a trial of volume administration to improve tissue perfusion
(2) rapid assessment of the etiology of shock
(3) assurance of adequate oxygen delivery
(4) administration of an α-adrenergic pressor drug to improve blood pressure

123. Manifestations of myocardial ischemia in the critically ill include

(1) an increase in airway pressure in a mechanically ventilated patient
(2) an increase in pulmonary artery diastolic pressure
(3) a *v* wave greater than 10 mm Hg above mean pulmonary capillary wedge pressure (PCWP)
(4) difficulty in discontinuing mechanical ventilation

124. Indications for transvenous pacing in acute myocardial infarction include

(1) type 1 second-degree AV block with a ventricular response of 55/min resulting in hemodynamic compromise that is unresponsive to atropine
(2) alternating left bundle branch block and right bundle branch block (LBBB and RBBB)
(3) new bifascicular block
(4) new first-degree AV block plus a preexisting bifascicular block

125. A 26-year-old woman, G_1P_0, presents at 26 weeks with complaints of headache, blurred vision, and bilateral lower extremity swelling. On examination, her blood pressure is 165/115 and her cardiac exam is notable for a hyperdynamic precordium with the presence of an S_4 and a II/VI systolic murmur. Auscultation of her chest reveals bibasilar crackles, and she has 2+ pitting edema in both lower extremities. Her hematocrit is 45, and the urine dipstick is notable for a specific gravity of 1.030 with 4+ protein. An appropriate antihypertensive regimen might include

(1) nitroprusside
(2) enalapril
(3) furosemide
(4) hydralazine

126. Properties of adenosine include

(1) coronary artery vasodilation
(2) AV nodal blockade
(3) decreased sinus node automaticity
(4) bronchospasm

127. In patients with right ventricular infarction

(1) right atrial pressure is low and pulmonary capillary wedge pressure (PCWP) is usually high
(2) pulmonary edema commonly develops
(3) right precordial leads typically show ST-segment depression
(4) a dual-chamber AV sequential pacemaker should be used when transvenous pacing is indicated

128. A 32-year-old woman is transferred by an outside physician for evaluation of breathlessness. She had previously been seen for complaints of fatigue and one episode of near syncope. She later presented with disturbing shortness of breath, especially with exertion, and also experienced dizziness, which correlated on examination with decreases in blood pressure to 90/60 mm Hg. An echocardiogram done at the outside medical center suggested pulmonary hypertension. She had duplex Doppler studies of the lower extremities, which were negative for deep-vein thrombosis, and she had a normal ventilation-perfusion scan. Other symptoms and findings consistent with primary pulmonary hypertension (PPH) as the etiology of her pulmonary hypertension would include

(1) rheumatoid arthritis
(2) a normal electrocardiogram
(3) atrial fibrillation on electrocardiography
(4) a mean pulmonary artery pressure in excess of 60 mm Hg

129. Inhaled nitric oxide has been shown to significantly improve hemodynamic function and gas exchange in

(1) the adult respiratory distress syndrome
(2) congestive heart failure
(3) acute right ventricular failure after cardiac transplantation
(4) aortic insufficiency

130. Which of the following may contribute to the hypoxemia seen in some patients with pulmonary embolism?

(1) Right-to-left shunt
(2) Decreased mixed venous oxyhemoglobin saturation
(3) Ventilation-perfusion mismatching
(4) Alveolar hypoventilation

131. Presentations of pulmonary embolism in the intensive care unit include

(1) sudden death
(2) unexplained fever
(3) increased Pa_{CO_2} in a muscle-relaxed, mechanically ventilated patient
(4) elevated hemidiaphragm on routine chest x-ray

132. A 65-year-old man presents with crushing substernal chest pain, shortness of breath, and light-headedness. ECG reveals 3-mm ST elevations throughout the precordium. His blood pressure is 85/65, and an ABG on 50% O_2 face mask reveals a pH of 7.24, Pa_{CO_2} of 25 mm Hg, and Pa_{O_2} of 75 mm Hg. His serum lactate is 6.8 mg/dL, and his urine output has decreased to 10 mL/h despite the infusion of 1.5 L of 0.9% normal saline. He continues to complain of chest pain and dyspnea despite therapy with aspirin and IV nitroglycerin. Appropriate interventions might include

(1) intraaortic balloon pump insertion
(2) intravenous morphine administration
(3) intubation and mechanical ventilation
(4) intravenous epinephrine administration

133. Digoxin administration is contraindicated in which of the following clinical situations?

(1) Irregular, wide-complex tachycardia in a young person
(2) Atrial fibrillation in a patient with mitral stenosis
(3) Congestive heart failure in a patient with systolic obliteration of the left ventricle on echocardiography
(4) Dilated cardiomyopathy in an alcoholic

134. Pericardial disease is associated with

(1) renal failure
(2) mediastinal radiation therapy
(3) bacterial endocarditis
(4) myocardial infarction

135. Symptoms of aortic stenosis include

(1) chest pain
(2) dyspnea on exertion
(3) syncope
(4) fatigue

136. A 57-year-old man with Ehlers-Danlos syndrome is admitted to the coronary care unit after a near-syncopal episode. His blood pressure is 105/45, and his pulse is 110. Transesophageal echocardiography reveals moderately severe aortic regurgitation. Initial management should include

(1) nitroprusside
(2) norepinephrine
(3) dobutamine
(4) immediate aortic valve replacement

137. A 65-year-old woman with idiopathic hypertrophic subaortic stenosis is transferred to the intensive care unit with complaints of dyspnea after an elective hip replacement. Her vital signs reveal a pulse of 124 beats per minute, blood pressure of 88/70, and a respiratory rate of 24. A chest x-ray demonstrates a diffuse four-quadrant infiltrate consistent with pulmonary edema. Appropriate therapeutic options include

(1) digoxin
(2) esmolol
(3) dobutamine
(4) saline infusion

138. Drugs associated with rebound hypertension after cessation of the medication include

(1) calcium channel blockers
(2) β blockers
(3) minoxidil
(4) clonidine

139. Potential complications of therapy with sodium nitroprusside include

(1) pancreatitis
(2) acute renal failure
(3) psychosis
(4) lactic acidosis

140. Complications of bronchial artery embolization include

(1) cerebrovascular accident
(2) paraplegia
(3) renal failure
(4) pulmonary infarction

141. As opposed to one- and two-dimensional echocardiography, Doppler echocardiography allows better assessment of

(1) cardiac chamber size
(2) cardiac output
(3) left ventricular aneurysm
(4) valve stenosis or regurgitation

142. In patients free of left ventricular disease, the echocardiographic signs of right ventricular pressure overload include

(1) right ventricular enlargement
(2) reduced transventricular septal pressure differential
(3) leftward deflection of the interventricular septum
(4) abnormalities of right ventricular regional wall motion

143. Technical advances offered by transesophageal echocardiography (TEE) include

(1) an accessible mode of echocardiographic monitoring that will not interfere with the surgical field
(2) better visualization of the intracardiac air to determine which patients are at risk for air embolism after cardiac and neurosurgical procedures
(3) better visualization of AV valves and valvular function
(4) a greater number of imaging locations than offered by the precordium

144. A 48-year-old man with leukemia presents with pneumonia. Blood cultures grow *Pseudomonas aeruginosa*. Because of hypotension refractory to vigorous fluid administration, a pulmonary artery catheter is inserted, yielding the following results: cardiac output = 10 L/min, Ppw = 18 mm Hg, mixed venous oxygen saturation = 78 percent, arterial blood gases are pH 7.25, Pa_{CO_2} 20 mm Hg, Pa_{O_2} 110 mm Hg, lactate = 8 mmol/L. Possible etiologies of this patient's lactic acidosis include

(1) inadequate oxygen delivery
(2) overabundance of pyruvate
(3) hypotension
(4) anaerobic metabolism

Questions 145–147.

145. A 27-year-old man with a history of rheumatic fever who is being treated for bacterial endocarditis is noted to become increasingly short of breath over a short period of time. Physical examination is notable for tachycardia, a blood pressure of 80/65, a respiratory rate of 40, and crackles to two-thirds bilaterally on auscultation of the chest. Cardiac examination reveals a jugular venous pulsation at the angle of the jaw while the patient is sitting at a 45-degree angle in bed. A soft S_1 is heard, with a loud III/VI holosystolic murmur, which radiates to the axilla and the apex of the heart. A flow-directed pulmonary artery catheter is placed with initial readings of right atrium 18 mm Hg, right ventricle 63/15 mm Hg, and pulmonary artery 63/31 mm Hg. Attempts to "wedge" the catheter resulted in the tracing below. True statements about the therapy for this patient's shock state include

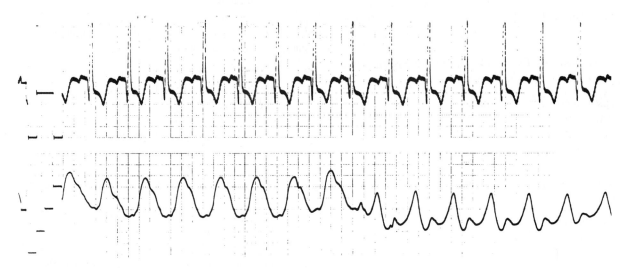

(1)   nitroprusside would be inappropriate given the patient's hypotension

(2)   consultation for cardiac surgery should be obtained immediately

(3)   α-adrenergic agents for the patient's hypotension are contraindicated

(4)   intraaortic balloon pumping would be indicated

146. The same patient undergoes replacement of the mitral valve. He does well postoperatively and is moving toward extubation when he develops bronchospasm. He is initially treated with diuretics for presumed pulmonary edema but becomes hypotensive. Review of the chart reveals a past history of asthma. On physical examination he is anxious, his heart rate is tachycardic, blood pressure is 95/68 mm Hg, and respirations are 32 per minute with recruitment of expiratory muscles. Chest examination reveals diffuse inspiratory and expiratory wheezes, with prolonged expiration. Heart sounds reveal well-heard metallic S_1 and S_2 without murmurs or rubs. The tracing below of the pulmonary artery occlusion pressure is obtained. Given your interpretation of the available data, the appropriate interventions include

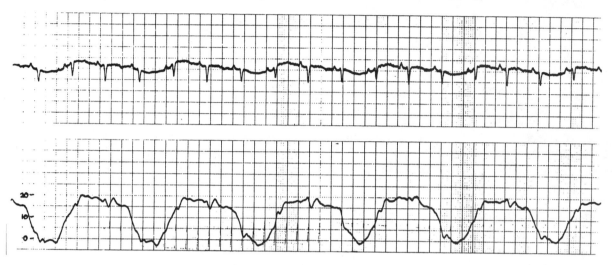

(1) emergent pericardiocentesis
(2) administration of further fluids
(3) administration of dobutamine and nitroprusside
(4) administration of inhaled bronchodilators

147. The same patient is treated with inhaled bronchodilators and then is sedated because of persistent hypotension. His blood pressure has fallen to 82/60 mm Hg. Airway pressures were noted to increase after sedation and muscle relaxation. Currently, the peak airway pressure is 52 cm H_2O, the plateau pressure is 24 cm H_2O, and the airway pressure after the insertion of an expiratory pause is 12 cm H_2O. The tracing below of the pulmonary artery occlusion pressure is obtained. Given the available hemodynamic data, the appropriate therapy might include

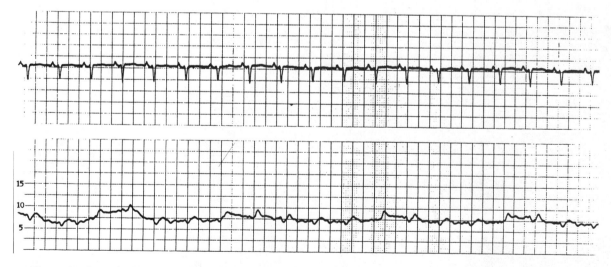

(1) reduction of minute volume
(2) further administration of a bronchodilator
(3) volume administration
(4) removal from mechanical ventilation for up to 1 minute after preoxygenation with 100% oxygen

148. Factors to be considered in evaluating the risk-benefit ratio of coronary angioplasty include

(1) presence of renal insufficiency
(2) ability to withstand coronary artery surgery
(3) history of previous cardiac surgery
(4) presence of significant left ventricular dysfunction

149. True statements about aortic valvuloplasty include

(1) severe coronary artery disease is a contraindication
(2) the prognosis of patients with left main coronary artery disease and symptomatic aortic stenosis probably is not improved by aortic valvuloplasty
(3) the majority of patients who experience perforation of the left ventricle during aortic valvuloplasty require surgical drainage and repair
(4) the long-term hemodynamic results of aortic valve replacement are much superior to those of balloon aortic valvuloplasty

150. True statements regarding ventricular assistance devices include which of the following?

(1) Most are used in the postcardiotomy state in patients with cardiac indices less than 2 L/min
(2) They have been shown to decrease infarct size but show no clear impact on mortality
(3) They have been shown to decrease left ventricular oxygen consumption when a ventricular bypass device is used
(4) When used as a bridge to transplantation, they have allowed most persons to be transplanted

151. Traumatic aortic rupture from acceleration-deceleration injury

(1) occurs most often just distal to the origin of the left subclavian artery
(2) can be treated medically if the hematoma appears to be contained within an intact adventitial layer
(3) may be evaluated further by placement of a nasogastric tube
(4) should be evaluated with CT before aortography in most cases

152. A 46-year-old woman is admitted to the emergency room with central chest pain of 90 minutes duration. Her examination is remarkable only for a sinus tachycardia of 100. Her electrocardiogram is shown below. Medications likely to be required in the first 24 hours of her management include

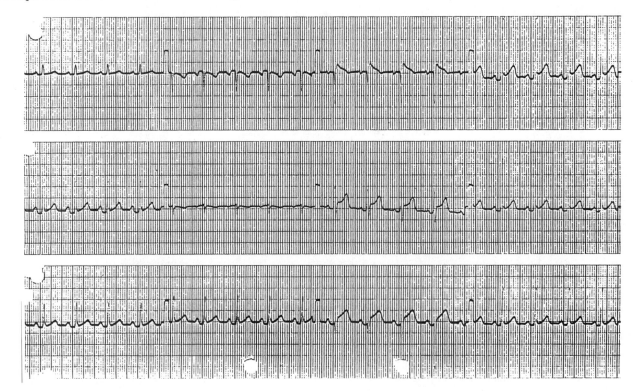

(1) thrombolytic agents
(2) calcium channel blockers
(3) intravenous nitroglycerin
(4) indomethacin (Indocin)

DIRECTIONS: Each group of questions below consists of lettered headings followed by a set of numbered items. For each numbered item select the one lettered heading with which it is **most** closely associated. Each lettered heading may be used **once, more than once, or not at all.**

Questions 153–156.

Match each clinical situation and treatment with the most likely result.

(A) Resolution of right ventricular (RV) ischemia
(B) Diminished right atrial (RA) filling resulting from increased pleural pressures with resultant elevations in RA pressure
(C) Decrease in mean systemic pressure and consequent diminished venous return
(D) Increased pulmonary hypertension leading to diminished left atrial (LA) filling
(E) Acute right ventricular infarction

153. A 58-year-old man experienced a pulmonary embolus 10 days after a right knee replacement procedure. He was subsequently mechanically ventilated and anticoagulated. He has been persistently hypotensive to 80/50 mm Hg over the last 4 hours with a progressive metabolic acidosis and a cardiac index of 2.0 L/min, and a PA pressure of 50/30 mm Hg. This hypoperfusion has been unresponsive to 2 L of intravenous saline and dobutamine. Norepinephrine was added as the attending physician was being contacted about possible thrombolytic therapy. With the addition of the norepinephrine, the patient's blood pressure rose to 100/70 mm Hg and his cardiac index increased to 3.0 L/min.

154. A patient with severe COPD and cor pulmonale is in respiratory failure from respiratory muscle fatigue. Upon being placed on the ventilator with positive-pressure ventilation, blood pressure precipitously fell from 140/70 to 90/60 mm Hg and he became confused and diaphoretic.

155. A 45-year-old woman develops pulmonary hypertension and acute right heart failure after a pneumonectomy. Inhaled nitric oxide (iNO) therapy results in a dramatic decrease in pulmonary hypertension with improved gas exchange. Within 30 seconds of discontinuation of iNO therapy the patient becomes cyanotic and unresponsive. Her mean systolic blood pressure drops to 50 mm Hg, and her mixed venous oxygen saturation declines to 52 percent.

156. A patient with cystic fibrosis, awaiting a lung transplant, experiences an exacerbation of bronchopneumonia and requires mechanical ventilation. On the initial settings his Pa_{CO_2} is 45 mm Hg. The minute ventilation is increased, and Pa_{CO_2} increases further to 50 mm Hg. The patient's blood pressure drops from 110/60 to 90/55 mm Hg. The patient's ventilator tubing is disconnected at end expiration, and a rush of air is heard from the patient's ET tube coincident with a return in blood pressure to the previous value.

Questions 157–160.

Match each medication with the most appropriate toxicity encountered in the intensive care setting.

(A) Esmolol
(B) Lidocaine
(C) Diltiazem
(D) Amiodarone
(E) Adenosine

157. Hypothyroidism

158. Hypoglycemia

159. Tonic-clonic seizures

160. Facial flushing

Questions 161–164.

For each drug listed, select the letter that best describes its effects.

	Vasodilation	Myocardial Depression	Depression of AV Conduction	Depression of SA Node
(A)	+ + +	+	0	0
(B)	+ + +	0	0	0
(C)	+ +	+ +	+	+ +
(D)	+ +	+ + +	+ +	+

0 = no effect; + = slight effect; + + = moderate effect; + + + = substantial effect

161. Verapamil

162. Nicardipine

163. Diltiazem

164. Nifedipine

Questions 165–169.

For each of the following clinical conditions, select the hemodynamic data that best support the diagnosis. (BP = blood pressure, RA = right atrial pressure, RV = right ventricular pressure, PA = pulmonary artery pressure, PCWP = pulmonary capillary wedge pressure, CO = thermodilution cardiac output, Sv_{O_2} = mixed venous oxyhemoglobin saturation)

	BP	RA	RV	PA	PCWP	CO	Sv_{O_2},%
(A)	95/63	18	32/16	33/20	19	6.4	80
(B)	92/59	19	53/17	53/35	16	2.7	52
(C)	85/42	16	36/9	36/14	14	9.2	78
(D)	89/64	18	33/17	33/19	18	2.5	61
(E)	76/40	17	65/15	66/44	24	5.4	68

165. Pericardial tamponade

166. Massive pulmonary embolism

167. Ruptured ventricular septum

168. Cor pulmonale with sepsis

169. Cirrhosis with acute renal failure

Questions 170–173.

Match the following rhythm strips or ECGs with the appropriate electrolyte abnormality.

(A) Hypokalemia
(B) Hyperkalemia
(C) Hypocalcemia
(D) Hypercalcemia

170.

171.

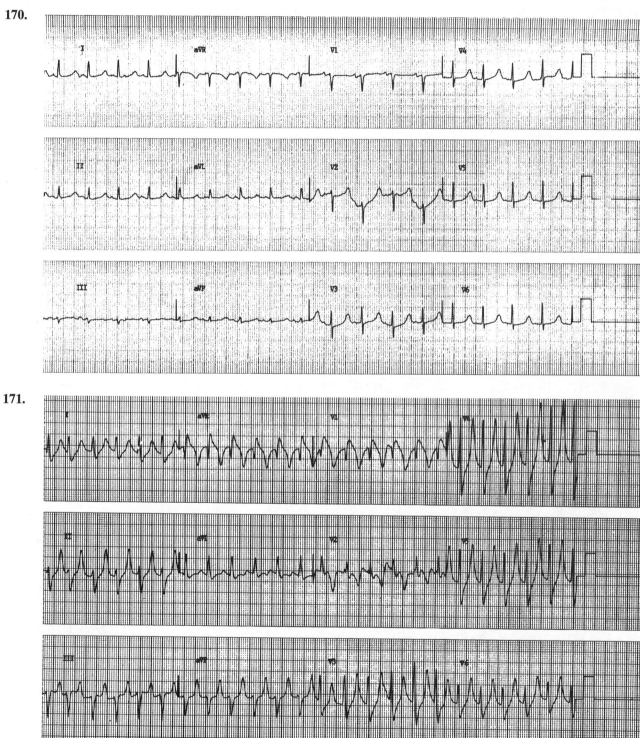

172.

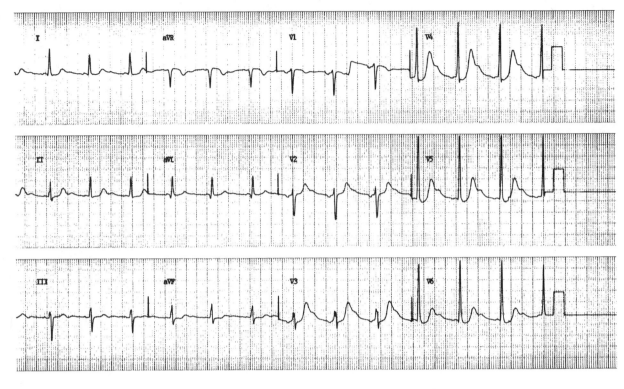

173.

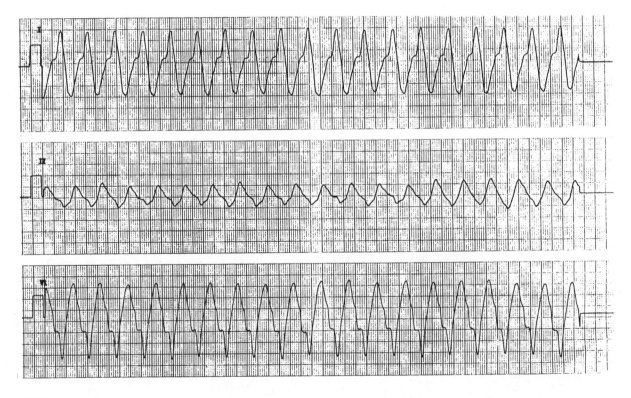

Questions 174–179.

Match the following rhythm strips and ECGs with the appropriate clinical condition.

(A) Myocardial infarction
(B) Pericarditis
(C) Pericardial effusion/tamponade
(D) Hypothermia
(E) Situs inversus
(F) Post-cardiac transplantation
(G) Flail chest

174.

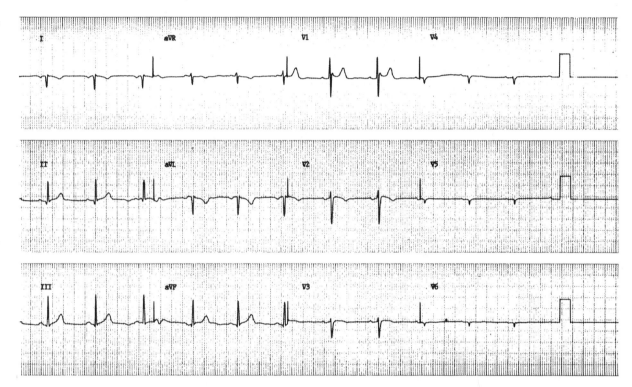

175.

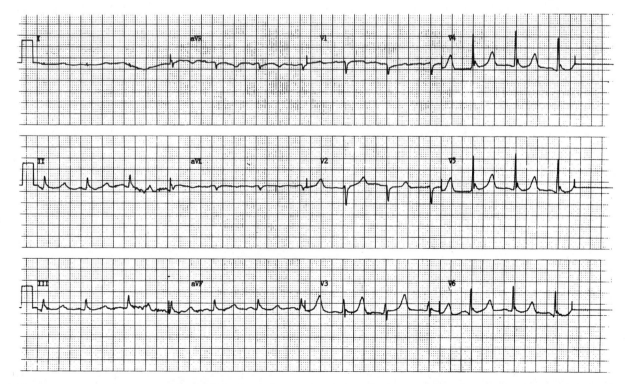

176.

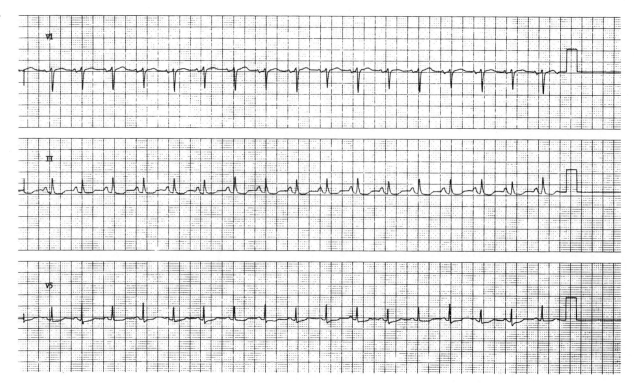

177.

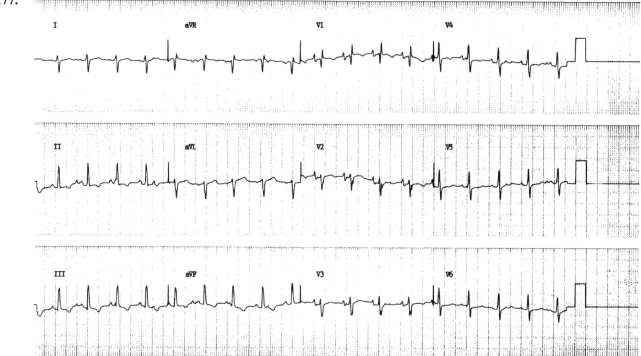

178.

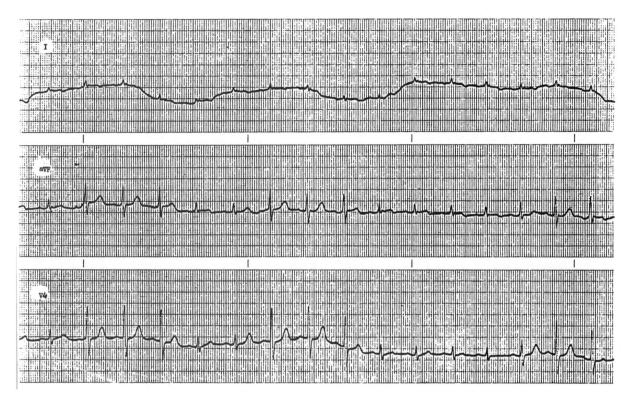

179.

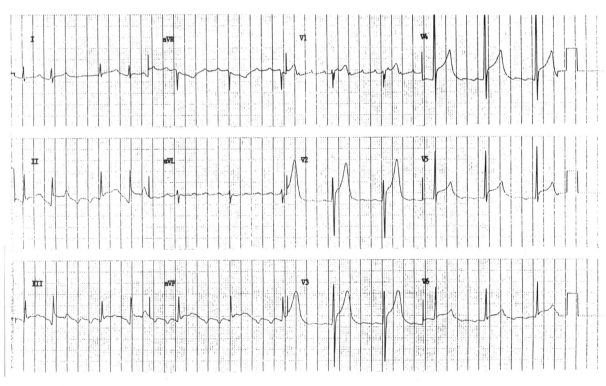

Questions 180–183.

Several left ventricular pressure-volume relationships are depicted below. Match the clinical situations listed with the pressure-volume relationship that best describes the expected pathophysiology.

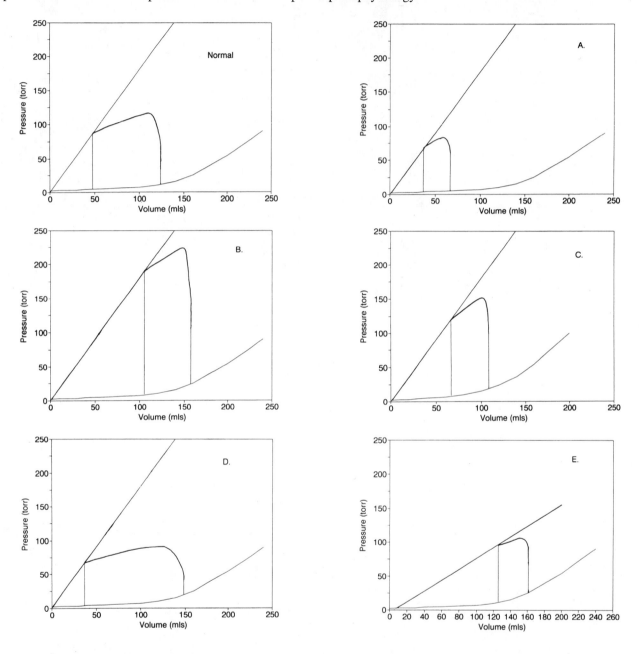

180.   A hypotensive patient with fulminant hepatic failure, a wide pulse pressure, and warm digits

181.   Hypotension in a patient with an acute gastrointestinal hemorrhage

182.   A young male with severe hypertension and pulmonary edema

183.   A middle-aged man with mild pulmonary edema after a large anterior myocardial infarction

Questions 184–187.

Illustrated at right are a series of venous return curves and points plotted along them corresponding to the venous return at a given right atrial pressure. Match the following clinical situations with the point on the venous return graph that best represents the ongoing pathophysiology.

184. An acute, hemodynamically significant pulmonary embolus

185. An acute gastrointestinal hemorrhage

186. The institution of positive-pressure ventilation with PEEP and the administration of morphine for sedation in a hypovolemic patient with acute hypoxemic respiratory failure

187. Compensated congestive heart failure

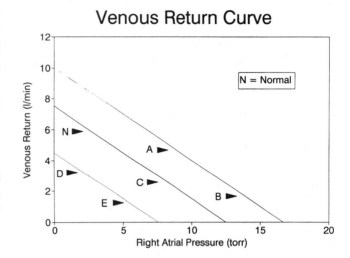

DIRECTIONS: Each group of questions below consists of four lettered headings followed by a set of numbered items. For each numbered item select

A   if the item is associated with   **(A) only**
B   if the item is associated with   **(B) only**
C   if the item is associated with   **both** (A) and (B)
D   if the item is associated with   **neither** (A) nor (B)

Each lettered heading may be used **once, more than once, or not at all.**

Questions 188–190.

  (A) Cardiac tamponade
  (B) Constrictive pericarditis
  (C) Both
  (D) Neither

188. Equal end-diastolic pressures in the right and left ventricles

189. Absence of ventricular filling early in diastole

190. Rapid x and y descent

Questions 191–192.

  (A) Mechanical heart valve
  (B) Bioprosthetic valve
  (C) Both
  (D) Neither

191. Requires anticoagulation therapy

192. Increased risk of developing endocarditis

Questions 193–194.

  (A) Sodium nitroprusside
  (B) Dobutamine
  (C) Both
  (D) Neither

193. Increased cardiac output

194. Decreased blood pressure

Questions 195–197.

  (A) Noncardiogenic pulmonary edema
  (B) Cardiogenic pulmonary edema
  (C) Both
  (D) Neither

195. Pleural effusions

196. Cardiomegaly

197. Infiltrates stable over days or even weeks

Questions 198–200.

  (A) Transthoracic echocardiography
  (B) Transesophageal echocardiography
  (C) Both
  (D) Neither

198. Reliable measure of left ventricular end-diastolic volume by short axis cross-sectional image

199. Reliable imaging of the left atrial appendage

200. Measurement of pressure differentials across restrictive orifices

Questions 201–203.

  (A) Cardiac tamponade
  (B) Constrictive pericarditis
  (C) Both
  (D) Neither

201. Right atrial tracing

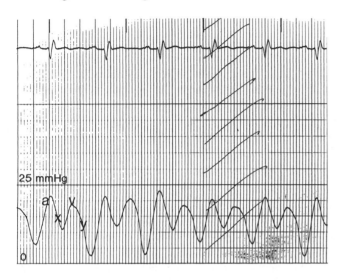

202. Right atrial tracing during mechanical ventilation

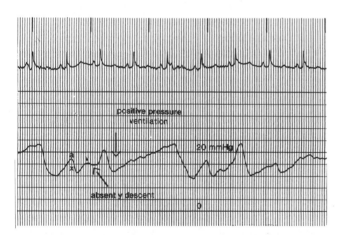

203. Left ventricular tracing

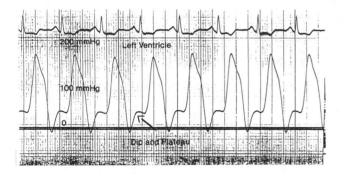

Questions 204–207.

  (A) Mitral valve replacement
  (B) Mitral valvuloplasty
  (C) Both
  (D) Neither

204. Useful in patients with a mitral valve area $< 1.5 \text{ cm}^2$

205. Useful in patients with severe mitral regurgitation

206. Contraindicated in patients with left atrial thrombus

207. Contraindicated in patients with thoracic spinal deformities

CARDIOVASCULAR DISORDERS IN THE CRITICALLY ILL

ANSWERS

95. The answer is E. *(Chapter 20)* Nitroprusside is metabolized by red cells to cyanide. The cyanide is then metabolized by the liver to thiocyanate. Thiocyanate is then excreted by the kidneys. Patients treated with high doses of nitroprusside over several days may be unable to metabolize the by-products of nitroprusside and so may develop thiocyanate or cyanide toxicity. Cyanide acts by binding to cytochrome aa3, thus impairing oxidative phosphorylation. The cells must therefore utilize the far less efficient anaerobic pathways to generate ATP. Therapy involves stopping the nitroprusside and, if toxicity is significant, administering cobalamin and considering the induction of methemoglobinemia.

96. The answer is A. *(Chapter 24)* The Second International Study of Infarct Survival (ISIS-2) concluded that daily aspirin therapy decreased mortality from acute MI by approximately 20 percent. In addition, the use of aspirin after an acute MI reduced the incidence of reinfarction and stroke by nearly 50 percent. To date, no studies have shown clear evidence of improved outcome in patients taking either warfarin or heparin with aspirin over aspirin alone. In the Global Utilization of Streptokinase and Tissue Plasminogen Activator for Occluded Coronary Arteries trial (GUSTO-1), comparisons of high-dose subcutaneous heparin and intravenous heparin failed to show any significant clinical difference. Although immediate institution of aspirin therapy is recommended in patients suffering an acute MI, delayed aspirin therapy confers a significant benefit over the absence of aspirin administration.

97. The answer is D. *(Chapter 25)* Whereas all the listed methods can suggest pulmonary hypertension, Doppler-aided echocardiography, especially with color flow, is the most sensitive and provides the most accurate quantification of the degree of pulmonary hypertension.

98. The answer is C. *(Chapter 20)* Shock is defined by evidence of multiple end-organ hypoperfusion. In this case, such evidence includes altered mental status and poor capillary refill on physical examination as well as laboratory evidence of poor perfusion, including a metabolic (lactic) acidosis and azotemia. Pulmonary edema, while suggestive of the etiology of the shock state, is not an example of end-organ hypoperfusion.

99. The answer is D. *(Chapter 20)* The left ventricular depression demonstrated here is due to markedly increased afterload and therefore, inotropic support with dobutamine will do little to increase forward flow. Agents or procedures that would decrease preload primarily—such as furosemide, nitroglycerin, and dialysis—might in fact reduce cardiac output by reducing the preload necessary to overcome the increased afterload. Nitroprusside, by vasodilating arterioles, will allow the ventricle to eject against a reduced afterload. This will improve forward flow and also will reduce the end-diastolic volume (as the end-systolic volume will be smaller), thus reducing end-diastolic pressure and pulmonary edema.

100. The answer is C. *(Chapter 24)* Patients with myocardial infarction often require a higher preload (usually about 18 mm Hg) to fill the stiff left ventricle. Hypotensive patients, including those with a high PCWP, should receive a volume challenge. Additionally, PCWP may fall when dobutamine is started, mandating further volume administration.

101. **The answer is B.** *(Chapter 26)* The utility of ventilation-perfusion scanning in patients with airway obstruction has been questioned. Areas of alveolar hypoventilation resulting from obstruction may cause hypoxic vasoconstriction, which in turn may cause perfusion defects. Consequently, unless the perfusion scan is completely normal, it offers no diagnostic information. In all the other situations described, the ventilation-perfusion scans offer significant additional information. In choice A the normal perfusion scan effectively excludes the diagnosis of pulmonary embolism. In choice C the perfusion scan strongly suggests a pulmonary embolus as the etiology of the shock state, and vena caval interruption is indicated. Whether pulmonary angiography and, if the angiogram confirms the proximal embolus, embolectomy should be performed depends on the center in which the patient is hospitalized. In choice D the correlation between the clinical findings and the chest x-ray abnormality is diagnostic of pneumonia. The absence of perfusion defects elsewhere argues against a diagnosis of superimposed pulmonary embolism. Unless there are compelling reasons to suspect pulmonary embolism, further workup is not necessary. Finally, in choice E the ventilation-perfusion scan suggests a high probability of pulmonary embolism in the correct clinical setting, and appropriate therapy should be instituted without further diagnostic studies.

102. **The answer is D.** *(Chapter 22)* In critically ill patients, arrhythmias may be precipitated by catecholamine excess, electrolyte abnormalities, or ischemia. Drug intoxication may complicate overdoses or may be iatrogenic in origin. Infiltrative cardiomyopathies, while a cause of arrhythmias, are relatively uncommon.

103. **The answer is E.** *(Chapter 26)* Patients who are morbidly obese and those with adenocarcinoma are at increased risk for thromboembolic events for unclear reasons. Those with lupus anticoagulant or anticardiolipin antibodies are also at increased risk for thrombosis, perhaps because of the effect of the anticardiolipin antibody on fibrinolysis or endothelial cell-platelet interactions. Patients with the nephrotic syndrome may lose antithrombin III as well as proteins C and S in the urine, predisposing them to thrombosis. Patients with chronic renal failure have a low incidence of venous thrombosis, perhaps owing to uremic platelet dysfunction or intermittent heparinization during dialysis.

104. **The answer is D.** *(Chapter 26)* There is no significant increase in the risk of bleeding in patients treated with subcutaneous heparin. However, because of the catastrophic consequences of bleeding in neurosurgical patients, alternative prophylaxis against venous thrombosis, such as pneumatic compression stockings, is recommended.

105. **The answer is D.** *(Chapter 21)* A recent study by the Digitalis Investigation Group revealed that the use of digoxin did not reduce overall mortality in patients with CHF who were receiving diuretics and ACE inhibitors. The study did reveal, however, a decrease in the rate of hospitalization in this population. The use of digoxin has been shown to increase the incidence of cardiac arrhythmias, including atrial and ventricular tachyarrhythmias and advanced atrioventricular block.

106. **The answer is D.** *(Chapter 28)* The common causes of aortic regurgitation include primary valvular disease—either congenital (bicuspid aortic valve) or acquired (rheumatic)—syphilis, infective endocarditis, and aortic dissection. Less common causes include hereditary disorders of connective tissue (Marfan and Ehlers-Danlos syndromes, osteogenesis imperfecta) and collagen vascular diseases (rheumatoid arthritis, systemic lupus erythematosus, Reiter syndrome). Scleroderma is associated with myocardial fibrosis and arrhythmias but not with aortic insufficiency.

107. **The answer is D.** *(Chapter 27)* The electrocardiogram reveals electrical alternans, and the postintubation chest radiograph reveals a "water bottle"–shaped heart, findings classic for a large pericardial effusion, which, when coupled to the clinical history, strongly suggests cardiac tamponade.

108. **The answer is D.** *(Chapter 21)* In malignant hypertension, funduscopic findings do not predict a patient's prognosis. An obvious reason for this is that the treatment of malignant hypertension has become so effective at preventing premature death that the condition of the fundi carries little long-term prognostic significance. The prognosis depends on the care with which the blood pressure is reduced acutely, the presenting serum creatinine, and long-term blood pressure control. Cerebral autoregulation is deranged with a shift to the right of the cerebral flow–pressure curve.

109. **The answer is C.** *(Chapter 21)*   Funduscopic examination revealed papilledema, one of the signs of malignant hypertension. This constitutes a hypertensive emergency that requires treatment in minutes to hours. To avoid reducing the blood pressure below the autoregulatory capacity of the patient's various vascular beds, most authorities suggest that the mean arterial pressure be reduced only about 15 percent during the first hour and reduced gradually thereafter to a diastolic blood pressure of 100 to 110 mm Hg or a reduction of 25 percent compared with initial baseline, whichever is higher. Rapid reduction of blood pressure to "normal," or even by as little as 35 percent, has been associated with major organ dysfunction.

110. **The answer is C.** *(Chapter 29)*   Luminal stresses and thus extension of the dissection are related both to the level of the systolic blood pressure and to the rate of rise of the blood pressure. Consequently, decreasing cardiac contractility as well as blood pressure is beneficial. CT scan is less sensitive than aortography or echocardiography. Transthoracic echocardiography is less accurate than transesophageal echocardiography in the diagnosis of aortic dissections. Transesophageal echocardiography has a sensitivity and specificity of > 98 percent. In about 40 percent of type A aortic dissections, chest radiography does not reveal a widened mediastinum.

111. **The answer is E.** *(Chapter 27)*   The clinical situation here strongly suggests pericardial tamponade. Pericardial tamponade is characterized by tachycardia, hypotension, pulsus paradoxus, and muffled heart tones, with low voltage and electrical alternans on ECG. Echocardiography would reveal a pericardial effusion, which results in diastolic collapse of the right atrium and right ventricle when it becomes hemodynamically significant. Diminished left ventricular systolic performance and acute papillary muscle rupture would be expected to cause dyspnea from pulmonary edema and would not cause pulsus paradoxus. Cor pulmonale would not cause pulsus paradoxus or electrical alternans. Left ventricular hypertrophy with systolic anterior motion of the mitral valve is characteristic of a hypertrophic cardiomyopathy, not of the clinical situation described here.

112. **The answer is A.** *(Chapter 24)*   The risk of death during coronary arteriography is less than 0.1 percent and has fallen in the last decade. Age over 60, New York Heart Association class IV congestive heart failure, and left main coronary artery stenosis are factors that increase the risk from the 0.1 to the 0.5 percent range.

113. **The answer is B.** *(Chapter 27)*   Acute accumulations of as little as 200 mL of fluid may cause tamponade because of the indistensibility of the pericardium, so that a normal cardiac silhouette is present in as many as 80 percent of cases. Jugular venous pressure may not be elevated, as blood may exit through a hole in the pericardium. Pericardiocentesis is an unreliable diagnostic procedure in acute tamponade and may be falsely positive or falsely negative in 50 percent of cases. Hypotension is absent in as many as 37 percent of these patients.

114. **The answer is B.** *(Chapter 24)*   Chronic total occlusions remain one of the major limitations of balloon angioplasty. The likelihood of success varies directly with their duration. Even more than a few weeks' duration results in a lower success rate. While intravenous thrombolytic therapy causes recanalization in 60 to 70 percent of patients, a patent infarct vessel may be achieved in over 90 percent with the combined approach of lysis and angioplasty. For patients with acute myocardial infarction and mitral regurgitation or shock caused by power failure, angioplasty even beyond 24 hours after the onset of infarct symptoms has been shown to be of benefit. Angioplasty is of benefit in patients who have previously undergone coronary artery bypass graft surgery with either saphenous vein or mammary artery grafts.

115. **The answer is C.** *(Chapters 19, 21, 27)* Pulmonary edema can occur when relief of tamponade increases venous return to the heart and results in an "internal" volume challenge. Contributing factors include an expanded circulating volume and an increase in afterload commonly seen in hypotensive patients with tamponade.

116. **The answer is A.** *(Chapters 20, 21)* Aortic insufficiency is an absolute contraindication to the use of an intraaortic balloon pump (IABP). Other ventricular assistance devices can be considered in this circumstance. IABP has been used successfully in the treatment of refractory angina, acute ventricular septal defect with shock, acute mitral regurgitation, and as a bridge to cardiac transplantation.

117. **The answer is C.** *(Chapter 23)* Direct-current cardioversion has the broadest spectrum of any antiarrhythmic therapy. It is most useful in rhythm disturbances that are due to re-entry and is not generally useful in those which are due to enhanced automaticity. Therefore, it is successful in the treatment of AV nodal reentrant tachycardia, reentrant tachycardia using a bypass tract, atrial flutter, paroxysmal atrial tachycardia, and paroxysmal ventricular tachycardia. It is ineffective in the treatment of sinus tachycardia, multifocal atrial tachycardia, and nonparoxysmal junctional tachycardia, in which enhanced automaticity underlies the disturbance. An exception to this general rule is torsade de pointes, a disturbance that arises from enhanced automaticity but responds to cardioversion.

118. **The answer is E.** *(Chapter 23)* When defibrillation is unsuccessful, it is important to consider factors involving the electrodes (e.g., improper paddle position, insufficient pressure, failure to use conductive gel), increased transthoracic impedance (e.g., pneumothorax), metabolic derangements (e.g., hypokalemia, hyperkalemia, hypomagnesemia, alkalosis, acidosis, hypoxemia), and drug effects (e.g., digitalis intoxication and a proarrhythmic effect of encainide or flecainide). The polarity of the paddles does not affect the efficacy of defibrillation.

119. **The answer is B.** *(Chapter 23)* The tracing demonstrates an intrinsic heart rate of 58 with failure to capture. Note the regular QRS complexes, which lack synchrony with the pacemaker spikes. No instances of ventricular capture are depicted.

120. **The answer is D.** *(Chapter 23)* After four captured beats, the tracing reveals a failure of the pacemaker to fire as a result of oversensing of the patient's atrial activity.

121. **The answer is A.** *(Chapter 20)* In cardiogenic shock, as oxygen delivery decreases, the extraction fraction increases to a critical value of 0.67. After this point, oxygen consumption becomes dependent on supply. This limit of aerobic metabolism appears to be associated with increased lactic acid production, an increase in the lactate-to-pyruvate ratio, and a decrease in the production of high-energy ATP bonds, all suggesting the onset of less efficient oxygen utilization associated with anaerobic metabolism and lactic acidosis. The normal oxygen extraction fraction is 0.25, which gives a mixed venous hemoglobin saturation of 0.75. This corresponds to a Pa_{O_2} of 40 mm Hg.

122. **The answer is A (1, 2, 3).** *(Chapter 20)* Shock is characterized by evidence of end-organ hypoperfusion, which may culminate in ischemic damage and organ failure. Initial therapy for shock should be directed at determining the origin of the shock state and moving to correct the treatable causes (e.g., cardiac ischemia, hemorrhage). The initial step in the resuscitation should focus on an adequate airway and respiration. Once these have been secured, steps to improve the circulation should be taken. Most forms of shock may be amenable to volume resuscitation; even cardiogenic shock may improve with further preload augmentation. A trial of volume is therefore appropriate in most cases of shock to test the hypothesis that the patient is relatively hypovolemic. If there is improvement, further trials of volume administration are attempted. α-adrenergic pressor therapy aimed at restoring the blood pressure, without better assessment of the etiology of shock and the hemodynamic effects of the drug administered, carries a significant risk. If these agents are administered to a hypovolemic patient, there may be "improvement" in the blood pressure

at the expense of cardiac output as peripheral resistance is increased, thus worsening the shock state. Similarly, in patients given β-adrenergic agonists in the setting of ischemia-induced cardiogenic shock with inadequate preload, the resultant increased myocardial oxygen consumption may outweigh the improvement in systolic performance.

123. The answer is E (all). *(Chapter 24)*   Myocardial ischemia may be difficult to detect in critically ill, ventilated patients. It may manifest as a change in vital signs, agitation, or increases in left ventricular diastolic pressure and thus pulmonary artery diastolic pressure and pulmonary capillary wedge pressure. A transient fourth heart sound or murmur of mitral regurgitation (which increases the *v* wave on the PCWP tracing) may be heard. Airway pressure may increase when myocardial ischemia causes pulmonary edema or "cardiac asthma." Myocardial ischemia also can thwart attempts at discontinuing mechanical ventilation, a process that adversely affects the myocardial oxygen supply:demand ratio.

124. The answer is E (all). *(Chapter 24)*   Any bradyarrhythmia unresponsive to atropine that results in hemodynamic compromise is an indication for pacing. New conduction disturbances such as those listed may progress to high-grade AV block and also require pacing.

125. The answer is D (4). *(Chapter 21)*   This patient has clinical and laboratory evidence supporting a diagnosis of preeclampsia. While delivery of the child is recommended after the thirty-sixth week of pregnancy, delivery of a viable fetus in this case is not likely. Hydralazine should be considered first-line therapy in the treatment of hypertension in a pregnant patient, given its record of safety and efficacy. The potential for serious fetal injury should discourage the use of nitroprusside and enalapril in this patient. Furosemide should be avoided in this patient because of evidence of the intravascular volume depletion that often accompanies preeclampsia.

126. The answer is E (all). *(Chapter 22)*   Adenosine is indicated for the treatment of paroxysmal supraventricular tachycardias. The primary mechanism of action involves slowing conduction through the AV node. Adenosine also has been shown to cause coronary vasodilation and decreased sinus node automaticity. Potential side effects of adenosine include prolonged AV nodal blockade, cardiac arrhythmias, and facial flushing. Adenosine also has been implicated in the development of bronchospasm in patients with hyperreactive airways.

127. The answer is D (4). *(Chapter 24)*   Right ventricular infarction is characterized by elevated right atrial pressure and normal to low PCWP. Right ventricular contractility is decreased, resulting in poor filling of the left ventricle. Consequently, pulmonary edema is rare. Right precordial leads may demonstrate ST-segment elevation, and echocardiography may show a dilated, poorly contracting right ventricle. Treatment consists of providing an adequate circulating volume and occasionally the administration of dobutamine. Since atrial contraction assumes greater importance in filling the stiff right ventricle, patients who require transvenous pacing should have a dual-chamber AV sequential pacemaker.

128. The answer is D (4). *(Chapter 25)*   The vast majority (85 percent) of patients with PPH will have abnormal ECG findings consistent with cor pulmonale, and very few will present with rhythms other than the normal sinus rhythm. When these patients are symptomatic, their pulmonary artery pressures are usually quite elevated. Rheumatoid arthritis may lead to secondary pulmonary hypertension resulting from extensive pulmonary manifestations but is not related to primary pulmonary hypertension.

129. The answer is B (1, 3). *(Chapter 19)*   Inhaled nitric oxide (iNO) is a selective pulmonary vasodilator that has been used therapeutically to reduce pulmonary hypertension and improve ventilation-perfusion matching. Clinical applications of inhaled NO have included treatment of ARDS and right heart failure secondary to pulmonary hypertension after cardiac transplantation. Nitric oxide is scavenged rapidly by red blood cells and inactivated before contact with the systemic circulation. There is no direct effect on left ventricular function or systemic vasculature, making iNO ineffective in the treatment of congestive heart failure and aortic insufficiency.

130. The answer is A (1, 2, 3). *(Chapter 26)* Pulmonary embolism may cause hypoxemia via right-to-left shunting through areas of lung atelectasis or potentially through a patent foramen ovale. These low ventilation-perfusion units return relatively desaturated blood to the left atrium that is not compensated for by the remaining high V/Q and normal V/Q units. The result is lower arterial saturation. Such low Sv_{O_2} saturations are commonly seen in the low-flow state associated with pulmonary embolism. Alveolar hypoventilation is not seen in patients with pulmonary embolism. There is an increase in dead space that may lead to an increase in Pa_{CO_2}, however, this usually is negated by increased alveolar ventilation.

131. The answer is E (all). *(Chapter 26)* The clinical manifestations of pulmonary embolism are protean, particularly in the critically ill. The most common chest radiographic finding in pulmonary embolism is, in retrospect, volume loss. Other radiographic signs of a pulmonary embolus include atelectasis, pleural effusion, and oligemia of the pulmonary vasculature. Pulmonary embolism is one of the many causes of fever in a critically ill patient. In a patient who suffers significant pulmonary embolism, the increase in dead space may lead to increased Pa_{CO_2} if the patient is unable to increase minute volume to compensate. If the pulmonary embolus is large enough, acute right ventricular failure and death may ensue.

132. The answer is A (1, 2, 3). *(Chapter 24)* This patient demonstrates an acute myocardial infarction complicated by severe cardiac dysfunction with end-organ hypoperfusion. Initial medical therapy with oxygen, aspirin, heparin, and nitroglycerin is appropriate. Pain that is unresponsive to escalating doses of nitroglycerin should be treated with morphine, as pain increases sympathetic discharge with resultant increases in myocardial work. In this patient, intubation and mechanical ventilation are indicated to diminish the work of breathing, further decreasing myocardial work. An intraaortic balloon pump should be considered in all patients with cardiogenic shock refractory to medical therapy. Definitive intervention, including cardiac catheterization with PTCA or coronary artery bypass grafting, should be considered. The use of epinephrine may increase blood pressure, although controversy remains regarding the ability of epinephrine to improve organ perfusion. In the setting of acute myocardial infarction or ischemia, the use of epinephrine should be discouraged because of the questionable benefit and the increase in myocardial oxygen consumption resulting from epinephrine administration.

133. The answer is B (1, 3). *(Chapter 22)* Digoxin administration is extremely useful in controlling heart rate in patients with atrial fibrillation. However, it may cause a catastrophic increase in heart rate in patients with Wolff-Parkinson-White syndrome by decreasing conduction through the AV node and increasing conduction through the bypass tract. This increased heart rate may lead to ventricular fibrillation. Digoxin is also a useful adjunct to the treatment of chronic dilated cardiomyopathy. However, in congestive heart failure caused by diastolic dysfunction with functional aortic outflow obstruction, the increase in systolic performance actually may decrease cardiac output and worsen the left ventricular dysfunction.

134. The answer is E (all). *(Chapter 27)* Pericardial disease is associated with mediastinal radiation therapy, renal failure, cardiac surgery, collagen vascular disease, and infection. Up to 40 percent of patients with chronic renal failure will develop pericardial effusions, which may occur before dialysis but also may develop or worsen during maintenance dialysis. The most common settings for purulent pericarditis are empyema, mediastinitis, endocarditis, burns, and the postpericardiotomy period. Pericarditis and effusion have been reported in 6 and 25 percent, respectively, of patients with acute myocardial infarction during the first week after infarction.

135. The answer is E (all). *(Chapter 28)* The classic triad of symptoms associated with aortic stenosis is angina, dyspnea on exertion, and syncope. Dizziness or fatigue may precede these symptoms. Angina may occur as a result of increased oxygen consumption, syncope from altered hemodynamics or arrhythmias, and dyspnea from left ventricular dysfunction.

136. **The answer is B (1, 3).**   *(Chapter 28)*   Management of aortic insufficiency consists of improving forward flow while reducing the regurgitant fraction. Afterload reduction with a short-acting agent such as nitroprusside is recommended. In addition to afterload reduction, cardiac output may be augmented by the use of ionotropic agents such as dobutamine. Norepinephrine should be avoided unless complete cardiovascular collapse occurs, as the increase in systemic vascular resistance will worsen the degree of insufficiency. Immediate aortic valve replacement is not indicated in moderately severe aortic regurgitation. Coronary angiography with left ventriculography should be performed before surgical intervention.

137. **The answer is C (2, 4).**   *(Chapter 28)*   The major hemodynamic abnormality in idiopathic hypertrophic subaortic stenosis (IHSS) is the prevention of adequate left ventricular filling caused by the inability of the ventricular muscle to relax. The basic principles of management include maximizing loading conditions while minimizing contractility. β blockers such as esmolol are the initial drugs of choice. Patients with IHSS and pulmonary edema or hypotension usually improve with saline and calcium channel or β blockers. Drugs that increase contractility—such as digoxin, epinephrine, dobutamine, and amrinone—should not be used.

138. **The answer is E (all).**   *(Chapter 21)*   All the drugs listed have been reported to cause rebound hypertension, which is most prominently seen with α-agonists (e.g., clonidine).

139. **The answer is E (all).**   *(Chapter 21)*   Limitations of nitroprusside therapy include its metabolic products, thiocyanate and cyanide, which can accumulate at high doses (> 8 μg/kg per minute) or during long infusion periods (> 24 hours). These accumulations are potentially fatal, particularly in patients with renal and hepatic disease and with Leber optic atrophy. Side effects may first be recognized by the patient (nausea, fatigue, muscle spasms) or the physician (widening anion gap, lactic acidosis, disoriented or psychotic mental status).

140. **The answer is A (1, 2, 3).**   *(Chapter 29)*   Cerebrovascular accidents resulting from the embolic complications of bronchial artery angiography have been well described. Spinal artery occlusion leading to paraplegia may further complicate this difficult procedure. Renal failure secondary to dye-induced acute tubular necrosis is a potential complication of all angiographic procedures. Pulmonary infarction is an uncommon complication of bronchial angiography because of the redundant pulmonary blood supply by pulmonary and bronchial arteries.

141. **The answer is C (2, 4).**   *(Chapters 21, 24)*   Doppler echocardiography provides physiologic data by allowing the detection and quantitation of flow velocities within the cardiovascular system. Cardiac output is calculated by multiplying Doppler-measured flow across the aortic root by the aortic root area. Valvular stenosis is identified by abnormally high velocities across the valve. Valvular regurgitation can be identified by the Doppler detection of flow across the valve when none should exist or by color-coding of the regurgitant stream. Anatomic information, such as chamber size and left ventricular aneurysm, is provided by one- and two-dimensional echocardiography.

142. **The answer is A (1, 2, 3).**   *(Chapter 25)*   Isolated pressure overload of the right ventricle occurs in primary pulmonary hypertension, pulmonary embolic disease, and pulmonary parenchymal disease with secondary pulmonary reduction in transventricular septal pressure differential, a leftward shift in the ventricular septum, and right ventricular enlargement. Abnormalities of regional wall motion usually are considered to be a result of ischemic heart disease.

143. **The answer is E (all).**   *(Chapter 21)*   TEE is a method that offers a less obstructed ultrasonic view of the heart in some patients. Better visualization of the left atrium, AV

valves, and intracardiac air has been reported. There is also evidence that TEE may provide a better index of right ventricular function than does precordial evaluation. Multiplanar transesophageal echocardiography allows multiple views of the heart in a 180-degree arc—many more than does conventional transthoracic echocardiography.

144. The answer is C (2, 4). *(Chapter 20)* With the elevated cardiac output and mixed venous saturation, the patient has adequate oxygen delivery. The problem in the sepsis may be an inability to extract the oxygen, resulting in anaerobic metabolism and subsequent lactic acidosis. Another possible explanation is that in sepsis there is excess generation of pyruvate. Instead of the lactate/pyruvate ratio rising, as it does in cardiogenic shock, it remains the same, with lactate rising in proportion to the excess pyruvate. Thus, instead of resulting from anaerobic metabolism, the increased lactate occurs secondary to the high levels of pyruvate. Hypotension in this situation is secondary to vasodilation and is simply a manifestation of the patient's septic state rather than a cause of his lactic acidosis.

145. The answer is E (all). *(Chapter 28)* The patient's hemodynamic compromise and increasing pulmonary edema are due to severe acute mitral regurgitation, as demonstrated by the large *v* wave on the pulmonary artery occlusion pressure tracing. Appropriate therapy would be directed at surgical correction of the valvular lesion. Attempts at medical management in this setting are often unsuccessful. Temporizing measures while awaiting surgical consultation include agents to unload the left ventricle, thus reducing the regurgitant fraction. Alpha-adrenergic agents would be strictly contraindicated, as increased afterload would simply increase the mitral regurgitation. Finally, an intraaortic balloon pump would be extremely useful in the management of the acute mitral regurgitation.

146. The answer is D (4). *(Chapter 14)* Pulmonary capillary wedge pressure is read at end expiration (functional residual capacity); however, if a patient is actively inspiring and expiring, it may be difficult to determine end expiration. Interpretation of the pulmonary capillary wedge pressure in this setting is extremely difficult. In addition, the patient's expiratory effort may artificially elevate the intravascular pressures at end expiration by increasing intrathoracic pressure. Resolution of the patient's bronchospasm may allow a more accurate interpretation of the pulmonary capillary wedge pressure tracing. Sedation followed by muscle relaxation (rarely necessary) may be used if the hemodynamic data are deemed crucial for patient management.

147. The answer is E (all). *(Chapter 14)* The patient's low pulmonary capillary wedge pressure in the face of significant PEEPi strongly suggests hypovolemia. Hypovolemic patients are at greatest risk for decreased cardiac output with PEEP. Therefore, therapy should be aimed at reducing PEEPi while volume repletion is ongoing. Furthermore, if hypotension is severe and does not respond adequately to volume infusion, disconnecting the patient from the ventilator allows (in a patient under sedation and muscle relaxation) the dissipation of the PEEPi by prolonging exhalation. This maneuver should be done only after preoxygenation with 100% oxygen to ensure that hypoxemia does not occur because of hypoventilation. Resolution of hypotension and tachycardia with this simple maneuver confirms that PEEPi is impeding venous return. Significant hypercapnia and acidosis would not be expected to occur within 1 min of apnea. Reduction of minute volume would help reduce PEEPi, as would relief of airflow obstruction.

148. The answer is E (all). *(Chapter 24)* Since a complication requiring emergency bypass surgery may occur during angioplasty (e.g., acute closure of a partially occluded coronary vessel), a patient undergoing angioplasty should be a good surgical candidate. Lesions that are likely to close acutely include those which are complicated by filling defects, those which are very long or extremely irregular or eccentric, stenoses at acutely angled bends in an artery, and subtotal stenoses. Preexisting left ventricular dysfunction or a large area of myocardium at risk of infarction in the event of acute vessel closure during angioplasty is associated with a higher risk. Because of the 200 to 500 mL of contrast dye given during angioplasty, preexisting renal insufficiency is a major consideration. Finally, adhesions resulting from previous cardiac operations would make emergency bypass surgery difficult after acute closure of a vessel during angioplasty.

149.   The answer is C (2, 4).   *(Chapter 28)*   Although there is increased risk for patients with severe coronary disease, the majority will tolerate valvuloplasty. Patients with left main or severe triple-vessel coronary artery disease and symptomatic aortic stenosis probably do not have an improved prognosis with valvuloplasty. In these patients, the procedure probably should be reserved for palliation of symptoms. While patients undergoing aortic valvuloplasty have a mean area of 1.1 cm^2 after the procedure, prosthetic valves have an in vivo area between 1.0 and 1.5 cm^2 with on average a greater increase in cardiac output and a fall in pulmonary capillary wedge pressure. In addition, the restenosis rate 1 year after balloon dilation is at least 50 percent and may be higher. Between 1 and 3 percent of patients experience catheter or guidewire perforations of the left ventricle. Although as many as two-thirds may be managed by pericardiocentesis, some will require surgical drainage of the pericardial space and repair of the ventricle.

150.   The answer is A (1, 2, 3).   *(Chapter 86)*   Ventricular assistance devices have been associated with a decrease in myocardial oxygen consumption when the left ventricular bypass rather than the left atrial device is used. This reduction in oxygen consumption may be the mechanism by which infarct size is decreased, although an overall reduction in mortality has not been demonstrated with the use of these devices. A reasonable indication for postcardiotomy use is a cardiac index < 2 L/min despite routine support. They provide an adequate bridge to transplantation in the vast majority of studies; however, current problems with organ availability result in a substantial number of patients dying before an organ is available.

151.   The answer is B (1, 3).   *(Chapter 91)*   Aortic rupture from an acceleration-deceleration injury occurs most commonly just distal to the origin of the left subclavian artery at the ligamentum arteriosum (which is the junction between the fixed and mobile parts of the aorta). It requires immediate surgical intervention. Most authorities recommend angiography over CT to make the definitive diagnosis. Placement of a nasogastric tube can show the degree of esophageal deviation and hematoma size on chest x-ray.

152.   The answer is D (4).   *(Chapter 22)*   The electrocardiogram reveals diffuse ST-segment elevation with upward concavity (seen best in leads V_1–V_6 and II, III, and aVF) as well as PR-segment depression. These changes are typical of acute pericarditis, which can be managed readily in most circumstances with indomethacin (Indocin).

153–156.   The answers are 153-A, 154-B, 155-D, 156-B.   *(Chapter 25)*   In the pressure-loaded right ventricle, decreases in systemic blood pressure have been associated with right ventricular ischemia in experimental models. Norepinephrine has been associated with increases in right coronary blood flow and right ventricular performance.

Positive-pressure ventilation, particularly in patients with airflow obstruction and gas trapping, increases pleural pressure and RA pressure. This can result in diminished venous return and hence diminished RV filling.

Rapid reversal of pulmonary vasodilation seen in withdrawal of inhaled nitric oxide may result in significant elevations in pulmonary artery pressures. An acute increase in right ventricular afterload can lead to rapid right ventricular failure manifested by decreased right ventricular systolic function and diminished left atrial filling. Systemic hypotension may result from diminished left ventricular filling in addition to deleterious right-left ventricular interaction.

The sequence of events in the patient with cystic fibrosis is consistent with the development of intrinsic PEEP in a mechanically ventilated patient with airflow obstruction. Intrinsic PEEP is a measure of the increase in intrathoracic and RA pressure under these circumstances and causes diminished venous return and potentially hypotension and hypoperfusion.

157–160. **The answers are 157-D, 158-A, 159-B, 160-E.** *(Chapter 22)* Amiodarone partially inhibits the peripheral conversion of thyroxine (T_4) to the active hormone, triiodothyroxine (T_3), which may lead to clinical hypothyroidism. Esmolol, like other β-blockers, may cause hypoglycemia by impairing the glycogenolytic process.

Lidocaine may lower the seizure threshold, thus predisposing certain patients to tonic-clonic seizure activity. Transient facial flushing has been reported in up to 18 percent of patients receiving adenosine.

161–164. **The answers are 161-D, 162-B, 163-C, 164-A.** *(Chapter 24)* Nicardipine and nifedipine are the least cardiodepressant of the calcium channel blockers. Diltiazem causes the most sinus node depression, and verapamil causes the most depression of AV node conduction. Since nifedipine has a dominant effect on the vasculature with little impact on the heart, it often is chosen to treat hypertension. However, verapamil is preferred in the treatment of paroxysmal supraventricular arrhythmias because these disturbances typically involve the AV node.

165–169. **The answers are 165-D, 166-B, 167-A, 168-E, 169-C.** *(Chapter 14)* Tamponade is a state of low cardiac output and hypoperfusion caused by impediment to filling of all chambers of the heart as a result of increased intrapericardial pressures. This reduction in transmural pressure is uniform throughout the pericardial space, and so there is equalization of all diastolic pressures.

Shock caused by massive pulmonary embolus is due to the inability of the right ventricle (RV) to maintain its output in the setting of an increase in pulmonary vascular resistance. This inability to maintain output results in dilation and ischemia, which cause further RV dysfunction. These changes may occur at relatively low pulmonary artery pressures, so that shock may occur with pulmonary artery systolic pressures in the 50s and mean pulmonary pressures in the 40s.

Ventricular septal defects may complicate acute myocardial infarction. The large left-to-right shunt may cause right ventricular failure, with resultant venous hypertension. The thermal dilution cardiac output may be artifactually high because of the dilution of cold saline by warm blood from the LV. Similarly, the inflow of oxygenated blood from the left side may increase the arterial saturation of blood sampled in the pulmonary artery. The diagnosis is confirmed by serial saturations from the right atrium to the pulmonary artery with the demonstration of such a "step-up."

Some patients are unable to increase cardiac output despite systemic vasodilation. These patients typically have one of several conditions, such as underlying heart disease, pericardial disease, and pulmonary vascular disease. Other potential causes include hypovolemia and adrenal insufficiency. In this example, the patient is unable to increase cardiac output because of severe pulmonary hypertension. The chronicity of the pulmonary hypertension is demonstrated by pressures well in excess of those capable of being generated by the normal right ventricle. The inability to increase cardiac output in the face of systemic vasodilation results in profound hypotension.

The peripheral vasodilation that occurs in cirrhosis results in a marked decrease in systemic vascular resistance. This fall in resistance is associated with a high-cardiac-output state. Because of the high cardiac output, the mixed venous oxygen saturation is usually high. In this case, the high filling pressures suggest some component of volume overload. This might be expected with acute renal failure from acute tubular necrosis or hepatorenal syndrome. Incidentally, the low-resistance, high-cardiac-output state with high mixed venous oxygen saturation is identical to that seen in sepsis, making it impossible to differentiate between the two by using hemodynamic criteria.

170–173. **The answers are 170-C, 171-B, 172-A, 173-B.** *(Chapter 22)* Hypocalcemia prolongs the QT interval, generally preserving both the shape and the polarity of the T wave. When hypocalcemia is gross, the T wave may invert. In hypokalemia, the specific ECG finding is U on T phenomenon. In hyperkalemia, the T wave becomes taller (best seen in V_4), and then QRS and P-wave durations become expanded. When the potassium level is greater than 7.5 mEq/L, the QRS is grossly widened. Hypercalcemia may shorten the QT interval at levels above 15 mg/dL.

174–179.   The answers are 174-E, 175-D, 176-C, 177-F, 178-G, 179-B. *(Chapter 22)* In pericarditis, the ST segment becomes elevated in leads II, III, aVF, I, and V_4–V_6. The PR segment is depressed in the same leads. The ST segment is invariably depressed in aVR, and in the same lead PR segment is elevated. PR-segment depression also is seen in atrial hypertrophy and in thyrotoxicosis. Electrical alternans occurs with pericardial effusions. In electrical alternans, the QRS voltage alternates with each beat. By contrast, in flail chest, the QRS voltage changes with the respiratory cycle. Hypothermia is characterized by the J wave (Osborne wave) after the QRS complex. In situs inversus, the lateral leads record diminishing voltages. Lead reversal in leads V_1–V_6 in this case gives a normal ECG (see figure opposite).

After heart transplantation, the ECG usually reveals two P waves, one from the native heart from the remaining part of the right atrium and the other from the transplanted heart.

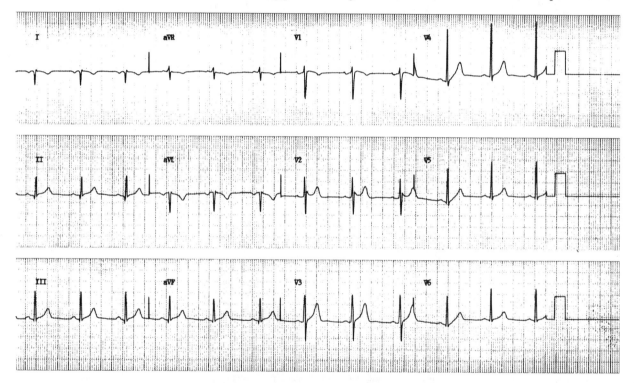

180–183.   The answers are 180-D, 181-A, 182-B, 183-E. *(Chapter 21)* The hypotension associated with liver failure usually is due to extreme vasodilatation (if the patient is volume replete). This vasodilatation allows rapid runoff of blood from the aorta with resultant low diastolic pressure. Consequently, the ventricle ejects against minimal load, allowing for a large stroke volume. The large stroke volume is manifest on examination by bounding pulses and a wide pulse pressure. These hemodynamics are similar to those seen in septic shock; however, some degree of systolic dysfunction also would be expected (although its effects usually are masked by the marked unloading of the left ventricle). Whether such systolic dysfunction occurs in hepatic failure is unknown.

In acute volume depletion there is a reduction of the mean systemic pressure despite compensatory mechanisms. This results in a fall in venous return to the heart. The left ventricle is inadequately filled, without cardiac impairment to filling. In this setting, the stroke volume and pulse pressure are low, and mean blood pressure falls despite reflex-increased systemic vascular resistance, which brings diastolic pressure up.

In severe hypertension, the left ventricle must eject against an abnormally high afterload. This causes an increase in the end-systolic volume. End-diastolic volume increases as peripheral reflexes try to maintain venous return and stroke volume. The increase in end-diastolic volume comes at the cost of an increase in end-diastolic pressure, with a resultant increase in pulmonary capillary pressure and the formation of pulmonary edema.

Loss of myocardium causes a reduction in the contractile function of the left ventricle. This is manifest as a shift of the end-systolic pressure-volume relationship downward and to the right: the ventricle ejects to a larger end-systolic volume at the same end-systolic pressure. The ventricle dilates at end diastole to accommodate venous return to the larger end-systolic volume, again at the cost of an increase in end-diastolic pressure and pulmonary capillary pressure. This effect may be exacerbated by an increase in left ventricular diastolic stiffness, which may occur in ischemic myocardium (not depicted here).

184–187. The answers are 184-B, 185-D, 186-E, 187-A. *(Chapters 19, 21)* An acute pulmonary embolus large enough to cause hemodynamic compromise would do so by causing acute right ventricular failure. This failure would be associated with an increase in right atrial pressure. Reflex venoconstriction would increase the stressed volume of the circulation, increasing the mean systemic pressure. This increase in mean systemic pressure is graphically demonstrated as a parallel shift of the venous return curve to the right (point B). The increase in right atrial pressure would result in a decrease in the gradient for venous return despite the compensatory rise in the mean systemic pressure. If resistance to venous return remains constant, as it does on these curves, venous return and cardiac output will fall.

Acute gastrointestinal hemorrhage results in an acute reduction in the intravascular volume, in particular from the stressed volume of the circuit. If venoconstriction is unable to compensate for this reduction in stressed volume, the mean systemic pressure will fall. This is graphically demonstrated as a parallel shift of the venous return curve to the left (point D). The fall in mean systemic pressure reduces the gradient for venous return despite a fall in the right atrial pressure. This reduction in the gradient for venous return causes a fall in venous return, since resistance to venous return does not change on these curves.

The institution of positive-pressure ventilation results in a change in intrathoracic and pleural pressures from negative to positive. This increase in pleural pressure raises the right atrial pressure. The addition of PEEP potentiates this effect. The administration of morphine will decrease the mean arterial pressure (MAP) in two ways. Both are more potent when MAP is maintained by sympathetic reflexes in hypovolemia. Morphine is a venodilator, and so its administration will result in a decrease in the stressed volume of the circulation with a consequent reduction in the mean systemic pressure. In addition to its direct venodilating effect, morphine decreases adrenergic tone through its sedating effects. This reduction in adrenergic tone causes further venodilation and a reduction in mean systemic pressure. The combination of reduction in the mean systemic pressure and increase in the right atrial pressure leads to a dramatic reduction in venous return (point E).

Heart failure leads to an elevation of the right atrial pressure, since the heart is unable to maintain output at lower pressures. In compensation for this elevated right atrial pressure, several mechanisms serve to increase the stressed volume of the circulation and increase the mean systemic pressure, thus maintaining the gradient for venous return. These mechanisms include increases in renin and aldosterone, which lead to increased fluid retention, and increased plasma catecholamines, which lead to venoconstriction. The increase in mean systemic pressure is demonstrated by a parallel shift of the venous return curve to the right (point A), leading to normalization of the venous return despite an elevated right atrial pressure.

188–190. The answers are 188-C, 189-A, 190-B. *(Chapter 27)* The hemodynamic effects of pericardial disease result entirely from interference with cardiac filling. Understanding the pathophysiology of disordered cardiac filling helps one distinguish between cardiac tamponade and constrictive pericarditis. In pericardial tamponade, pericardial fluid is free-flowing and distributes pericardial pressure among all chambers, with resultant equalization of intracavitary pressures during diastole on both sides of the heart. Because of this, there is no pressure gradient between the chambers in diastole (except during atrial systole) and early ventricular filling does not occur, as reflected in the absence of the *y* descent in the atrial tracings. In constrictive pericarditis, the pericardium encases the heart like a rigid box. Filling occurs rapidly in early diastole until the limits of dispensability of the constricted pericardium are met. This results in rapid *y* descent with an early nadir and a sharp rise in atrial pressure as the ventricle cannot expand further. Similarly, after atrial systole the fall in atrial pressure, or *x* descent, is rapid. Because the volume of the pericardium is constricted, ventricular interdependence will result in equalization of right and left ventricular diastolic pressures once their volume is such that they are encroached on by the rigid pericardium.

191–192. The answers are 191-A, 192-C. *(Chapter 28)*   The choice of mechanical valve versus bioprosthesis is influenced by a number of factors, including the risk of anticoagulation and the expected duration of the replaced valve. Mechanical valves routinely require anticoagulation to prevent valvular stenosis and the formation of a thombus. In general, bioprosthetic valves do not require anticoagulation and are the valves of choice in patients in whom anticoagulation is not desired. Both mechanical valves and bioprosthetics carry a significantly increased risk of developing endocarditis, thus necessitating antibiotic prophylaxis during certain procedures.

193–194. The answers are 193-C, 194-C. *(Chapter 20)*   Dobutamine is primarily a stimulant of β_1-adrenergic receptors, which accounts for its positive inotropic effect (increased cardiac output). Its mild β_2 effects can result in vasodilation and a fall in blood pressure.

Sodium nitroprusside is an arterial and venous vasodilator that can increase cardiac output by decreasing afterload. Arterial vasodilation can result in hypotension.

195–197. The answers are 195-C, 196-B, 197-A. *(Chapters 21, 33)*   The distinction between cardiogenic and noncardiogenic pulmonary edema cannot be made reliably on portable films. Cardiomegaly suggests cardiogenic edema. Pleural effusion is present in both disorders, though large effusions easily seen on portable radiographs are more characteristic of cardiogenic edema. One feature suggestive of noncardiogenic pulmonary edema is an infiltrate that is stable over many days to weeks.

198–200. The answers are 198-C, 199-B, 200-D. *(Chapter 21)*   Both transthoracic and transesophageal echocardiography can provide reliable short axis cross-sectional images of the left ventricle. This allows real-time assessment of ventricular function and allows one to identify regional wall motion abnormalities—a sign of myocardial ischemia or infarction. Left ventricular cavity size also allows a subjective assessment of intravascular volume status. The left atrial appendage often is interrogated for the presence of clot and can be seen reliably only with transesophageal echocardiography. Doppler echocardiography is required to measure pressure differentials across restrictive orifices.

201–203. The answers are 201-B, 202-A, 203-B. *(Chapters 14, 27)*   The right atrial tracing indicates the prominent and rapid *x* and *y* descents, also termed the "M" wave, characteristic of constrictive pericarditis and restrictive cardiomyopathies.

The right atrial tracing during mechanical ventilation demonstrates the nearly absent *y* descent and "blurred" waveform during positive-pressure breaths that are typical of cardiac tamponade.

The left ventricular tracing demonstrates a distinct dip and plateau during diastole that is typical of pericardial constriction or restrictive cardiomyopathy. This may be detected in either left or right ventricular tracings.

204–207. The answers are 204-C, 205-A, 206-B, 207-B. *(Chapter 28)*   Most patients with symptomatic mitral stenosis have a mitral valve area between 0.5 and 1.5 cm² and will benefit from mitral valvuloplasty or mitral valve replacement. In patients with more than moderate mitral regurgitation, mitral regurgitation rather than mitral stenosis may be the predominant lesion. These patients are unlikely to benefit from balloon valvuloplasty, which also may make the mitral regurgitation worse. Contraindications to transseptal puncture include left atrial thrombus and severe thoracic spinal deformity. The latter obscures the landmarks necessary for safe transseptal puncture.

PULMONARY DISORDERS IN THE CRITICALLY ILL

QUESTIONS

DIRECTIONS: Each question below contains four or five suggested responses. Select the **one best** response to each question.

208. Causes of acute ventilatory failure include all the following EXCEPT

(A) phrenic nerve paralysis
(B) postictal edema
(C) botulism
(D) myasthenia gravis
(E) upper airway obstruction

209. A mechanically ventilated patient with a 50 percent intrapulmonary shunt has a Pa_{O_2} of 60 mm Hg (92 percent saturation), a Pv_{O_2} of 40 mm Hg (75 percent saturation) on 100% oxygen, and a hemoglobin of 15 g/dL. Assuming that blood flowing through normal lung units achieves 100 percent saturation and no other variables change, approximately what arterial oxygen saturation (Sa_{O_2}) would result from a fall in Pv_{O_2} to 27 mm Hg (50 percent saturation)?

(A) 95%
(B) 90%
(C) 80%
(D) 70%
(E) 50%

210. A 44-year-old woman with multiple sclerosis is intubated and mechanically ventilated for respiratory failure caused by neuromuscular weakness. Her chest x-ray reveals right lower lobe collapse. PEEP is added sequentially in an effort to reexpand the collapsed lobe. The static airway pressure is recorded for each incremental increase in PEEP. Choose the level of PEEP that corresponds to successful reexpansion of the right lower lobe.

	Static Airway Pressure (cm H$_2$O)	PEEP (cm H$_2$O)
(A)	20	5.0
(B)	22	7.5
(C)	25	10.0
(D)	22	12.5
(E)	26	15.0

211. What is the cardiac output of a patient with an oxygen consumption of 250 mL/min and an arterial-venous oxygen content difference (Ca−Cv) of 5 mL/dL?

(A) 2.5 L/min
(B) 3.0 L/min
(C) 4.5 L/min
(D) 5.0 L/min
(E) 7.5 L/min

212. What is the Pa_{CO_2} at sea level of a patient with a carbon dioxide production of 200 mL/min, tidal volume of 500 L, respiratory rate of 14/min, and V_D/V_T of 0.5?

(A) 30 mm Hg
(B) 35 mm Hg
(C) 40 mm Hg
(D) 45 mm Hg
(E) 50 mm Hg

213. With regard to diaphragmatic function in acute-on-chronic respiratory failure, all the following statements are true EXCEPT

(A) aminophylline may enhance the strength and endurance of respiratory muscles
(B) diaphragmatic function is independent of the oxygen saturation of blood
(C) pulmonary mechanical abnormalities can place the diaphragm at a mechanical disadvantage for optimal function
(D) hypophosphatemia may cause a decrease in the strength of muscles
(E) intraabdominal pathologic conditions can affect diaphragmatic function

214. Clinical signs of severe asthma include all the following EXCEPT

(A) absence of wheezing
(B) subcutaneous emphysema
(C) pulsus paradoxus > 15 mm Hg
(D) dyspnea that precludes speech
(E) metabolic alkalosis

Questions 215–217.

215. A 40-kg woman with AIDS and a CD4 count of 121 presents with a 5-day history of a nonproductive cough and severe dyspnea. Her chest x-ray reveals a diffuse four-quadrant infiltrate, and she requires intubation and mechanical ventilation for acute hypoxemic respiratory failure. An ABG reveals a pH of 7.37, Pa_{CO_2} of 30 mm Hg, and Pa_{O_2} of 50 mm Hg. Serum LDH is 554, and you suspect *Pneumocystis carinii* pneumonia. Initial evaluation should include

(A) repeat CD4 count
(B) sputum gram stain
(C) bronchoscopy with bronchoalveolar lavage
(D) bronchoscopy with transbronchial biopsy
(E) infused CT of the chest

216. While awaiting diagnostic results, the patient is started on empiric antimicrobial therapy. The following medications are indicated for the treatment of presumed PCP in this patient EXCEPT

(A) trimethoprim-sulfamethoxazole (TMP-SMX)
(B) dapsone
(C) azithromycin
(D) pentamidine
(E) prednisone

217. An appropriate dosing schedule of TMP-SMX for this patient would be

(A) one double-strength tablet (TMP = 800 mg) PO three times per week
(B) two double-strength tablets PO BID
(C) 100 mg TMP IV every 6 hours
(D) 200 mg TMP IV every 6 hours
(E) 400 mg TMP IV every 6 hours

218. Of the following, the LEAST common clinical presentation of sleep-disordered breathing is

(A) daytime hypersomnolence
(B) pulmonary edema
(C) personality changes
(D) systemic hypertension
(E) morning headache

219. The scoliotic angle of curvature in the following figure is

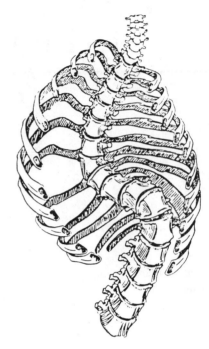

(A) 60 degrees
(B) 90 degrees
(C) 120 degrees
(D) 150 degrees
(E) unobtainable without a lateral view

220. Which of the following statements about the role of empiric antibiotics in the setting of aspiration is most accurate?

(A) Bacterial superinfection is such a common occurrence after aspiration that empiric antibiotics are indicated
(B) Bacterial superinfection is such an uncommon occurrence after aspiration that empiric antibiotics are not indicated
(C) Empiric antibiotics are indicated only when a patient is known to have aspirated fecal material
(D) Empiric antibiotics are indicated for intubated patients who have aspirated

221. When massive hemoptysis is fatal, what is the most common cause of death?

(A) Myocardial infarction
(B) Asphyxiation
(C) Hypovolemia secondary to hemorrhage
(D) Underlying disease

222. A 68-year-old man with a past medical history notable for adenocarcinoma of the lung and hypertension presents with the acute onset of severe left-sided chest pain and dyspnea. He denies a history of chest trauma. He is hemodynamically stable with a physical examination notable for dullness over the lower third of the left lung. The ECG shows a sinus tachycardia, and chest x-ray reveals an enlarged aortic knob with a pleural effusion occupying one-third of the left side of the chest. Thoracentesis yields bloody fluid. Repeat thoracentesis reveals a pleural fluid hematocrit of 25 (serum Hct = 40). Which of the following causes of bloody pleural fluid is least likely?

(A) Aortic dissection
(B) Pleural metastasis
(C) Pulmonary emboli
(D) Traumatic thoracentesis

223. A 65-year-old woman with chronic atrial fibrillation on coumadin, multiple CVAs, and baseline dementia is admitted to the ICU after the staff on the medical ward notes her to be coughing up blood. Her vital signs are temperature 36.9°C (98.4°F), heart rate 110 and irregular, blood pressure 105/78, and respiratory rate 26. Physical exam reveals an elderly cachectic woman who answers to her name only. Gag reflex is intact. Lungs show coarse bilateral breath sounds without crackles. Abdominal exam is normal. Her prothrombin time is 22 seconds (INR 2.3), and hematocrit is 21 (decreased from 33 yesterday). Chest x-ray shows diffuse interstitial markings, and no focal opacities. All the following are true EXCEPT

(A) a nasogastric tube should be placed to empty the stomach and look for a bleeding source
(B) evaluation should include esophagogastro-duodenoscopy (EGD)
(C) early bronchoscopy to localize a bleeding source is indicated
(D) evaluation should include inspection of the oro-/nasopharynx to identify a possible bleeding source

224. A 58-year-old man presents with complaints of nausea and vomiting with the sudden onset of excruciating, "tearing," left lower precordial chest pain, and moderately severe dyspnea on exertion. His past medical history is notable for a long history of smoking and alcohol abuse and a deep venous thrombosis diagnosed by venography 2 years ago and treated for 6 months with warfarin (Coumadin). Physical examination was notable only for dullness to percussion at the left base, one-third of the way up the lung field, and epigastric tenderness on deep palpation but no rebound. Chest x-ray revealed a left-sided pleural effusion one-third of the way up the lung field. Thoracentesis showed WBC 18,000 with 88 neutrophils, 9 lymphocytes, 2 eosinophils, no mesothelial cells, RBC 4500, protein 4.1, LDH 880, amylase 612, and pH 6.8. The most likely etiology of this patient's pleural effusion is

(A) tuberculosis
(B) pulmonary embolus
(C) esophageal rupture
(D) pancreatitis
(E) pneumonia

225. A 48-year-old man with acute myelogenous leukemia is transferred to the ICU from the medical ward. He is status post-allogeneic bone marrow transplantation and has had neutropenic fevers for 6 days. He is tachypneic and hypoxemic with diffuse crackles on lung exam. Sp_{O_2} is 88 percent on 100% nonrebreather face mask. He is mask ventilated and intubated for acute hypoxemic respiratory failure. Initial ventilatory settings are assist control mode at a rate of 14, tidal volume of 500 mL, FI_{O_2} of 100 percent, and PEEP of 5 cm H_2O. His spontaneous respiratory rate is 34, and he is dysynchronous with the ventilator, appearing to take a second breath immediately after the first breath is delivered ("stacking breaths"). Initial strategies to improve synchrony between the patient and the ventilator include all the following EXCEPT

(A) auscultate the chest and obtain a chest x-ray to ensure that the endotracheal tube is properly placed in the trachea
(B) insert an orogastric tube to decompress the stomach
(C) assure adequate sedation, analgesia, and relief from air hunger with appropriate pharmacologic intervention
(D) administer a paralytic agent

226. A 51-year-old woman is admitted to the ICU with a chief complaint of worsening shortness of breath. On physical exam she is morbidly obese (450 pounds) and has decreased breath sounds bilaterally in the bases but no audible wheezes or crackles. An arterial blood gas shows pH 7.07, Pa_{CO_2} 105 mm Hg, Pa_{O_2} 92 mm Hg, and Sa_{O_2} 96 percent on a 60% face mask. An intubation for ventilatory failure is planned, and the endotracheal tube is secured after several attempts. One hour after mechanical ventilation is instituted, the patient's blood pressure suddenly drops to 70/50 with a heart rate of 150. A chest x-ray is obtained (figure). Peak airway pressure is 80 cm H_2O. The next appropriate step is

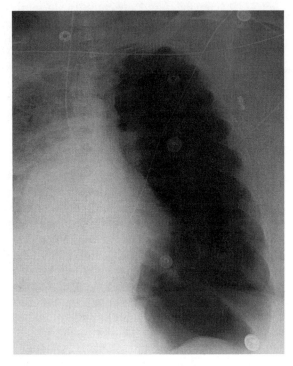

(A) rapid administration of 1L of 0.9% normal saline
(B) insertion of a catheter into the left pleural space
(C) pulling back the endotracheal tube 3 cm
(D) beginning dopamine at 10 μg/kg per minute for hypotension

227. Noninvasive mask ventilation may be used to improve oxygenation in patients with

(A) heroin-induced ARDS
(B) lobar pneumonia
(C) pulmonary hemorrhage
(D) aspiration pneumonitis
(E) congestive heart failure secondary to acute anterior wall myocardial infarction

228. The pulse oximeter of an intubated 65-kg patient in the ICU shows a sudden desaturation from 95 to 80 percent. Coincident with this decline in saturation, the peak pressure alarm on the ventilator sounds. At this time, the peak pressure is 80 cm H_2O (up from 30) and the plateau pressure is 20 cm H_2O (unchanged). The ventilator settings are assist/control at 20 breaths per minute, tidal volume 600 mL, $F_{I_{O_2}}$ 50 percent, PEEP 5 cm H_2O. The most appropriate response to this situation would be to

(A) decrease the tidal volume setting on the ventilator to 450 mL
(B) disconnect the ventilator and provide hand-bag ventilation with oxygen
(C) administer a sedative and a muscle relaxant
(D) administer a nebulized bronchodilator H_2O
(E) increase the inspired oxygen concentration

229. In pressure support ventilation

(A) the patient receives a mandatory minute ventilation
(B) the patient receives a set tidal volume after initiation of the respiratory cycle
(C) tidal volume depends on respiratory system compliance and patient effort
(D) respiratory rate is set by the ventilator

230. A young woman with steroid-dependent asthma has a respiratory arrest immediately on arrival in the emergency room. She is intubated without difficulty with no loss of pulse. After intubation there are bilateral breath sounds with moderate resistance to ventilation with an Ambu-bag. Blood pressure is 150/90, and pulse is 115. After 10 minutes on 100% oxygen, the arterial Pa_{O_2} is 59 mm Hg and the Pa_{CO_2} is 39 mm Hg. A likely finding on chest radiography to explain the gas-exchange abnormality is

(A) esophageal intubation
(B) pneumonia or lung collapse
(C) large lung volumes and flattened diaphragms
(D) tension pneumothorax
(E) pneumomediastinum

231. The major hazard of prolonged endotracheal intubation is

(A) tracheoesophageal fistula
(B) laryngeal damage with resultant upper airway obstruction
(C) patient depression resulting from inability to eat or talk
(D) aspiration around the endotracheal tube
(E) potential for accidental dislodgment of the endotracheal tube

232. In patients with increased airway resistance, gas trapping may result in the development of intrinsic positive end-expiratory pressure (PEEPi). Which of the following statements is true regarding the monitoring of airway function when PEEPi is present?

(A) Normal calculation of the "peak-to-plateau gradient" no longer accurately reflects airway resistance

(B) PEEPi is best determined by the airway pressure measured during an inspiratory pause

(C) Normal calculation of static compliance no longer accurately reflects the elastic properties of the lung

(D) PEEPi is independent of variations in minute ventilation or flow

(E) PEEPi would not be expected to have an effect on oxygenation

233. A 29-year-old man suffered multisystem trauma in a motor-vehicle accident and required laparotomy. After surgery he developed adult respiratory distress syndrome (ARDS) and required mechanical ventilatory support for 5 days. He was extubated yesterday and has been maintained on a 60% face mask, which he wears regularly. Over the course of the day his vital signs have been stable with a respiratory rate of 22 to 26, pulse 110 to 118, and blood pressure 120/75 to 130/85, and he notes no change in his breathing and no chest pain. He is generally immobilized owing to orthopedic injuries. Arterial blood gases are drawn every 4 hours, and although the Pa_{CO_2} varies only between 32 and 33 mm Hg, the recorded Pa_{O_2} measurements are 55, 85, 60, and 98 mm Hg. The likely explanation for this variation in Pa_{O_2} is

(A) hypoventilation in association with his pain medications

(B) recurrent pulmonary emboli

(C) fluctuations in the fraction of inspired oxygen

(D) varying degrees of intrinsic PEEP

(E) alterations in cardiac output

234. A 26-year-old homosexual man with *Pneumocystis carinii* pneumonia diagnosed by bronchoalveolar lavage (BAL) develops hypoxemic respiratory failure. His ventilator management includes the use of inverse ratio ventilation (IRV). All the following statements about this mode of ventilation are true EXCEPT

(A) improved oxygenation may result from improved ventilation of lung units with slower time constants

(B) lower mean airway pressure may reduce barotrauma

(C) flooded alveoli may be opened by the prolonged inspiratory time

(D) functional residual capacity (FRC) is reduced, and so there is less risk of barotrauma

(E) IRV may be used in either pressure-cycled or volume-cycled ventilatory modes

235. From which of the following causes of pleural effusion is closed pleural biopsy MOST likely to aid in making a diagnosis?

(A) Asbestos-related pleural effusion

(B) Viral pleurisy

(C) Tuberculosis

(D) Systemic lupus erythematosus

(E) Drug-induced pleural disease

236. This chest radiograph is most consistent with

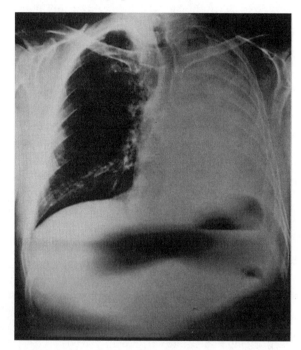

(A) massive left pleural effusion

(B) left thoracoplasty

(C) complete collapse of the left lung

(D) massive cardiomegaly

(E) right tension pneumothorax

237. Open-lung biopsy is characterized by which of the following statements?

(A) It is unsafe in patients with severe thrombocytopenia

(B) It is contraindicated in patients receiving mechanical ventilation

(C) It requires that the patient be well oxygenated without the use of PEEP

(D) It is helpful in diagnosing pulmonary infiltrates that are causing acute respiratory failure once pulmonary edema has been excluded

(E) It is most useful in patients with myeloproliferative disorders and pulmonary infiltrates

238. All the following statements are true regarding portable chest radiographs EXCEPT

(A) the heart appears larger
(B) the mediastinum appears larger
(C) the vascular pedicle appears distended
(D) the image quality is inferior because of radiation scatter
(E) there is a longer distance between x-ray source and patient

239. All the following statements regarding pulmonary contusion are true EXCEPT

(A) the clinical picture is usually more impressive than the radiographic findings
(B) rib fractures are usually absent
(C) it usually appears as a nonsegmental airspace infiltrate
(D) infiltrates appear immediately after trauma
(E) infiltrates should start to resolve after 48 hours

240. Which of the following statements about inferior vena caval filter placement is true?

(A) It is recommended only for a patient with pulmonary embolus complicated by shock
(B) It has been associated with a decreased incidence of femoral vein thrombosis with the newer filter design (bird-nest filter)
(C) It is often only a temporary procedure because of filter drift
(D) It is still associated with recurrent pulmonary emboli at a rate of 10 to 15 percent
(E) It is contraindicated with anticoagulation

241. A 35-year-old woman is treated for adult respiratory distress syndrome (ARDS) complicating an obstetric catastrophe. She requires an inspired oxygen concentration of 100% and positive end-expiratory pressure (PEEP) of 15 cm H_2O to maintain an arterial oxygen saturation of 82 percent. A pulmonary artery catheter is inserted, and the following data are obtained: RA = 10, RV = 35/8, PA = 34/22, PCWP = 14, CO = 4.4 L/min, Sv_{O_2} = 70 percent. All the following interventions are likely to improve oxygenation EXCEPT

(A) ventilation of the patient in the prone position
(B) delivery of inhaled nitric oxide at 20 ppm
(C) reduction of PEEP to 10 cm H_2O to improve venous return and cardiac output
(D) sedation and muscle relaxation to decrease oxygen consumption
(E) further reduction of the pulmonary capillary wedge pressure by diuresis while maintaining cardiac output with dobutamine

242. A 34-year-old woman with end-stage renal disease secondary to systemic lupus erythematosus develops hypoxemia during hemodialysis. The most likely etiology of this patient's hypoxemia is

(A) pulmonary edema
(B) pulmonary embolism
(C) atelectasis
(D) hypoventilation

243. In patients with adult respiratory distress syndrome (ARDS)

(A) noninvasive mask ventilation constitutes inappropriate therapy
(B) diuretic therapy may improve oxygenation significantly
(C) high levels of PEEP (> 10 cm H_2O) frequently cause barotrauma
(D) alveolar edema fluid typically has a low protein content
(E) all of the above

244. Which of the following interventions is most useful in determining whether the cause of hypoxemia is ventilation-perfusion mismatch or shunt?

(A) Determining the response to an $F_{I_{O_2}}$ of 100 percent
(B) Insertion of a pulmonary artery catheter
(C) Performance of a ventilation-perfusion scan
(D) Measurement of static and dynamic compliance on the ventilator

Questions 245–248.

A 70-year-old man with an unknown medical history is intubated because of hypoxemia refractory to a 100% nonrebreather mask. On assist control with $F_{I_{O_2}}$ of 40 percent, tidal volume (V_T) of 500 mL, respiratory rate (R) of 15 breaths per minute, and inspiratory flow (IF) of 40 L/min, the arterial blood gas (ABG) is pH 7.36, Pa_{CO_2} 50 mm Hg, Pa_{O_2} 120 mm Hg. Peak pressure is 60 cm H_2O, inflation hold pressure is 30 cm H_2O, and intrinsic PEEP (PEEPi) is 15 cm H_2O.

245. This patient's calculated elastance is

(A) 60 cm H_2O/L
(B) 50 cm H_2O/L
(C) 30 cm H_2O/L
(D) 20 cm H_2O/L

246. This patient's calculated resistance is

(A) 60 cm H_2O/Lps (liters per second)
(B) 45 cm H_2O/Lps
(C) 30 cm H_2O/Lps
(D) 15 cm H_2O/Lps

247. Given the above data, the most likely explanation for this patient's respiratory mechanics and arterial blood gas is

(A) pulmonary edema
(B) pneumonia
(C) pulmonary embolism
(D) bronchospasm

248. After 10 days of intensive therapy, the patient has the following ventilatory parameters: assist control, FI_{O_2} of 25 percent, VT = 500 mL, RR = 15 breaths per minute, PEEP = 5 cm H_2O, IF = 60 L/min. Peak pressure = 20 cm H_2O, inflation hold pressure = 15 cm H_2O, PEEPi = 0, negative inspiratory pressure (NIP) = −20 cm H_2O. ABG measures are pH 7.41, Pa_{CO_2} 42 mm Hg, Pa_{O_2} 120 mm Hg. A trial using continuous positive airway pressure (CPAP) of 5 cm H_2O was terminated abruptly after 60 minutes because the patient became progressively more diaphoretic, hypertensive, and tachypneic. Just before reinstitution of the assist control mode of ventilation, physical examination revealed clear lungs, II/VI systolic ejection murmur (SEM), and no cyanosis or edema. ECG was unchanged except for a sinus tachycardia. An ABG done at this time shows pH 7.26, Pa_{CO_2} 60 mm Hg, Pa_{O_2} 90 mm Hg. Possible explanations for this patient's CPAP trial failure might include all the following EXCEPT

(A) hypothyroidism
(B) malnutrition
(C) hypomagnesemia
(D) pulmonary edema

249. The expected bicarbonate level in a patient with compensated respiratory acidosis and a Pa_{CO_2} of 61 mm Hg is

(A) 25
(B) 27
(C) 29
(D) 31
(E) 33

250. All the following are causes of hypophosphatemia EXCEPT

(A) administration of glucose
(B) respiratory acidosis
(C) hypomagnesemia
(D) administration of β-adrenergic agonists
(E) administration of antacids containing magnesium and aluminum hydroxide

DIRECTIONS: Each question below contains four suggested responses of which **one or more** is correct. Select

A	if	**1, 2, and 3**	are correct
B	if	**1 and 3**	are correct
C	if	**2 and 4**	are correct
D	if	**4**	is correct
E	if	**1, 2, 3, and 4**	are correct

Questions 251–253.

A 56-year-old man requires mechanical ventilation for influenza pneumonia complicated by nosocomial pneumonia. Ventilator settings are F_{IO_2} 0.8, tidal volume 550 mL, respiratory rate 23 per minute, and PEEP 10 cm H_2O. Arterial blood gases are pH 7.24, Pa_{CO_2} 33 mm Hg, and Pa_{O_2} 54 mm Hg. Blood pressure is 85/55 mm Hg, pulse is 123 per minute, and urine output is 15 mL/h.

251. At this point, the next appropriate action(s) would include

(1) increasing PEEP
(2) giving furosemide to decrease lung water
(3) increasing tidal volume to normalize pH
(4) measuring Sv_{O_2}

252. A pulmonary artery catheter is placed. Pulmonary capillary wedge pressure (PCWP) is 14 mm Hg, and Pv_{O_2} is 27 mm Hg (50 percent saturation) with an arterial-venous oxygen content difference (Ca−Cv) of 8.9 mL/dL. Assuming normal oxygen consumption, explanations for these measurements include

(1) myocardial dysfunction
(2) anemia
(3) hypovolemia
(4) sepsis

253. The patient is started on dobutamine. The next day, on the same F_{IO_2}, Sv_{O_2} increases to 65 percent, but Pa_{O_2} has not increased. Explanations include

(1) worsening anemia
(2) worsening left ventricular function
(3) pericardial tamponade
(4) worsening pneumonia

254. A 54-year-old alcoholic man aspirates and develops ARDS. Initial ventilator settings are F_{IO_2} 1.0, tidal volume 550 mL, respiratory rate 25/min, and PEEP 5 cm H_2O. Arterial blood gases 20 minutes later are pH 7.39, Pa_{CO_2} 39 mm Hg, and Pa_{O_2} 54 mm Hg. White cell count is 18,000/mm^3 and hemoglobin is 10 g/dL. Strategies that could allow for a nontoxic F_{IO_2} (less than 0.6) include

(1) sedation and paralysis
(2) increasing PEEP
(3) treating fever
(4) transfusion

255. Characteristics of patients who present with acute-on-chronic respiratory failure include

(1) a decrease in drive to breathe
(2) an increase in Pa_{O_2} and Pa_{CO_2} with the application of supplemental oxygen therapy
(3) a decrease in respiratory drive and minute ventilation with the application of supplemental oxygen
(4) increased resistive loads from increased airway resistance

256. A 60-year-old man with long-standing COPD associated with hypercapnia and pulmonary hypertension presents with increasing peripheral edema, fatigue, and shortness of breath, along with a Pa_{O_2} of 45 mm Hg. Your evaluation also discloses an irregular pulse, and the electrocardiogram reveals an irregular rhythm at a rate of 120 beats per minute with varying P-wave morphologies and PR and RR intervals. Correct treatment for this disturbance would include

(1) digoxin
(2) bronchodilator therapy
(3) avoidance of supplemental oxygen because of the risk of worsened respiratory acidosis
(4) intravenous diltiazem

Questions 257–258.

257. A 25-year-old woman who weighs 50 kg presents with severe status asthmaticus. Despite high doses of β agonists and corticosteroids, she requires intubation and mechanical ventilation for impending respiratory failure. Appropriate initial ventilator settings include

(1) tidal volume of 350 mL
(2) respiratory rate of 16 breaths per minute to maintain adequate minute ventilation
(3) inspired gas of 20% oxygen and 80% helium
(4) PEEP of 10 cm H_2O

258. The patient is placed on initial ventilator settings of assist-control mode, rate of 22 breaths per minute, tidal volume of 400 mL, PEEP of 0 cm H_2O, and a helium/oxygen mixture of 80/20. Her initial blood gas on these settings is pH 7.28, Pa_{CO_2} 55 mm Hg, Pa_{O_2} 68 mm Hg and Sa_{O_2} 91 percent. Peak airway pressure is measured at 65 cm H_2O, and plateau pressure is 30 cm H_2O. PEEPi is 18 cm H_2O. Appropriate ventilator changes include

(1) discontinue the helium/oxygen and increase the F_{IO_2} to 60 percent
(2) increase the tidal volume to 500 mL
(3) increase the respiratory rate to 28 breaths per minute
(4) decrease the respiratory rate to 12 breaths per minute

259. The differential diagnosis of severe dyspnea with wheezing includes

(1) upper airway obstruction
(2) foreign body
(3) left ventricular failure
(4) ARDS

260. A 30-year-old man is intubated for status asthmaticus. Arterial blood gas measurements on F_{IO_2} of 0.4, V_T 600 mL, rate 18 bpm, and inspiratory flow rate of 60 L/min reveal a pH 7.16, Pa_{CO_2} 70 mm Hg, and Pa_{O_2} 95 mm Hg. Peak airway pressure is 80 cm H_2O. The intrinsic PEEP is 25 cm H_2O, and further adjustments in tidal volume or rate fail to improve Pa_{CO_2} or intrinsic PEEP. Appropriate measures include

(1) sedation and muscle relaxation
(2) PEEP, 10 cm H_2O
(3) helium/oxygen mixture (80%/20%)
(4) reduction of inspiratory flow rate

261. A 55-year-old man with interstitial pulmonary fibrosis and pneumonia develops progressive hypercapnia during mechanical ventilation. Strategies that could lower Pa_{CO_2} include

(1) avoiding nutrients high in calories and carbohydrates
(2) decreasing PEEP
(3) sedation and paralysis
(4) fluid challenge

262. Noninvasive mask ventilation can be used in which of the following situations?

(1) Sepsis-induced ARDS with hypotension and refractory hypoxemia
(2) Pulmonary edema related to tocolytic therapy for preterm labor
(3) Acute exacerbation of COPD with respiratory distress
(4) Postictal state with neurogenic pulmonary edema

263. Interstitial pulmonary fibrosis (IPF) is characterized by

(1) predominance of radiologic abnormalities in upper lobe
(2) hilar adenopathy
(3) early and uniform honeycombing
(4) clubbing of fingers and toes

264. Electrolyte disturbances associated with decreased respiratory muscle strength include

(1) hypophosphatemia
(2) hypomagnesemia
(3) hypokalemia
(4) hypernatremia

265. Heliox (a mixture of helium and oxygen gases) is useful for treatment of

(1) upper airway obstruction resulting from acute epiglottitis while awaiting a response to antibiotics
(2) upper airway obstruction caused by laryngeal edema in recently extubated patients in conjunction with racemic epinephrine
(3) upper airway obstruction caused by involvement of the trachea by a tumor while awaiting a response to radiation therapy
(4) severe status asthmaticus with inability to ventilate with conventional therapy

266. Conditions that may precipitate or worsen sleep apnea include

(1) upper airway infection
(2) congestive heart failure
(3) general anesthesia
(4) alcohol

267. A 38-year-old man suffers a sharp blow to the neck during a basketball game. Shortly afterward he presents to the emergency room with mild dyspnea and stridor. The appropriate diagnostic or therapeutic maneuvers should include

(1) endotracheal intubation
(2) emergent cricothyroidotomy
(3) trial of dexamethasone and racemic epinephrine
(4) fiber-optic direct laryngoscopy

268. A 24-year-old employee of a power company is admitted directly to the intensive care unit after an electrical injury. He is believed to have contacted a high-voltage line while climbing a pole and was found unconscious at its base. In the intensive care unit his breathing is labored and stridorous. Burns of the right hand and middle upper back are noted. The appropriate airway management could include

(1) administration of heliox
(2) immediate oral endotracheal intubation
(3) nasotracheal intubation
(4) cricothyroidotomy

269. A 65-year-old morbidly obese man presents with altered mental status. His family reports that he has a history of cigarette use and daytime hypersomnolence. On examination he is afebrile with respiratory rate of 20 breaths per minute, pulse of 115 beats per minute, and blood pressure of 160/105 mm Hg. Lung examination is notable for elevated jugular venous pulsation and pitting edema of the lower extremities. Laboratory data include a hematocrit of 50 and arterial blood gas measurements on room air of pH 7.34, Pa_{CO_2} 65 mm Hg, and Pa_{O_2} 45 mm Hg. Appropriate management would include

(1) digoxin
(2) thyroid function tests
(3) diuretic therapy
(4) oxygen

270. Conditions predisposing to aspiration syndromes include

(1) seizure disorders
(2) multiple sclerosis
(3) pregnancy
(4) use of a nasogastric tube

271. Aspiration of noxious materials may have which of the following outcomes?

(1) Upper airway obstruction
(2) Bronchospasm
(3) Adult respiratory distress syndrome (ARDS)
(4) Minimal symptoms

272. An 82-year-old man admitted for right hip arthroplasty is transferred to the intensive care unit after a witnessed aspiration. His temperature is 37°C (98.6°F), blood pressure is 150/80, pulse is 96, and respiratory rate is 30. He has crackles in the lower half of his right hemithorax with a corresponding opacity in this region on chest x-ray. Pulse oximetry reveals an Sp_{O_2} of 78 percent on room air. On 100% nonrebreather face mask, Sp_{O_2} is 87 percent. Potentially useful therapies include

(1) early use of empiric antibiotics
(2) positive end-expiratory pressure (PEEP)
(3) steroids
(4) reduction of intravascular volume

273. True statements about the evaluation of hemoptysis include which of the following?

(1) The ability to determine the site of bleeding is improved when bronchoscopy is done early
(2) Patients with a nonfocal chest x-ray and normal findings on bronchoscopy need no further immediate evaluation
(3) In the setting of rapid bleeding, rigid bronchoscopy is preferable to flexible bronchoscopy in allowing optimal visualization of endobronchial anatomy
(4) The clinical outcome is improved when bronchoscopy is done early

274. In the setting of hemoptysis, appropriate initial interventions might include

(1) correcting the underlying bleeding diathesis
(2) placing the bleeding lung in the dependent position
(3) placing a double-lumen endotracheal tube
(4) administering codeine

Questions 275–276.

A 60-year-old man with a 50-pack-year smoking history, an unknown PPD status, and an otherwise unremarkable past medical history presents with a 5-day history of progressively increasing dyspnea on exertion. Chest x-ray reveals a completely opacified right hemithorax.

275. Radiographic signs that may help differentiate collapse from massive pleural effusion include

(1) shift of mediastinal structures
(2) herniation of the lung
(3) distance between adjacent ribs
(4) presence of air bronchograms

276. Thoracentesis yielded the following results: protein 4.0 g/dL, LDH 312, glucose 115, amylase 25, pH 7.32, WBC 22,600 cells/mL with 85 neutrophils, 7 lymphocytes, 3 macrophages, 1 eosinophil, and 4 mesothelial cells, RBC 350 cells/mL. Cytology was negative. Based only on the results of thoracentesis, possible causes of this pleural effusion include

(1) tuberculosis
(2) pulmonary embolism
(3) intraabdominal abscess
(4) pneumonia

277. A closed pleural biopsy should be considered when one suspects a diagnosis of

(1) tuberculosis
(2) mesothelioma
(3) carcinoma
(4) rheumatoid arthritis

Questions 278–279.

278. A 62-year-old man with a history of colon cancer is admitted to the ICU for gastrointestinal bleeding. In the morning he was noted to have one bowel movement with bright red blood, and he has had two recurrences in the afternoon. The patient was recently in the ICU for a similar problem and required five units of packed red blood cells before the bleeding ceased spontaneously. No bleeding source has been identified. He has a history of mild COPD treated with an ipratropium inhaler. He has never been hospitalized for COPD. On physical exam he is in moderate respiratory distress. His temperature is 37.8°C (100.0°F), heart rate is 127, blood pressure is 72/42, and respiratory rate is 32. His lung exam reveals coarse breath sounds bilaterally in the lower lung fields without wheezing. Cardiac exam is normal. Abdominal exam reveals mild, diffuse tenderness to deep palpation without rebound tenderness. There are no abdominal masses and no organomegaly. His abdominal aorta is palpable and not enlarged. Arterial blood gas on room air shows pH 7.24, Pa_{CO_2} 42 mm Hg, Pa_{O_2} 52 mm Hg, Sa_{O_2} 86 percent. On a 40% face mask his ABG shows pH 7.23, Pa_{CO_2} 45 mm Hg, Pa_{O_2} 87 mm Hg, Sa_{O_2} 94 percent. His hematocrit has decreased from 30 to 21 despite transfusion of three units of packed red blood cells. He is not passing any blood per rectum at present. His chest x-ray shows minimal left lower lobe atelectasis but is otherwise clear. The first steps in this patient's management include

(1) surgical consultation for ongoing bleeding and possible surgical intervention
(2) arrangement for colonoscopy to identify the bleeding source
(3) radionuclide bleeding scan to attempt to localize the source of gastrointestinal bleeding
(4) intubation and mechanical ventilation

279. Causes of increased load on the respiratory muscles include

(1) bronchospasm
(2) heart failure
(3) pleural effusion
(4) pulmonary embolus

280. The vast majority of undiagnosed pleural effusions in patients in the ICU require diagnosis with a thoracentesis. Exceptions include

(1) pleural effusion associated with pneumococcal pneumonia convincingly diagnosed by blood cultures and Gram stain of sputum
(2) small pleural effusion in an afebrile patient who has undergone cholecystectomy within the past 24 hours
(3) small right-sided pleural effusion in an afebrile patient with congestive heart failure by history and physical examination
(4) small bilateral pleural effusions in an afebrile patient with adult respiratory distress syndrome (ARDS)

281. A 37-year-old woman is admitted to the intensive care unit in respiratory failure. Two months ago she noted arthralgias and wrist swelling. One month ago she developed a facial rash. For 1 week she has had an unproductive cough, shortness of breath, and pleuritic chest pain. She takes no medications and has had no prior health problems. On examination the pulse is 142, respirations are 34, and temperature is 38.9°C (102°F) orally. There are crackles and dullness at both lung bases and a normal cardiac examination. There is also a malar rash. On room air the pH is 7.49, Pa_{CO_2} is 28 mm Hg, and Pa_{O_2} is 38 mm Hg. On a rebreather mask the Pa_{O_2} is 60 mm Hg. The chest radiogram reveals diffuse alveolar infiltrates and bilateral pleural effusions. The urinalysis and creatinine level are unremarkable. True statements concerning this disorder include

(1) endomyocardial biopsy is often more specific than is lung biopsy
(2) a high titer of serum antinuclear antibody strongly supports the diagnosis
(3) hemoptysis strongly suggests complicating, infectious cavity lung disease
(4) when the likelihood of infection has been excluded, high-dose immunosuppressive therapy is appropriate

282. In normal subjects, an 8.0 endotracheal tube will cause which of the following alterations in pulmonary function?

(1) A decrease in peak flow
(2) A decrease in maximum voluntary ventilation (MVV)
(3) An increase in resistance
(4) A decrease in slow vital capacity

283. Indications for tracheostomy include

(1) to overcome upper airway obstruction
(2) to provide airway access in patients who require long-term mechanical ventilation
(3) to facilitate weaning from mechanical to spontaneous ventilation in patients with marginal ventilatory function
(4) to provide airway access for the maintenance of tracheobronchial toilet

284. Late complications of tracheostomy include

(1) tracheoeosophageal fistula
(2) pneumothorax
(3) hemorrhage of the innominate artery
(4) hemorrhage of the lowest thyroid artery (arteria thyroidea ima)

285. Indications for split-lung ventilation include

(1) airway hemorrhage
(2) bronchopleural fistula
(3) bronchopulmonary lavage
(4) adult respiratory distress syndrome (ARDS)

286. Complications of hyperbaric oxygen therapy include

(1) air embolism
(2) tympanic membrane rupture
(3) pneumothorax
(4) claustrophobia

287. Indications for hyperbaric oxygen therapy include

(1) carbon monoxide poisoning
(2) air embolism
(3) decompression sickness
(4) anaerobic pneumonia

288. Sources of error for in vitro blood-gas analysis include

(1) a varying electrode temperature
(2) heparin-induced changes in Pa_{CO_2}
(3) air bubbles causing a lower Pa_{CO_2} reading
(4) failure to place samples on ice if the analysis is delayed by more than 2 minutes

289. True statements concerning pulse oximetry include

(1) oximetry depends on a spectrophotometric measurement
(2) accuracy may be confounded by a low intravascular volume status
(3) shivering and other movements of the patient often confound measurement
(4) pulse oximetry will still be accurate in cases of carboxyhemoglobinemia

290. Thoracentesis in a mechanically ventilated patient with a massive pleural effusion would be expected to

(1) relieve dyspnea
(2) improve oxygenation
(3) improve respiratory system compliance
(4) improve ventilation

291. Indications for tube thoracostomy in a mechanically ventilated patient include

(1) pneumothorax
(2) hemothorax
(3) empyema
(4) rib fracture

292. Indications for surgical obliteration of the pleural space (pleurodesis) include

(1) recurrent unilateral pneumothorax
(2) bilateral pneumothorax
(3) persistent air leak
(4) malignant pleural effusion

293. Closed pleural biopsy is useful in the diagnosis of

(1) tuberculosis
(2) lung cancer
(3) coccidioidomycosis
(4) renal cell cancer

294. Patients in whom one would perform prompt thoracentesis include

(1) a patient admitted with substernal chest pain and nausea, an enlarged heart on x-ray, and small bilateral pleural effusions who has a prothrombin time of 16 seconds (INR 1.8) and a BUN of 70 mg/dL
(2) an asymptomatic patient with a small unilateral pleural effusion after sclerotherapy for esophageal varices who has a prothrombin time of 16 seconds (INR 1.8)
(3) a patient with a normal preoperative chest x-ray who develops an isolated small right-sided pleural effusion 6 hours after liver transplantation and a fever of 38.3°C (100.9°F) and a prothrombin time of 16 seconds (INR 1.8)
(4) a mechanically ventilated febrile patient on PEEP with pneumonia of the left lower lobe and left-sided pleural effusion who has a prothrombin time of 16 seconds (INR 1.8)

295. Fiber-optic bronchoscopy is a reasonable first-choice procedure for which of the following?

(1) Retrieval of foreign bodies
(2) Evaluation of airways in trauma victims
(3) Evaluation of inhalation airway injury
(4) Treatment of lobar collapse

296. In interpreting a portable chest radiograph, the patient's actual position (i.e., erect, sitting, supine) can be estimated by which of the following?

(1) An opaque inclinometer
(2) The appearance of the gastric air bubble
(3) The position of the breasts in females
(4) The appearance of small-bowel gas

297. A positive cytology or culture from bronchoalveolar lavage would be diagnostic in which of the following disease entities?

(1) Bronchoalveolar cell carcinoma
(2) Tuberculosis
(3) Blastomycosis
(4) Infection with *Pseudomonas*

298. A patient developed acute opacification of the left hemithorax. Which of the following would favor atelectasis as the primary cause?

(1) Rotation of the patient to the right on an anteroposterior portable film
(2) An elevated right hemidiaphragm
(3) Mediastinal shift away to the right
(4) Narrowing of rib interspaces on the left

299. A 56-year-old man with cardiogenic pulmonary edema required intubation and mechanical ventilation for refractory hypoxemia. After 24 hours of diuresis and afterload reduction, lung compliance increased and oxygenation improved. Ventilator settings were changed from F_{IO_2} 0.6, V_T 700 mL, RR 20 breaths per minute, and PEEP 12.5 cm H_2O to Fo_2 0.6, V_T 500 mL, RR 16 breaths per minute, and PEEP 7.5 cm H_2O. Repeat chest x-ray showed increased "whiteness." Possible explanations include

(1) worsening pulmonary edema
(2) decreased PEEP
(3) decreased V_T
(4) decreased x-ray penetration

300. A 26-year-old pregnant (30 weeks) patient with steroid-dependent asthma is intubated and ventilated with 50% oxygen at a rate of 16/min and a tidal volume of 600 mL for status asthmaticus. A right internal jugular cannulation was attempted, but access was not obtained after 1 hour. Arterial blood gases are stable for 12 hours at pH 7.40, Pa_{CO_2} 32 mm Hg, and Pa_{O_2} 90 mm Hg. During the next 6 hours, on the same ventilator settings, Pa_{O_2} falls to 42 mm Hg, Pa_{CO_2} increases to 49 mm Hg, and peak airway pressure increases from 58 to 68 cm H_2O. A portable anteroposterior chest radiograph is obtained (see figure) and is compared with her admitting x-ray, which showed bilateral equal hyperinflation with no lung infiltrates. On the basis of the abnormal findings in the figure, appropriate interventions include

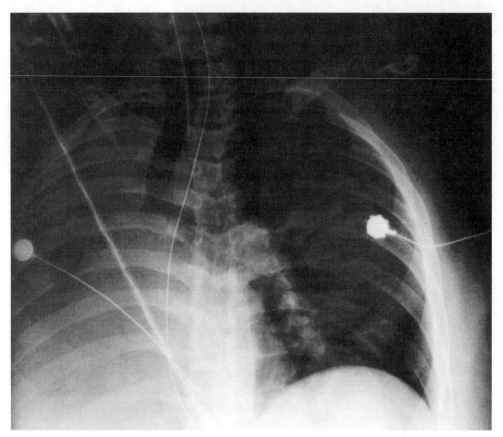

(1) thoracentesis and examination of the pleural fluid, including white cell count and differential, pH, and hematocrit
(2) broad-spectrum antibiotics for rapidly progressing hospital-acquired pneumonia after sputum and blood samples are obtained for culture and sensitivity
(3) insertion of a chest tube on the right side
(4) fiber-optic bronchoscopy to exclude or remove a right bronchial plug, followed by placement of the patient in the lateral decubitus position (left side down) and provision of increased tidal volume, end-inspiratory pause, and PEEP until the measured respiratory compliance increases or until hypotension or end-inspiratory pause pressure is excessive

301. Correct statements regarding the placement of a tracheostomy tube include

(1) small amounts of air in the subcutaneous tissues of the neck are common and should be watched carefully
(2) the tip of the tracheostomy tube is generally at the level of the clavicles
(3) air dissecting inferiorly into the mediastinum suggests a significant air leak
(4) tracheostomy tubes projecting above the level of the clavicles (and angulated) on an anteroposterior film can result in a tracheal–innominate artery fistula

302. A patient with ARDS attributed to cytomegalovirus (proved by lung biopsy) has been ventilated adequately for a week with 60 percent F_{IO_2} at a tidal volume of 500 mL, rate of 30/min, and PEEP of 12 cm H_2O. Arterial blood gases this morning reveal little change (pH 7.42, Pa_{CO_2} 44 mm Hg, and Pa_{O_2} 62 mm Hg), and the peak and static airway pressures are unchanged at 42 and 32 cm H_2O, respectively. The daily erect anteroposterior chest x-ray (see figure) suggests which of the following interventions?

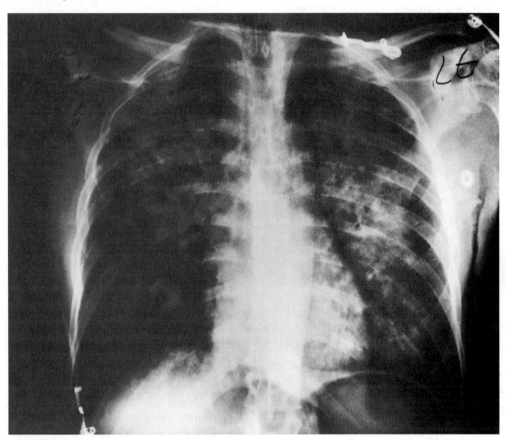

(1) Repeat the chest x-ray with less penetration
to exclude a loculated pneumothorax at the right base
(2) Place a nasogastric tube
(3) Consider the patient's need for nutritional supplementation
(4) Reposition the endotracheal tube

303. True statements concerning nosocomial pneumonias in the ICU setting include

(1) they often are diagnosed on clinical grounds, and treatment is largely empiric
(2) alkalinization of the stomach may predispose to aspiration of pathogenic organisms
(3) colonization of the oropharynx with pathogenic bacteria is felt to be a predisposing condition for the development of nosocomial pneumonias
(4) all organisms cultured from a protected brush catheter are pathogenic, and antibiotic coverage should be adjusted appropriately

Questions 304–305.

A 76-year-old man with chronic obstructive pulmonary disease of moderate severity is recovering after an elective herniorrhaphy. Two days after surgery he abruptly complains of dyspnea and substernal pressure. On examination, he responds to voice and has a blood pressure of 90/65, a heart rate of 115, and respirations of 28. The neck veins are elevated, the peripheral pulses are barely palpable, there is central cyanosis, and adequate bilateral breath sounds are heard. Face-mask oxygen at 50% is given, and two peripheral intravenous lines are begun. He is subsequently noted to be obtunded, with a blood pressure of 80/60. A 1-L fluid bolus is given with no improvement in blood pressure. The face mask is replaced by a Venturi mask at 24% oxygen. Transport to the intensive care unit is begun, during which the patient becomes bradycardic and then asystolic. Cardiopulmonary resuscitation (CPR) is initiated, and the patient is intubated, ventilated, and given 2 mg of atropine intravenously, followed by 1 mg of epinephrine and 10 mL of 10% calcium gluconate. Sinus tachycardia is noted on the monitor, the blood pressure is 150/100, and the patient is admitted to the ICU. A presumptive diagnosis of pulmonary embolism is made, and heparin is begun. The blood pressure stabilizes at 110/80 with a heart rate of 110 and urine output of 15 mL/h. Dopamine, 2 μg/kg per minute, is begun to improve urine output. The next morning, the patient responds sluggishly to voice and the abdomen is found to be distended and diffusely tender. Over the next several hours, metabolic acidosis develops, and a diagnosis of mesenteric infarction is made. At laparotomy, 20 cm of infarcted mid small intestine is resected.

304. In this man's initial resuscitation, management errors included

(1) the administration of calcium
(2) the use of an initial dose of atropine of 2 mg
(3) an unacceptable delay in intubation
(4) delivery of a fluid bolus in the setting of elevated neck veins

305. Since this patient had chronic obstructive pulmonary disease (COPD),

(1) the reduction in F_{IO_2} represented a reasonable attempt to avoid intubation
(2) it was best to avoid early intubation since he might have become ventilator-dependent
(3) a loading dose of aminophylline should have been given for respiratory distress, before he went into cardiac arrest
(4) it was important to exclude tension pneumothorax as a contributor to his deterioration

306. A 49-year-old woman with a history of pulmonary fibrosis is admitted with pneumococcal pneumonia. Because of hypoxemia refractory to a 100% nonrebreathing mask, the patient is intubated and eventually paralyzed. Despite no changes being made on the ventilator, the patient's Pa_{CO_2} increases from a baseline of 38 mm Hg to 48 mm Hg. Possible etiologies of this patient's rising Pa_{CO_2} include

(1) change in nutrition
(2) high fevers
(3) pulmonary embolism
(4) onset of bronchospasm

DIRECTIONS: Each group of questions below consists of lettered headings followed by a set of numbered items. For each numbered item select the **one** lettered heading with which it is **most** closely associated. Each lettered heading may be used **once, more than once, or not at all.**

Questions 307–311.

For each of the following clinical conditions, select the pleural fluid analysis with which it is most consistent.

	pH	Glucose	Protein	LDH	Amylase
(A)	7.32	64	3.8	357	356
(B)	6.83	86	1.2	23	35
(C)	7.33	76	4.1	227	25
(D)	6.54	37	5.9	765	1227
(E)	7.38	95	1.2	44	56

307. Congestive heart failure

308. Ureteral tear after major abdominal trauma

309. Esophageal rupture

310. Pulmonary embolus

311. Pancreatitis

Questions 312–315.

Match each description below with the appropriate procedure.

(A) Bronchoalveolar lavage
(B) Transbronchial biopsy
(C) Sterile brush
(D) None of the above

312. Most useful in the diagnosis of bacterial pneumonias

313. Most useful in the diagnosis of lymphangitic spread of malignancy

314. Can be performed safely in patients with clotting abnormalities

315. Absolutely contraindicated in patients on mechanical ventilation

Questions 316–319.

Match each maneuver that probably will improve oxygenation with the appropriate radiograph.

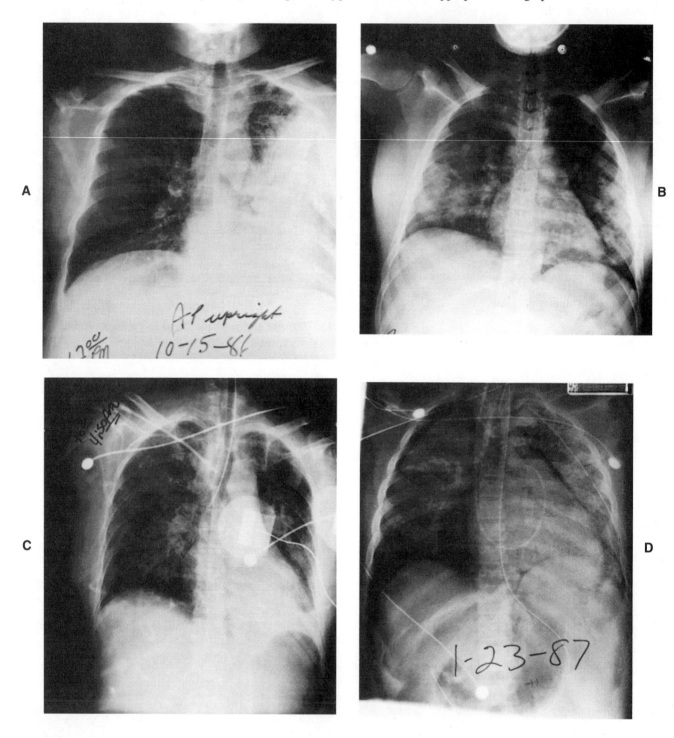

316. Right lateral decubitus positioning

317. PEEP

318. Withdrawal of the endotracheal tube 2 cm toward the mouth

319. Chest tube placement

DIRECTIONS: Each group of questions below consists of four lettered headings followed by a set of numbered items. For each numbered item select

A   if the item is associated with   **(A) only**
B   if the item is associated with   **(B) only**
C   if the item is associated with   **both** (A) and (B)
D   if the item is associated with   **neither** (A) nor (B)

Each lettered heading may be used **once, more than once, or not at all.**

Questions 320–323.

(A) Acute hypoxemic respiratory failure
(B) Acute ventilatory failure
(C) Both
(D) Neither

320. Therapy with PEEP

321. Postictal pulmonary edema

322. Polymyositis

323. Hypermagnesemia during the treatment of eclampsia

Questions 324–329.

(A) Noninvasive mask ventilation
(B) Endotracheal intubation with mechanical ventilation
(C) Both
(D) Neither

324. A 65-year-old woman with hypertension who presents with severe congestive heart failure

325. A 55-year-old man with severe COPD. Respiratory rate is 30, and ABG shows pH 7.34, Pa_{CO_2} 60 mm Hg, Pa_{O_2} 58 mm Hg, and Sa_{O_2} 90 percent

326. A 17-year-old man after a motor vehicle accident with facial trauma and stridor

327. An 84-year-old man with a metastatic prostate who develops pulmonary edema after fluid resuscitation for urosepsis

328. A 24-year-old woman, 20 weeks pregnant, who presents dyspneic after a witnessed aspiration

329. A 36-year-old woman with active tuberculosis who presents with hemoptysis. Her chest x-ray reveals dense infiltrates throughout the right hemithorax, and her Sp_{O_2} is 95 percent

Questions 330–333.

(A) Bronchial artery embolization
(B) Surgery
(C) Both
(D) Neither

330. Appropriate treatment for a patient with hemoptysis and a history of systemic lupus erythematosus

331. Appropriate treatment for a patient with hemoptysis and a chest x-ray that demonstrates diffuse scarring from sarcoidosis

332. Appropriate treatment for a patient with emphysema and bronchiectasis who presents with hemoptysis and an FEV_1 of 0.75 L

333. Appropriate treatment for a 50-year-old man with a 60-pack-year history of tobacco use and a solitary mass of 2 to 3 cm in the right middle lobe who develops hemoptysis. FEV_1 is 1.8 L, and D_LCO is 65 percent of predicted for his age, sex, and body surface area

Questions 334–335.

(A) Inspired oxygen fraction ($F_{I_{O_2}}$)
(B) Hemoglobin concentration
(C) Both
(D) Neither

334. Calculation of the alveolar partial pressure of oxygen (Pa_{O_2}) for determination of the alveolar-arterial oxygen difference is dependent on

335. Calculation of arterial oxygen content would require Pa_{O_2} and

Questions 336–338.

(A) Bronchoalveolar lavage
(B) Transbronchial biopsy
(C) Both
(D) Neither

336. Can demonstrate proof of tissue invasion

337. May be complicated by pneumothorax

338. Can aid in the diagnosis of lung disease in an immunocompromised host

PULMONARY DISORDERS IN THE CRITICALLY ILL

ANSWERS

208. The answer is B. *(Chapters 30, 34)* Acute ventilatory failure results from diminished drive to breathe, neuromuscular weakness, or increased mechanical load. Diminished drive to breathe can result from a head injury, an ischemic insult, or sleep apnea. Neuromuscular weakness can result from spinal cord injury, phrenic nerve paralysis, motor end-plate disease or blockade (myasthenia gravis, botulism), motor neuron degeneration (ALS), and muscular weakness (polymyositis, muscular dystrophies). Flail chest can result in hypoventilation, since the bellows action of the chest wall is interrupted. Increased resistive loads from bronchospasm or upper airway obstruction can result in ventilatory failure. Postictal edema usually results in hypoxemia with tachypnea and hyperventilation. The rapid improvement in gas exchange that is typical of this disorder usually allows clearing of the alveolar edema before fatigue of respiratory muscles develops.

209. The answer is C. *(Chapter 33)* Fifty percent of cardiac output perfuses normal lung units and leaves the capillaries with an oxygen content of 22.8 mL/dL [oxygen content = $(1.39 \times Hg \times Sa_{O_2} / 100) + Pa_{O_2} \times .003$]. (Hg is 15 g/dL, saturation is 100 percent, Pa_{O_2} is about 650 mm Hg). Fifty percent of cardiac output perfuses nonventilated units and leaves the capillaries with the same oxygen content as mixed venous blood, or 15.6 mL/dL (Hg 15 g/dL, saturation 75 percent, Pa_{O_2} of 40 mm Hg; therefore, $1.39 \times 15 \times 0.75$). In this case, the arterial oxygen content reflects the equal mixture of these two flows, resulting in an oxygen content of $(22.8 + 15.6) / 2 = 19.2$ mL/dL. This results in an arterial saturation of about 92 percent ($19.2 = 1.39 \times 15 \times N$; $N = .92$) or a Pa_{O_2} of 60 mm Hg. When Pv_{O_2} falls to 27 mm Hg (saturation 50 percent), venous oxygen content falls to 10.4 mL/dL ($1.39 \times 15 \times 0.5$). Arterial oxygen content reflects the equal mixture of these two flows, resulting in an oxygen content of $(22.8 + 10.4) / 2 = 16.6$ mL/dL, and arterial saturation falls to approximately 80 percent, which corresponds to a Pa_{O_2} of 50 mm Hg.

210. The answer is D. *(Chapter 32)* One strategy to reexpand collapsed lung segments or lobes is to add PEEP sequentially to patients requiring mechanical ventilation. The end-expiratory pressure will often succeed in "popping open" collapsed lung units. With reexpansion of collapsed lung units, the same ventilator-delivered tidal volume is distributed to an increased lung capacity. Therefore, the static airway pressure is noted to decrease—an improvement in lung compliance. In this example the static pressure actually decreased, as PEEP was increased from 10 to 12.5 cm H_2O, and the right lower lobe reexpanded.

211. The answer is D. *(Chapter 33)* Oxygen consumption (mL/min) = cardiac output (dL/min) $\times$ (Ca−Cv) (mL/dL); 250 mL/min divided by 5 mL/dL = 50 dL/min, or 5 L/min.

212. The answer is B. *(Chapter 33)* Pa_{CO_2} is determined by carbon dioxide production divided by alveolar ventilation: Pa_{CO_2} = dry barometric pressure (760 mm Hg − 47 mm Hg) $\times$ 0.863 $\times$ CO_2 production (mL/min) / $[V_T \times RR \times (1 - V_D / V_T)]$; $(760 - 47) \times 0.863 \times 200 / [500 \times 14 \times (1 - 0.5)] = 35.2$ mm Hg.

213. **The answer is B.** *(Chapter 34)*   Aminophylline and other inotropic agents have been found by some investigators to have a positive inotropic effect on the diaphragm, but the clinical utility of these agents is not well defined. Hypoxia and other metabolic irregularities, including hypophosphatemia, impair diaphragmatic function. Both hyperinflation and intraabdominal processes can markedly affect diaphragmatic function.

214. **The answer is E.** *(Chapter 35)*   Patients with severe asthma initially manifest tachypnea, tachycardia, and wheezing. Respiratory muscle fatigue and ventilatory failure may be heralded by accessory muscle use, dyspnea that precludes speech, or a rising Pa_{CO_2}. Barotrauma, which is common, may manifest by chest pain, asymmetric breath sounds, or subcutaneous emphysema and correlates with progression to ventilatory failure. Pulsus paradoxus > 15 mm Hg indicates marked swings in intrathoracic pressure resulting from increased respiratory efforts. Wheezing may be absent in the late stages of status asthmaticus as air movement decreases as a result of respiratory muscle fatigue. Respiratory alkalosis, lactic acidosis, and respiratory acidosis are the acid-base disturbances that can be found with severe asthma.

215. **The answer is C.** *(Chapter 44)*   The diagnosis of *Pneumocystis carinii* pneumonia is made by examining specimens from the lung with silver stain techniques. Bronchoalveolar lavage (BAL) fluid is more sensitive than sputum. Transbronchial biopsy only minimally increases the diagnostic yield above BAL. In addition, there is a risk of pneumothorax that can progress to tension pneumothorax during mechanical ventilation. Therefore, BAL is the best choice for this patient.

216. **The answer is C.** *(Chapter 44)*   The first-line drug for PCP is TMP-SMX. In patients with severe PCP with a Pa_{O_2} less than 70 mm Hg or an A−a gradient greater than 35 mm Hg, prednisone therapy is recommended to decrease inflammation seen in response to organism destruction. The use of prednisone in this setting is associated with an improved outcome. Dapsone and pentamadine are alternatives if patients cannot tolerate TMP-SMX. Azithromycin is ineffective against PCP.

217. **The answer is D.** *(Chapter 44)*   The appropriate dose of TMP-SMX is 5 mg/kg of TMP. In severe PCP, initially it should be given parenterally.

218. **The answer is B.** *(Chapter 37)*   Most of the adverse consequences of sleep-disordered breathing result from apnea-induced recurrent hypoxemia. Hypoxemia stimulates arousal and interrupted sleep, with consequent daytime hypersomnolence and personality changes. Autonomic discharge during episodes of obstruction produces tachycardia and systemic hypertension. Morning headache results from apnea-related hypercapnia. Significant inspiratory efforts against an obstructed upper airway can result in large negative pleural pressures that increase left ventricular afterload and cause pulmonary edema on rare occasions.

219. **The answer is B.** *(Chapter 36)*   The scoliotic deformity consists of a primary initiating curve and a secondary compensatory curve. The scoliotic angle is determined by the intersection of lines estimating the position of the upper and lower components of the primary curve.

220. **The answer is C.** *(Chapter 47)*   Although bacterial superinfection complicates aspiration quite frequently (20 to 30 percent of cases), empiric antibiotics usually are not indicated because of the possible emergence of resistant organisms. The only exception is a patient with paralytic or obstructive ileus who aspirates fecal material. Broad-spectrum antibiotic therapy against gut pathogens should be instituted immediately, although survival after such episodes is poor. Bacterial superinfection usually does not occur until several days after the aspiration, and the best approach is to withhold antibiotics until an actual infection is documented.

221. **The answer is B.** (*Chapter 30*)   Most commonly, death from hemoptysis occurs when the volume of blood being produced cannot be cleared and is aspirated diffusely. The patient dies of hypoxia. Although volume depletion is a common problem, it is rarely the primary cause of death.

222. **The answer is B.** (*Chapters 13, 15, 26, 29*)   The most common entities that cause a bloody pleural effusion are hemothorax, either traumatic or nontraumatic, malignancy, pulmonary embolus, and traumatic thoracentesis. All bloody pleural effusions should be investigated with measurement of pleural fluid hematocrit. If it is greater than 50 percent that of blood, the patient has a hemothorax and insertion of chest tubes and further diagnostic workup should be considered. If it is more than 1 percent but less than 50 percent, the patient most likely has malignant pleural disease, a pulmonary embolus, or a traumatically induced pleural effusion. If it is less than 1 percent, the blood in the pleural fluid has no clinical significance. Even if the blood is insignificant, the patient's pain and dyspnea require further evaluation.

223. **The answer is C.** (*Chapter 15*)   The patient in this case has suffered a significant blood loss with a history of "coughing up blood." In this situation it is important to distinguish hemoptysis from hematemesis, since both can give the appearance of coughing up blood. Hemoptysis severe enough to cause a 12 percent decrease in hematocrit over less than 24 hours would be associated with focal abnormalities on the chest x-ray. Investigation for gastrointestinal and pharyngeal sources of blood loss should ensue.

224. **The answer is C.** (*Chapters 53, 78*)   An elevated pleural fluid amylase indicates esophageal rupture, pancreatic disease, or malignancy. The acuteness of the patient's symptoms favors either pancreatitis or esophageal rupture. However, the low pleural fluid pH makes esophageal rupture the most likely diagnosis.

225. **The answer is D (4).** (*Chapter 10*)   Dysynchrony with the ventilator during mechanical ventilation occurs commonly in critically ill patients. Initial interventions should be directed at reversing causes of distress such as malpositioned endotracheal tube or orogastric tube, gastric distention, and pain or anxiety. Ventilator settings that are insufficient to meet the needs of the patient (e.g., respiratory rate setting much lower than patient's spontaneous respiratory rate) commonly lead to ventilator dysynchrony. Neuromuscular blockade should be used only when all the above issues have been addressed and ventilator dysynchrony remains. Most patients can be adequately sedated during mechanical ventilation and do not require paralysis.

226. **The answer is B.** (*Chapters 15, 30, 32*)   This patient has a left mainstem intubation and a left-sided pneumothorax. The widened rib spaces and hemodynamic compromise are diagnostic of a tension pneumothorax that requires immediate evacuation. This can be done quickly with a large-bore venous catheter and later followed up with tube thoracostomy. The endotracheal tube should be pulled back, but this should not take precedence over evacuation of the tension pneumothorax.

227. **The answer is D (4).** (*Chapter 31*)   Noninvasive ventilation is useful in the treatment of many types of respiratory failure. The benefits include avoidance of endotracheal intubation with its inherent complications, increased patient acceptance and comfort, and increased likelihood of more rapid liberation from mechanical ventilation. Acute hypoxemic respiratory failure from many different causes can be treated with noninvasive ventilation (ARDS, focal pneumonia, pulmonary hemorrhage). Noninvasive ventilation also serves to decrease left ventricular afterload and may improve low-output left ventricular failure. The inability to protect the airway from aspiration is a contraindication to noninvasive ventilation.

228.   **The answer is B.**   *(Chapters 11, 15, 32)*   The increased gradient between peak and plateau pressures indicates that increased resistance is the likely etiology of the patient's sudden oxygen desaturation. Possible causes include bronchospasm, excessive secretions or mucous plugging in the peripheral airways, and obstruction of the endotracheal tube secondary to biting, kinking of the tube, or luminal obstruction with mucus, vomitus, or a blood clot. The first response of any evaluating physician should be to disconnect the ventilator and provide hand-bag ventilation. This simultaneously isolates a likely problem source (the ventilator) and provides a much better sense of the mechanical situation than does auscultation alone. The addition of auscultation will inform the examiner of bronchospasm and right (or left) main stem intubation. Changes in ventilator settings and other therapeutic interventions should be done only after initial assessment with the hand-bag ventilation maneuver.

229.   **The answer is C.**   *(Chapter 32)*   In pressure support ventilation the patient initiates each breath; therefore, respiratory rate is set by the patient. Since the ventilator assists only by delivering a flow to maintain a predetermined airway opening pressure, the tidal volume received by the patient is determined by the patient's respiratory system compliance and effort.

230.   **The answer is B.**   *(Chapter 30)*   Airflow obstruction often produces radiologic evidence of air trapping (such as large lung volumes and flattened diaphragms), but the associated gas-exchange abnormality is that of ventilation-perfusion mismatch, not intrapulmonary shunt, as indicated by the data in this case. It is likely that a large region of lung is atelectatic or consolidated, as one would encounter with lung collapse or pneumonia. Pneumomediastinum causes no gas exchange abnormality, and esophageal intubation would be expected to result in hypoventilation. The clinical data do not support a diagnosis of tension pneumothorax.

231.   **The answer is B.**   *(Chapters 11, 15)*   The most serious consequence of prolonged endotracheal intubation is laryngeal injury from endotracheal tube pressure or abrasion that leads to mucosal denudation and perichondritis. This may result in upper airway obstruction from posterior commissural stenosis, posterior cordal synechiae, arytenoid fixation, or subglottic stenosis. Tracheoesophageal fistula is an extraordinarily rare complication of translaryngeal intubation. Aspiration around and accidental dislodgement of the tracheal tube may occur with either endotracheal or tracheostomy tubes and usually can be minimized by close medical attention.

232.   **The answer is C.**   *(Chapters 30, 32, 34)*   Because the measured PEEP during airflow obstruction does not reflect PEEPi, the calculation of compliance [C = V_T (Pstatic − PEEP)] may underestimate true compliance. Thus, compliance should be calculated by using the measured PEEPi. The development of PEEPi during airflow obstruction may result in increases in both peak and plateau pressures but should not affect the inspiratory flow-related pressure drop, which is reflected in the peak-to-plateau gradient. It is determined by evaluation of airway pressure during a pause at end expiration (or by the assessment of persistent expiratory flow at the time inspiration would normally begin). The development of PEEPi is exquisitely sensitive to changes in minute ventilation and, to a lesser degree, to inspiratory and expiratory flow rates. Finally, the increase in functional residual capacity that results from increased PEEPi may improve oxygenation in alveolar flooding or may worsen hypoxemia by reducing venous return and thereby also reducing mixed venous oxygen saturation.

233.   **The answer is C.**   *(Chapter 30)*   It is important to note that any patient receiving supplemental oxygen by mask or nasal cannula breathing with a tachypneic pattern is likely to entrain variable amounts of room air and thus have wide variation in the fraction of inspired oxygen. Accordingly, judgments regarding changes in alveolar-arterial oxygen gradient must be made on room air or in the intubated patient. The relatively constant Pa_{CO_2} excludes hypoventilation, and recurrent pulmonary emboli would be expected to cause

symptoms or cardiovascular changes. Intrinsic PEEP affecting gas exchange would be unlikely in a patient recovering from ARDS. Alterations in cardiac output certainly cause changes in arterial Pa_{O_2} in patients with lung disease, but there is little to suggest large changes in perfusion in this patient. Such frequent blood-gas sampling in a stable patient often yields data that are more confounding than helpful. It would be appropriate to monitor such a patient noninvasively with pulse oximetry alone.

234. **The answer is D.** (*Chapter 33*)   Inverse ratio ventilation is used in patients with acute hypoxemic respiratory failure. It is hypothesized to improve oxygenation in several ways. The slower inspiratory flow rates may allow the recruitment of flooded alveoli as well as the distribution of flow to lung units with slower time constants. In addition, these low inspiratory flow rates and the subsequent decreased expiratory time cause the development of intrinsic positive end-expiratory pressure (PEEPi). This increase in PEEPi causes an increase in FRC, with an improvement in oxygenation. It is not known which of these effects predominates.

235. **The answer is C.** (*Chapters 15, 47*)   Closed pleural biopsy is most useful when tuberculosis or cancer is the cause of pleural effusion. Pleural coccidioidomycosis and rheumatoid arthritis pleurisy also have been diagnosed by closed pleural biopsy, but other conditions are diagnosed only rarely.

236. **The answer is C.** (*Chapters 13, 15*)   It is important to distinguish between massive pleural effusion and complete lung collapse in the evaluation of an opacified hemithorax. In this case the deviated trachea, mediastinal shift, high gastric air bubble, and narrowing of the intercostal spaces on the left all point to complete collapse of the left lung.

237. **The answer is D.** (*Chapters 15, 33*)   Open-lung biopsy is the most accurate diagnostic procedure in patients with pulmonary infiltrates that result in acute respiratory failure. It is the preferred procedure in patients with coagulation abnormalities, since it allows direct control of bleeding. It does not result in a significant decrement in Pa_{O_2} and thus can be performed in patients with severe hypoxemia without fear of worsening the gas-exchange abnormality. Nondiagnostic biopsies are more likely to be seen in patients with myeloproliferative rather than lymphoproliferative and nonhematologic disorders.

238. **The answer is E.** (*Chapters 13, 15*)   The anteroposterior projection, combined with a shorter distance between the x-ray source and the patient, results in mediastinal and cardiac magnification. If the patient is not fully erect, the vascular pedicle may be distended. Image quality is diminished because an antiscatter grid is not typically placed between the patient and portable film, so that scattered radiation reaches the film and appears as a diffuse gray density.

239. **The answer is A.** (*Chapter 88*)   Pulmonary contusion typically results in a nonsegmental airspace infiltrate. Infiltrates usually appear immediately after trauma and start to resolve within 48 hours. Radiographic findings are often more impressive than the clinical picture.

240. **The answer is B.** (*Chapter 97*)   The bird-nest filter does not require as much venous dilation for cannulation and placement and has decreased the rate of femoral vein thrombosis. Recurrent pulmonary emboli have been reported in 2 percent of patients with vena caval filters in place. Anticoagulation certainly can be used with the filter, although many filters are placed because the patient has a contraindication to anticoagulation or has bled after anticoagulation. The indications for filter placement include failure of anticoagulation (or unacceptable complications) and an unacceptably high risk of death after recurrent embolization.

241. **The answer is C.** (*Chapter 33*)   Although reducing PEEP might increase cardiac output, it probably would cause life-threatening aggravation of arterial hypoxemia. Increasing PEEP is appropriate in this situation. In patients whose lung disease is characterized by shunt (or severe V/Q inhomogeneity), changes in the mixed venous oxygen saturation can have a profound effect on arterial saturation. Therefore, in such patients every effort should be made to increase oxygen delivery to the periphery and decrease oxygen consumption. Thus, if oxygen consumption remains constant or decreases, the mixed venous saturation will be expected to increase. Reduction of the level of applied PEEP also would increase mixed venous oxygen saturation. However, the resulting alveolar flooding and increase in shunt might overwhelm the expected increase in Pa_{O_2}. Inhaled nitric oxide has been shown to improve oxygenation in ARDS by improving ventilation-perfusion matching. Prone ventilation also improves oxygenation in ARDS. Speculated mechanisms include reduction of atelectatic lung regions and improved ventilation of the posterior portions of the lung where blood flow is increased, even in the prone position (i.e., it is not gravity-dependent).

242. **The answer is D.** (*Chapter 72*)   Hemodialysis removes about half the CO_2 produced by the body. In order for Pa_{CO_2} to remain constant, alveolar ventilation must be reduced by 50 percent in these patients, yet the oxygen uptake from the lungs remains the same. Accordingly, Pa_{O_2} falls during dialysis because twice as much oxygen is removed from inspired air as CO_2 is added to it.

243. **The answer is B.** (*Chapter 33*)   Even though ARDS causes a low-pressure pulmonary edema, diuretic therapy can significantly decrease alveolar edema and improve oxygenation. Noninvasive mask ventilation is a reasonable first step in patients who can protect the airway and may obviate intubation in some patients. Though PEEP may be associated with barotrauma in some patients, high levels can be used safely in most if plateau airway pressures remain below 30 to 35 cm H_2O. Alveolar edema in ARDS typically has a high protein content because of disruption of endothelial integrity.

244. **The answer is A.** (*Chapters 30, 33*)   Exposure to an Fi_{O_2} of 100 percent will completely correct hypoxemia secondary to ventilation-perfusion mismatch but not shunt, thus allowing differentiation between these two causes of hypoxemia. Right heart catheterization and sampling of arterial and mixed venous blood allow calculation of shunt but usually are not indicated for the simple distinction between the mechanisms of hypoxemia. Ventilation-perfusion scanning or lung mechanical measurements would be of little assistance in this setting.

245. **The answer is C.** (*Chapters 30, 34*)   The patient's elastance is calculated as follows: elastance = (inflation hold pressure − PEEP or PEEPi / V_T = (30 − 15) / 0.5 = 30 cm H_2O / L.

246. **The answer is B.** (*Chapters 30, 34*)   The patient's resistance is calculated as follows: resistance = (peak pressure − inflation hold pressure) / IF = (60 − 30) / 0.67 = 45 cm H_2O/Lps. In the question, the inspiratory flow (IF) is given as 40 L per minute. This must be converted to liters per second to match the units in the answer.

247. **The answer is D.** (*Chapters 30, 34*)   The patient has a normal elastance (upper limit of normal = 20 cm H_2O/L) but a markedly abnormal resistance (normal with a size 8 to 9 endotracheal tube = 10 cm H_2O/Lps). The high value of PEEPi provides evidence of extreme air trapping. Both of these phenomena could be explained by severe asthma. A patient with pulmonary edema or pneumonia usually has an abnormal elastance and normal resistance. A patient with pulmonary embolism usually has normal respiratory mechanics.

248.   The answer is D. *(Chapters 30, 34)*   The reasons for failure to liberate a patient from mechanical ventilation can be divided into excessive respiratory muscle load (e.g., pulmonary edema) and decreased respiratory muscle strength (e.g., myasthenia gravis). With normal peak and inflation hold pressures, this patient does not have an excessive respiratory load. The NIP of -20 cm H_2O (normal is >100 cm H_2O) documents that the patient's respiratory muscles are weak. Possible etiologies include hypocalcemia, hypophosphatemia, hypomagnesemia, hypothyroidism, protein-calorie malnutrition, neuromuscular disease, subclinical status epilepticus, and hypoperfusion states.

249.   The answer is D. *(Chapter 74)*   In patients with compensated (chronic) respiratory acidosis, the expected increase in plasma bicarbonate can be predicted by the following equation: predicted $[HCO_3] = (Pa_{CO_2} - 40)/3 + 24$.

250.   The answer is B. *(Chapter 73)*   Administration of glucose, especially after starvation, draws phosphate into the production of phosphorylated intermediates and high-energy phosphates as glycolysis resumes. Respiratory alkalosis, not acidosis, also can cause hypophosphatemia on the basis of stimulation of glycolysis. Hypomagnesemia leads to impaired conservation of phosphate, antacids containing magnesium and aluminum hydroxide bind phosphate in the gut, and β-adrenergic agonists probably cause internal shifts of phosphate.

251.   The answer is D (4). *(Chapter 33)*   Hypotension with a narrow pulse pressure, tachycardia, and low urine output suggests an inadequate cardiac output from causes such as hypovolemia, myocardial dysfunction, and pericardial tamponade. In this setting, Sv_{O_2} may be low and may constitute a circulatory component to arterial hypoxemia. Characterizing the circulation with a pulmonary artery catheter allows measurement of central pressures and determination of Sv_{O_2}, which then helps direct further therapy. Increasing PEEP, promoting diuresis, or increasing tidal volume may lower cardiac output by decreasing preload and result in deterioration. An assessment of cardiac function and oxygen delivery is necessary before further therapeutic interventions are undertaken.

252.   The answer is B (1, 3). *(Chapter 33)*   There are four causes of a low Pv_{O_2}: low Sa_{O_2}, anemia, inadequate cardiac output, and high oxygen consumption. Only the latter two result in a widened Ca−Cv. Inadequate cardiac output results from hypovolemia, myocardial dysfunction, pericardial tamponade, or stenotic or regurgitant heart valves. It is important to remember that despite what appears to be an adequate PCWP, patients may still need more volume when the heart is noncompliant or when PEEP artificially elevates the measured pulmonary capillary wedge pressure.

253.   The answer is D (4). *(Chapter 33)*   If the Sv_{O_2} is greater for a given Pa_{O_2}, intrapulmonary shunt is greater. Intrapulmonary shunt results when alveoli are collapsed or filled with water, pus, or blood. Left ventricular dysfunction from any etiology (including pericardial tamponade) can cause a decrease in Sv_{O_2} and a resulting decrease in Sa_{O_2}. Worsening anemia will decrease both arterial and mixed venous oxygen content but will not lead to an increase in the arterial-venous oxygen content difference.

254.   The answer is E (all). *(Chapter 33)*   In this patient all the listed interventions should decrease the oxygen requirement: sedation and paralysis by decreasing oxygen consumption, increased PEEP by decreasing intrapulmonary shunt, and transfusion by increasing Pv_{O_2}.

255.   The answer is C (2, 4). *(Chapter 34)*   Most of these patients actually present with an increased drive to breathe. Respiratory drive and minute ventilation have not been decreased by supplemental oxygen in a number of studies. However, increases in both Pa_{O_2} and Pa_{CO_2} do usually occur. The rise in Pa_{CO_2}, which is due to a worsening in V/Q mismatch, should not defer one from applying needed oxygen.

256. **The answer is C (2, 4).** (*Chapter 34*)   This rhythm disturbance is multifocal atrial tachycardia, which is not uncommon in this patient population. It is typically refractory to digoxin therapy but can respond to correction of hypoxemia and other metabolic disturbances. Aggressive treatment of COPD with bronchodilators may improve the rhythm disturbance. Theophylline toxicity should be excluded. Diltiazem and selective β-blocking agents can provide rate control and conversion to sinus rhythm, but the β-blockers may have adverse effects in this patient population.

257. **The answer is A (1, 2, 3).** (*Chapter 35*)   The goals of mechanical ventilation in a patient with status asthmaticus are adequate alveolar ventilation at an acceptable peak airway pressure (< 55 cm H_2O), with least intrinsic PEEP (< 15 cm H_2O) and a stable circulation. Small tidal volumes and high inspiratory flow rates minimize dynamic hyperinflation and intrinsic PEEP (PEEPi). Low respiratory rates will allow more time for exhalation, though an increase in Pa_{CO_2} may be seen. PEEP should not be used initially since it can result in dangerous increases in lung and airway pressure with resulting hypotension, hypoperfusion, and barotrauma.

258. **The answer is D (4).** (*Chapter 35*)   The patient has significant air trapping with a high intrinsic PEEP level and increased peak to pause airway pressure gradient. These airway pressures put the patient at risk for barotrauma. Further decreasing the respiratory rate will allow more time for exhalation and probably decrease PEEPi. Respiratory acidosis should be tolerated ("permissive hypercapnia") because barotrauma carries a substantially higher risk to the patient. The relative hypoxemia is expected because of the low FI_{O_2} in the setting of asthma (V / Q mismatch). A Pa_{O_2} of 68 mm Hg with an Sa_{O_2} of 91 percent is acceptable in this patient. The helium/oxygen mixture can decrease air trapping and should not be discontinued at this time.

259. **The answer is E (all).** (*Chapters 11, 21, 33, 35*)   The differential diagnosis of wheezing is broad. Wheezing can be a sign of upper airway obstruction, in which case wheezing may be localized or an inspiratory stridor may be heard over the trachea. It also may result from a foreign body, especially in children; cardiac asthma from left ventricular failure; COPD; and noncardiogenic pulmonary edema (ARDS).

260. **The answer is B (1, 3).** (*Chapter 35*)   Management of respiratory acidosis on the ventilator in patients with status asthmaticus focuses on setting a tidal volume and respiratory rate to allow adequate alveolar ventilation at an acceptable peak airway pressure (< 55 cm H_2O) with the least intrinsic PEEP possible (< 15 cm H_2O). When respiratory acidosis persists and cannot be corrected by increasing ventilation, sedation and muscle relaxation minimize airway pressures and lower carbon dioxide production. At this time, PEEP will be of no benefit, and the reduction of inspiratory flow will increase inspiratory time, decrease expiratory time, and cause further gas trapping with more intrinsic PEEP (PEEPi). A helium/oxygen gas mixture allows more complete emptying of trapped gas, thereby decreasing PEEPi. This low-density gas appears to improve airflow through narrowed distal airways.

261. **The answer is E (all).** (*Chapter 32*) Pa_{CO_2} may be reduced at a constant minute ventilation by lowering dead space or decreasing carbon dioxide production. Both volume challenge and lowering alveolar pressure may decrease dead space, while sedation and avoiding excessive carbohydrate and caloric intake decrease carbon dioxide production.

262. **The answer is B (1, 3).** (*Chapter 31*)   Noninvasive mask ventilation can be used safely and effectively for both acute hypoxemic respiratory failure and ventilatory failure. Unresponsive patients, such as those in a postictal state, and pregnant women are at significant risk for aspiration and should not be managed with mask ventilation.

263.   The answer is D (4).   *(Chapter 36)*   IPF is a disorder predominantly of the lower lobes that is associated with clubbing. Adenopathy is rare. Cystic spaces (honeycombing) are distributed unevenly within areas of fibrosis and are a late finding.

264.   The answer is A (1, 2, 3).   *(Chapters 30, 34)*   Disturbances in sodium balance have not been correlated with respiratory muscle weakness, but deficiencies of phosphate, magnesium, calcium, and potassium have all been reported to cause respiratory muscle weakness and ventilatory failure.

265.   The answer is C (2,4).   *(Chapters 11, 35)*   The administration of heliox in upper airway obstruction is solely a temporizing measure that should be used only in situations in which there is a high likelihood of rapid reversal of the process. Situations in which there is a significant chance of deterioration before improvement, such as epiglottitis and compression of the trachea by a tumor, probably should be managed with control of the airway. Finally, heliox has been demonstrated to be useful in patients with severe asthma by allowing effective ventilation at lower airway pressures.

266.   The answer is E (all).   *(Chapter 37)*   A number of conditions may precipitate or worsen sleep apnea by increasing airway narrowing. These conditions include acute upper airway infection, renal failure with edema, and congestive heart failure. Alcohol, sedatives, and general anesthesia selectively depress the activity of upper airway muscles, central control, or both, compounding airway obstruction in susceptible patients.

267.   The answer is D (4).   *(Chapter 11)*   Laryngeal trauma may result in hemorrhage and submucosal edema. Early evaluation is indicated to assess the degree of injury and airway compromise. If there is significant injury, stenting of the airway is appropriate. If there is only mild edema and hemorrhage, close observation is indicated. Endotracheal intubation is not indicated with mild dyspnea and stridor. Given that a significant component of the laryngeal obstruction is probably due to hemorrhage, there is little role for steroids or racemic epinephrine.

268.   The answer is D (4).   *(Chapters 11, 91, 93)*   This patient almost certainly fell from the pole after contacting the high-voltage line and should be evaluated for traumatic injury caused by the fall. In particular, the cervical spine should be assumed to be unstable until proved otherwise by radiologic investigation. While these studies usually are performed in the emergency department, it is unwise for a critical care physician to make such an assumption. Since this patient was admitted directly to the ICU, he must undergo radiologic evaluation of his spine before hyperextension of the neck. For this reason, oral endotracheal intubation is relatively contraindicated. Nasotracheal intubation is also relatively contraindicated because of concern over possible head trauma and basilar skull fracture. The safest method of urgently securing the patient's airway is cricothyroidotomy. Fiber-optically assisted intubation is an alternative when done by experienced personnel with stabilization of the cervical spine. While heliox will reduce the work of breathing, it does not constitute definitive management of the airway. As edema from the presumed injury to the airway progresses, respiratory arrest is likely. Finally, the upper airway should be evaluated for the presence of a foreign body.

269.   The answer is C (2, 4).   *(Chapter 37)*   The patient presented with cardiorespiratory failure. Morbid obesity, decline in cognitive function, daytime hypersomnolence, polycythemia, and compensated respiratory acidosis suggest chronic alveolar hypoventilation from disordered breathing during sleep. Systemic hypertension is found in 50 percent of these patients. The initial therapy is supplemental oxygen to reverse hypoxemia, which is the cause of most of the adverse effects of disordered breathing during sleep. A hypoventilatory response to supplemental oxygen may occur in patients with sleep apnea and may require mechanical ventilation to allow time for oxygen and restoration of normal sleep to reverse the cardiorespiratory failure. When the patient is stable, a diagnosis can be made by a polysomnogram and definitive therapy can be prescribed. Thyroid function tests should be administered to rule out hypothyroidism as a cause of disordered breathing during sleep. Digoxin and diuretic therapy are usually unnecessary because spontaneous diuresis occurs as oxygen therapy reverses hypoxic vasoconstriction and thus improves cardiac output. Diuretic therapy may in fact be harmful by decreasing venous return and thus cardiac output in patients who may have cor pulmonale and require positive-pressure ventilation.

270. The answer is E (all). (*Chapters 30, 57, 60*)   The protective mechanism that the body has to minimize the risk of aspiration of noxious substances involves the complex integration of central nervous system input with the peripheral neuromuscular system. Conditions that predispose to aspiration include those which depress central nervous system reflexes (seizures, head trauma, meningitis), interfere with the nerves to the pharyngeal muscles (multiple sclerosis, trauma to the neck and pharynx), interfere with the pharyngeal muscles or esophageal muscles themselves (myasthenia gravis, Guillain-Barré syndrome, dermatomyositis), interfere with the normal passage of materials into the stomach (scleroderma, achalasia), or promote reflux of gastric contents into airways (nasogastric tube). The hormonal changes that occur during pregnancy decrease gastric motility and lower esophageal sphincter tone. These factors, combined with the growing uterus, increase the risk of aspiration.

271. The answer is E (all). (*Chapters 30, 33*)   The clinical presentation of patients who have aspirated is quite variable, ranging from minimal symptoms to acute hypoxemic respiratory failure (ARDS). Possible results range from acute upper airway obstruction by large, solid materials to chronic bronchiolitis, chronic pneumonitis, bronchiectasis, granuloma formation, and atelectasis from aspiration of small, nonacidic particulate matter. Bronchospasm and bacterial superinfection are other possible outcomes.

272. The answer is C (2, 4). (*Chapters 30, 33*)   Although bacterial superinfection complicates aspiration in 20 to 30 percent of cases, empiric antibiotics usually are not indicated because of the possible emergence of resistant organisms. Bacterial superinfection usually does not occur until several days after the aspiration, and the best approach is to withhold antibiotics until an infection is apparent. One of the possible complications of aspiration is pulmonary capillary leak. In this setting, PEEP, lowering the pulmonary capillary wedge pressure, or both may be required to achieve adequate oxygenation. Steroids do not have significant beneficial effects on aspiration injury and have many adverse effects.

273. The answer is A (1, 2, 3). (*Chapters 15, 30*)   For most patients, bronchoscopy should be carried out without waiting for the hemoptysis to stop. Although the clinical outcome may be unaffected, the ability to determine the site of bleeding is markedly improved. This information may be very important if urgent therapeutic interventions are needed. The suction channel of most fiber-optic bronchoscopes is only 2 to 3 mm in diameter, making it difficult to remove large volumes of blood rapidly. Therefore, when the rate of bleeding is brisk, straight or rigid bronchoscopy is the procedure of choice. For patients with hemoptysis in the setting of a nonfocal chest x-ray and normal findings on bronchoscopy, the hemoptysis resolves before discharge in more than 50 percent of patients and within 6 months in 90 percent and recurs in less than 5 percent.

274. The answer is E (all). (*Chapter 11*)   Since asphyxiation is the most common cause of death in patients with hemoptysis, measures should be taken to assure adequate oxygenation, improve clearance of the massive bleeding, and protect the normal lung from aspiration of blood. Correction of any underlying bleeding diatheses is important in the initial management. If the site of bleeding is known, placing the bleeding lung in the dependent position may help protect the other lung. Intubating the mainstem bronchus of the normal lung or placing a double-lumen endotracheal tube may help protect the good lung and provide tamponade of the lung that is bleeding. In the appropriate dose, codeine, by decreasing cough, can decrease bleeding without depressing respiration or increasing the risk of aspiration.

275. **The answer is A (1, 2, 3).** (*Chapter 30*)   A pleural effusion would shift the mediastinal structures away from the side of the opacified hemithorax; lung collapse would have the opposite effect. If the opacified hemithorax were due to collapse, the interspaces between the ribs on the involved side would be closer together compared with the rib interspaces of the opposite hemithorax. Also, if the opacification is due to collapse, the contralateral lung may herniate to the opposite side.

276. **The answer is E (all).** (*Chapters 26, 47, 53*)   Thoracentesis demonstrated an exudative pleural effusion with an elevated white blood cell count that had a predominance of neutrophils. Pleural effusions contain predominantly neutrophils when they are due to an acute disease process such as pneumonia, esophageal rupture, pulmonary embolization, pancreatitis, collagen vascular disease, intraabdominal abscess, early tuberculosis, and rarely malignancy. Chronic pleural effusions usually have a predominance of lymphocytes.

277. **The answer is B (1, 3).** (*Chapters 15, 101*)   Although cytology is more sensitive, pleural biopsy does add to the diagnostic workup of malignant pleural effusions. Because of the low yield of pleural cultures, pleural biopsy is the diagnostic procedure of choice when tuberculosis is in the differential diagnosis. Because the sample size is too small with a closed biopsy, an open pleural biopsy is the procedure of choice for the diagnosis of mesothelioma.

278. **The answer is D (4).** (*Chapter 30*)   This patient has hemorrhagic shock and type IV respiratory failure. Intubation and mechanical ventilation to decrease the work of breathing are an essential part of his resuscitation while blood transfusion and attempts to identify and stop the bleeding are under way. At rest, the respiratory muscles require approximately 5 percent of the cardiac output. Patients in respiratory distress can require up to 40 to 50 percent of the cardiac output. The patient has a metabolic acidosis, probably secondary to tissue hypoperfusion, which is contributing to his increased work of breathing. COPD leaves him with limited pulmonary reserve. Noninvasive ventilation would be an option as long as airway protection was not a concern. The other diagnostic and therapeutic interventions listed may play a role in the management of this patient but only after his respiratory failure has been stabilized.

279. **The answer is E (all).** (*Chapter 34*)   Bronchospasm leads to increased airway resistance, increasing the work of breathing. In addition, intrinsic PEEP (PEEPi) puts the respiratory muscles at a mechanical disadvantage, thus increasing their load. Heart failure may lead to increased airway resistance ("cardiac asthma") and increase load in a similar way. Pleural effusion puts an increased elastic load on the chest wall. Pulmonary embolus leads to an increase in dead space and thus an increased minute ventilation requirement which increases the respiratory muscle load.

280. **The answer is E (all).** (*Chapters 21, 30, 33, 47*)   A pleural effusion associated with pneumococcal pneumonia occurs frequently and rarely requires tube thoracostomy. A small pleural effusion occurs commonly immediately after upper abdominal surgery and requires investigation only if there is suspicion of another etiology (e.g., pulmonary embolus). In the obvious case of uncomplicated congestive heart failure, a small right-sided pleural effusion need not be tapped. Factors that would necessitate a diagnostic thoracentesis in the setting of congestive heart failure include the presence of fever, the presence of only a left-sided pleural effusion, and a large inequality of right- and left-sided pleural effusions.

281. **The answer is C (2, 4).** *(Chapter 101)* This patient's history and presentation strongly suggest systemic lupus erythematosus (SLE) with acute lupus pneumonitis. Other lung-renal syndromes are somewhat less likely in view of the normal creatinine and lack of abnormalities on urinalysis. Lung biopsy is nonspecific, revealing alveolitis, edema, and lung hemorrhage. Nonetheless, it is often necessary to exclude infection, particularly in a patient with known SLE who is receiving immunosuppressives. A positive antinuclear antibody test would strongly support the diagnosis. Hemoptysis is typical in lupus pneumonitis itself. Endomyocardial biopsy would be of little value based on the data presented.

282. **The answer is A (1, 2, 3).** *(Chapters 11, 30, 39)* In normal subjects, functional residual capacity, total lung capacity, and slow vital capacity are unchanged, while forced vital capacity is diminished by the presence of an endotracheal tube. Anatomic dead space is reduced slightly by the substitution of an endotracheal tube for the nasopharynx. Although the cross-sectional area of an 8.0 endotracheal tube is similar to that of a normal adult glottis, the tube is much longer than the glottis, thus increasing resistance. In addition, the presence of a foreign body in the trachea, such as an endotracheal tube, may cause bronchospasm. Peak flow is decreased on average by 20 percent, while MVV is diminished by 35 percent.

283. **The answer is E (all).** *(Chapter 11)* Although the only absolute indication for the establishment of a tracheostomy is to overcome upper airway obstruction, providing airway access for long-term mechanical ventilation, promoting tracheobronchial toilet, and aiding weaning from mechanical to spontaneous ventilation are all felt to be important reasons to perform a tracheostomy. Since the risk of laryngeal damage that leads to obstruction or dysphonia is related to the length of time the endotracheal tube remains in place, tracheostomy is necessary in patients requiring long-term mechanical ventilation. Weaning from mechanical ventilation with a tracheostomy is easier than it is with an endotracheal tube owing to the decrease in nonelastic load related to the shorter length and larger diameter of a tracheostomy tube. This may be important in patients whose spontaneous ventilatory capability is marginal. Finally, tracheobronchial toilet is easier to maintain through a tracheostomy, since it provides a more direct route to the lower airway.

284. **The answer is B (1, 3).** *(Chapters 11, 39)* While tracheostomy performed by experienced personnel is a relatively minor procedure, late complications do occur, including tracheoesophageal fistula, hemorrhage of the innominate artery from tube erosion into the artery, and tracheal stenosis after decannulation. Complications that may occur immediately after tracheostomy include pneumothorax from inadvertent dissection into the pleural space during surgery and hemorrhage of the arteria thyroidea ima as a result of improper ligation of this vessel.

285. **The answer is A (1, 2, 3).** *(Chapter 11)* Split-lung ventilation can be used for airway hemorrhage, bronchopleural fistula, bronchopulmonary lavage, drainage of communicating empyema, protection from contamination, and thoracoscopy. The technique requires special competence and can be difficult to apply in the critical care setting. The use of split-lung ventilation protects the "good" lung from soilage in cases of airway hemorrhage and facilitates selective ventilation and the application of PEEP. The technique would not be of use in homogeneous lung diseases such as ARDS.

286. **The answer is E (all).** *(Chapter 99)* The complications of hyperbaric oxygen (HBO) therapy include ear or sinus trauma, tympanic membrane rupture, pneumothorax, air embolism, central nervous system toxic reactions, pulmonary toxic reactions, fire, reversible visual changes, and claustrophobia. Routine HBO therapy at 2 atmospheres for 90 minutes is relatively safe, with seizures occurring at an estimated rate of 1 in 10,000 cases.

287. **The answer is A (1, 2, 3).** (*Chapter 99*)   Decompression sickness, air embolism, and carbon monoxide poisoning are indications for hyperbaric oxygen (HBO) therapy. While HBO is a standard approach to decompression sickness and air embolism, the precise benefits derived from its use after carbon monoxide poisoning and the optimal schedule of use are under investigation. There is no clinical use of HBO in anaerobic pneumonia.

288. **The answer is A (1, 2, 3).** (*Chapters 13, 32*)   Even though putting samples on ice is a good policy when feasible, samples analyzed within 10 to 15 minutes should have little change in measured values. Changes that do occur over time are most often related to metabolism in blood, mainly by leukocytes. Heparin lowers Pa_{CO_2} mainly by dilution, whereas Pa_{CO_2} is lower in samples with air bubbles owing to the diffusion of CO_2 into the bubbles.

289. **The answer is A (1, 2, 3).** (*Chapters 13, 32*)   Carboxyhemoglobin is measured as saturated hemoglobin by the pulse oximeter, which therefore gives false values of hemoglobin oxygen saturation. The pulse oximeter cannot distinguish hemoglobin molecules saturated with oxygen from those saturated with carbon monoxide. The pulse oximeter spectrophotometrically determines arterial oxygen saturation and has proved very useful for the management of ventilated and unstable patients in the ICU. Hypovolemia may lead to peripheral vasoconstriction and decreased perfusion of the digits. In this situation, the oximeter probe may be unable to detect an accurate pulse signal and arterial saturation.

290. **The answer is B (1, 3).** (*Chapters 15, 36*)   Pleural effusions appear to cause dyspnea by displacing the chest wall from its position of optimal mechanical advantage. Removal of pleural fluid returns the chest wall toward its normal configuration and thus relieves dyspnea. This improvement in chest wall position, as well an increase in available intrathoracic volume, may lead to an increase in respiratory system compliance. However, this effect is usually not significant. There is usually little gas-exchange abnormality associated with even massive pleural effusions. Thus, removal of fluid has little effect on ventilation or oxygenation. In fact, Pa_{O_2} sometimes may decrease after fluid removal in patients with large effusions.

291. **The answer is A (1, 2, 3).** (*Chapter 15*)   In a critically ill patient, tube thoracostomy can be a lifesaving procedure when respiratory or circulatory stability is compromised by an abnormal accumulation of gas or fluid in the pleural space. In addition, tube thoracostomy allows quantitation of the rate of hemorrhage in patients with a hemothorax. Tension pneumothorax or a large pleural effusion may raise right atrial pressure and decrease venous return. Empyema in a mechanically ventilated patient requires a tube thoracostomy for adequate drainage in addition to antibiotic therapy for the eradication of infection. A simple rib fracture without pulmonary contusion or flail chest that necessitates mechanical ventilation does not require tube thoracostomy.

292. **The answer is A (1, 2, 3).** (*Chapter 30*)   Surgical obliteration of the pleural space (pleurodesis) should be considered in patients with pneumothorax and certain pleural effusions that are unresponsive to chemical pleurodesis. A single recurrence of an ipsilateral pneumothorax necessitates pleurodesis because of the greater than 50 percent incidence of a third event. Bilateral pneumothoraces, whether synchronous or metachronous, are an absolute indication. Patients with persistent air leaks do better with surgical pleurodesis unless they are too ill to undergo surgery. Malignant pleural effusions that are initially unresponsive to chemical pleurodesis may be considered for pleurodesis.

293. **The answer is A (1, 2, 3).** (*Chapters 15, 30*)   Pleural biopsy increases the yield in the diagnosis of pleural tuberculosis from approximately 60 percent to 85 percent. It is also useful in the diagnosis of pleural malignancies. However, the vascular lesions of metastatic renal cell cancer are probably unsafe to biopsy without better control of bleeding.

294. **The answer is D (4).** *(Chapter 15)* Thoracentesis is indicated to diagnose most newly discovered pleural effusions unless the effusion is small, its cause is clear, or the risk outweighs the benefit of knowing the composition of the pleural fluid. Relative contraindications include prolonged PT or PTT, platelet counts less than 20,000 per cubic millimeter of blood, and BUN greater than 60 mg/dL (which impairs platelet function). In patient 1 with probable congestive heart failure, the risk of bleeding outweighs the benefits of the procedure. Similarly, in patient 2, the common appearance of small pleural effusions after sclerotherapy makes the risk greater than the benefit. The same is true in patient 3, in whom abdominal surgery, not infection, is the likely cause of the effusion. Only in patient 4 is immediate thoracentesis warranted because of possible empyema. Rapid correction of the coagulopathy and minimization of airway pressures are desirable before thoracentesis, though these maneuvers should not prevent or unduly delay thoracentesis if they are not possible.

295. **The answer is A (1, 2, 3).** *(Chapter 15)* In general, lobar collapse is not associated with substantially worsened hypoxemia or patient discomfort, and it has been shown that bronchoscopy is not more effective than respiratory therapy in the treatment of acute lobar collapse. Bronchoscopy would be indicated if vigorous suctioning, respiratory therapy, and ventilatory maneuvers failed to remove the obstruction. In contrast, total lung collapse typically requires bronchoscopy.

296. **The answer is A (1, 2, 3).** *(Chapter 13)* Correct interpretation of portable chest radiographs requires knowledge of the patient's position. The patient's position sometimes is written on the film by the technician, but this may not be accurate. The patient's actual position can be estimated by an inclinometer, the position of the gastric air bubble (air collects in the fundus when the patient is erect, and in the antrum when the patient is supine), and the breast position in females.

297. **The answer is A (1, 2, 3).** *(Chapter 47)* Currently, the greatest utility of bronchoalveolar lavage in ICU patients is its ability to detect the presence of malignancy, tuberculosis, fungal infection, and *Pneumocystis carinii*. Sometimes viral pneumonia also can be diagnosed. Bronchoalveolar lavage normally is contaminated with small numbers of bacteria from the upper airway and should be used for aerobic or anaerobic bacterial culture only if quantitative cultures are performed. The sterile brush technique is much more useful for the diagnosis of bacterial diseases, except for infection by *Legionella*.

298. **The answer is D (4).** *(Chapters 13, 30)* Acute opacification of one hemithorax is more commonly due to total pulmonary atelectasis than to pleural effusion. Factors favoring atelectasis include a shift of the trachea and mediastinum toward the affected side and narrowing of the rib interspaces surrounding the atelectatic lung. Patients tend to rotate toward the side of the collapsed lung on an anteroposterior portable film, and this sometimes leads to misinterpretation of the mediastinal shift as being due to rotation alone.

299. **The answer is E (all).** *(Chapter 33)* Worsening edema or exudation will increase the density of infiltrates. However, decreased pulmonary inflation (as occurs when V_T or PEEP is lowered or when patients are extubated) produces a similar effect. Decreased x-ray penetration also results in a "whiter" film. However, increased pulmonary inflation or increased x-ray penetration may be wrongly interpreted as improvement.

300. **The answer is D (4).** *(Chapters 13, 32, 35)* The shift of the trachea and mediastinum toward the opacified right hemithorax confirms the diagnosis of right lung collapse during the last 6 hours. In status asthmaticus, this is often due to a bronchial plug, which should be removed by a focused bronchoscopy despite the acknowledged risk of aggravating bronchospasm before attempting to reinflate the lung. Usually the lung can be

reinflated with a larger tidal volume, PEEP to maintain a larger end-expired volume, and an end-inspiratory pause to sustain end-inspiratory volume long enough to allow inflated units in the right lung to reopen the collapsed units. Of course, the adverse effects of such hyperinflation are pulmonary barotrauma and hypotension, and so these ventilatory gymnastics should be performed within airway and blood pressure limits. The left lateral decubitus position focuses the favorable effects on the collapsed right lung while minimizing the hypotensive effects of the pregnant uterus on the inferior vena cava. Thoracentesis, chest tube insertion, and antibiotics are diagnostic and therapeutic procedures aimed at the wrong radiologic diagnosis.

301. The answer is B (1, 3). (*Chapter 11*)   After the placement of a tracheostomy tube, it is common to see small amounts of air in the subcutaneous tissues of the neck. Large amounts of air or air dissecting inferiorly into the mediastinum is an abnormal finding that is suggestive of a significant air leak. The tip of the tracheostomy tube should be one-half to two-thirds of the way between the stoma and the carina (usually below the clavicles). Low placement and angulation of the tube can lead to erosion of the tip through the tracheal wall, with the formation of a tracheal–innominate artery fistula.

302. The answer is E (all). (*Chapter 15*)   This critically ill patient is set up for an aspiration pneumonitis. The balloon of the endotracheal tube is at the vocal cords, and the stomach is massively distended in a ventilated patient who does not have a nasogastric tube. Further, no parenteral nutrition line is evident at 1 week of ventilator therapy, a reminder to ensure adequate nutrition. This routine chest radiograph is compatible with, but not diagnostic of, a right pneumothorax. This is not excluded by the lack of change in blood gases and mechanics, and so a repeat examination is indicated.

303. The answer is A (1, 2, 3). (*Chapter 47*)   Nosocomial pneumonias are difficult to diagnose. Coverage is empiric and includes coverage for gram-negative bacteria that colonize the oropharynx of hospitalized patients. Alkalinization of the stomach is reported to increase the colonization of the oropharynx with pathogenic bacteria. The protected brush continues to be studied as a diagnostic tool for accurate diagnosis of nosocomial pneumonia, but quantitative culture is required—usually 10^3 colony-forming units per milliliter (cfu/mL) is considered significant. Treatment is not necessarily altered by these data.

304. The answer is B (1, 3). (*Chapter 8*)   Calcium is of no demonstrated benefit in resuscitation except in settings of severe ionized hypocalcemia (e.g., after massive blood transfusion) or toxicity-related injury; it should not be given routinely during asystole or electromechanical dissociation. While the dose of atropine recommended by the American Heart Association is 1 mg, this is based on minimal evidence. Many experts advise giving a fully vagolytic dose (2 mg) on the grounds that there is nothing to be gained by the stepwise elimination of vagal tone. A hemodynamically unstable, obtunded patient should be intubated promptly, before respiratory failure becomes obvious. This generally can be done on clinical grounds and does not require evidence of deteriorating arterial blood gases. A fluid bolus should be part of the initial resuscitation of nearly all hypotensive patients. Even though the venous pressures were presumably elevated, additional volume administration might have increased cardiac output in this case.

305. The answer is D (4). (*Chapter 34*)   High concentrations of oxygen are mandatory in the setting of respiratory distress with cyanosis and hemodynamic instability. The reduction in F_{IO_2} risked hypoxemia with consequent injury to the heart, brain, and other organs. There was nothing to be gained from this maneuver. When respiratory failure is imminent, it is best to intubate and ventilate early, with a goal of preventing complications of frank respiratory failure such as aspiration, anoxia, and cardiac arrest. Early control of the airway and provision of ventilation may bring about stabilization of the circulation. All these factors argue for early intubation as a means of preventing ventilator dependence. Aminophylline is a weak bronchodilator and is of little utility in the acute setting. Moreover, a common side effect is hypotension, a complication that might have proved fatal in this patient. Elevated neck veins in the setting of acute hypoperfusion raise several diagnostic possibilities, including tension pneumothorax, cardiac tamponade, myocardial infarction, and pulmonary embolism. Each of these possibilities should be considered in this patient. Since tension pneumothorax is reversible and given the underlying COPD, it is particularly important to exclude this possibility.

306.   The answer is E (all).   *(Chapters 32, 74)*   Arterial carbon dioxide tension is determined by the following formula: $Pa_{CO_2} = k \times V_{CO_2} / V_T \times RR \times (1 - V_D / V_T)$, where k is a constant, V_{CO_2} is carbon dioxide production, V_T is tidal volume, RR is respiratory rate, and V_D / V_T is the ratio of dead space to tidal volume. Since the patient is paralyzed on a ventilator and no changes have been made, RR remains constant. Thus, factors that would increase V_{CO_2} or dead space would result in an increased Pa_{CO_2}. An increase in the amount of carbohydrate in the diet and fever are two etiologies of an increased V_{CO_2}. In a patient with pulmonary fibrosis and probable high airway pressures, either a further increase in airway pressure, as might occur with the onset of bronchospasm, or a lowering of pulmonary arterial perfusion, as might occur with pulmonary embolus, could result in more West's zone I lung (alveolar pressure greater than pulmonary arterial pressure) and therefore more dead space.

307–311.   The answers are 307-E, 308-B, 309-D, 310-C, 311-A.   *(Chapter 13)*   Congestive heart failure typically causes a transudative effusion with a normal pH.

Urinothorax may complicate disruption of the ureters. It is the only cause of an acidic transudative effusion.

Esophageal rupture may complicate vomiting (Boerhaave syndrome) or endoscopic procedures. The pH typically is very low, as is the glucose. A key diagnostic feature is a very high amylase, which is of salivary origin.

The effusion associated with a pulmonary embolus may be transudative, but most of these are exudative and many are bloody.

The pleural effusions associated with pancreatitis are usually exudates with moderately elevated amylases. If there is any question of the differentiation between pancreatitis and esophageal rupture, pleural fluid amylase isoenzymes may be determined. The amylase seen in effusions associated with pancreatitis is of pancreatic origin, while that seen in esophageal perforation is of salivary origin.

312–315.   The answers are 312-C, 313-B, 314-A, 315-D.   *(Chapter 15)*   Since samples are not contaminated by upper airway organisms, cultures of specimens obtained via the sterile brush technique are most useful in the diagnosis of bacterial pneumonias. Since transbronchial biopsy is the only technique that samples the lung interstitium, it has an excellent diagnostic yield in patients with lymphangitic spread of malignancy. Both the sterile brush technique and transbronchial biopsies can cause excessive bleeding in patients with clotting abnormalities. Although both transbronchial biopsy and a sterile brush can cause pneumothoraces and an open-lung biopsy is frequently preferred over transbronchial biopsy in patients on mechanical ventilation, both have been performed successfully with minimal complications.

316–319.   The answers are 316-A, 317-B, 318-C, 319-D.   *(Chapters 15, 33)*   PEEP is effective in improving oxygenation by redistributing the alveolar edema away from the alveoli and thus recruiting alveoli. When unilateral pneumonia is present, application of PEEP can redistribute blood from the uninvolved lung to the inflamed areas and thus increase the shunt fraction. In this situation, positioning the patient with the good lung down will improve V/Q matching and therefore oxygenation. In right main stem intubation, withdrawing the endotracheal tube toward the mouth will improve oxygenation. The evacuation of a pneumothorax may improve oxygenation.

320–323. **The answers are 320-A, 321-A, 322-B, 323-C.** (*Chapter 30*) Acute hypoxemic respiratory failure results when disease processes cause airspace filling or collapse (pulmonary edema, hemorrhage, pneumonia, or atelectasis). Despite the administration of high fractions of inspired oxygen, relatively small increases in Pa_{O_2} result. The administration of PEEP, however, may improve the hypoxemia seen with this disorder. Postictal pulmonary edema results in hypoxemic respiratory failure that usually improves quickly; thus, ventilatory failure rarely occurs. Acute ventilatory failure results from a diminished drive to breathe, neuromuscular weakness, or an increased mechanical load. Pa_{CO_2} rises and results in a mild hypoxemia, which is easily corrected by small increases in inspired oxygen. Polymyositis may result in myopathic weakness with resultant ventilatory failure. While eclampsia can be associated with pulmonary edema and hence acute hypoxemic respiratory failure, severe hypermagnesemia causes muscle weakness and thus ventilatory failure.

324–329. **The answers are 324-C, 325-C, 326-B, 327-C, 328-B, 329-D.** (*Chapters 30, 31, 33, 34*) Patients with heart failure, COPD exacerbations, and ARDS are all candidates for noninvasive ventilation. When airway protection cannot be assured (e.g., facial trauma and stridor, aspiration), the airway should be secured with an endotracheal tube. The patient with tuberculosis demonstrates no current need for mechanical ventilation of any variety.

330–333. **The answers are 330-D, 331-A, 332-A, 333-C.** (*Chapters 15, 47, 101*) Before surgery, one must establish whether a patient's pulmonary reserve is sufficient to tolerate surgery and whether the cause of hemoptysis is amenable to surgical correction. Patients with diffuse lung disease such as that which can occur secondary to tuberculosis, COPD, cystic fibrosis, and sarcoid frequently have inadequate pulmonary function to tolerate resection. The patient with emphysema and bronchiectasis has an FEV_1 that probably would prohibit pulmonary resection. The patient with a 2- to 3-cm mass in the right middle lobe has an FEV_1 adequate to tolerate surgical resection (predicted postoperative FEV_1 greater than 0.8 L). His $D_L CO$ is decreased but is not prohibitive. Intervention also should not be considered in patients with systemic diseases associated with hemoptysis (e.g., collagen vascular diseases). Localized diseases such as lung abscesses, tumors, pulmonary infarcts, and AV malformations can be removed surgically. Except for patients with pulmonary hemorrhage secondary to a systemic disease, bronchial artery embolization can be performed in most patients as long as the vascular anatomy allows a specific feeding vessel to be found with a low risk of spinal artery embolization.

334–335. **The answers are 334-A, 335-B.** (*Chapter 19*) Pa_{O_2} is determined by F_{IO_2}, barometric pressure, respiratory quotient, and Pa_{CO_2}. Arterial oxygen content (Ca_{O_2}) is equal to the sum of dissolved and hemoglobin-bound oxygen, or 1.39 mL O_2 × Hgb (g/dL) × Hgb saturation + (0.0031 mL O_2 / dL × mm Hg Pa_{O_2}).

336–338. **The answers are 336-B, 337-B, 338-C.** (*Chapter 15*) Bronchoalveolar lavage and transbronchial biopsy are both useful techniques in the diagnosis of pulmonary infiltrates in an immunocompromised host. Bronchoalveolar lavage can suggest a diagnosis of bacterial, fungal, mycobacterial, viral (especially CMV), and *Pneumocystis* pneumonias. Since lung tissue is obtained only with transbronchial biopsy and not with bronchoalveolar lavage, pathologic proof of tissue invasion can be demonstrated only by this method. The finding of an organism in bronchoalveolar lavage fluid does not document tissue invasion and may not correlate with true disease, especially when a fungus or CMV is noted. Bronchoalveolar lavage fluid that is positive for mycobacteria or *Pneumocystis* correlates well with true infection. Bronchoalveolar lavage, however, is a relatively low-risk procedure even in mechanically ventilated patients. The risks of transbronchial biopsy include pneumothorax and hemorrhage.

INFECTIOUS DISORDERS IN THE CRITICALLY ILL

QUESTIONS

DIRECTIONS: Each question below contains four or five suggested responses. Select the **one best** response to each question.

339. Accurate statements regarding the incidence of nosocomial infections in critically ill patients include all the following EXCEPT

(A) nosocomial infections occur twice as often in intensive care units as in general wards

(B) one-third of patients in surgical intensive care units develop infections

(C) the lowest rate of infection in intensive care units occurs in the general medical intensive care unit

(D) indwelling catheters increase the incidence of nosocomial infections

(E) infections with organisms with unusual resistance patterns occur with increased frequency in intensive care units

340. True statements regarding combination antimicrobial therapy include all the following EXCEPT

(A) it improves the outcome in polymicrobial sepsis

(B) it may prevent the emergence of antimicrobial resistance

(C) antagonistic effects are most important in normal hosts

(D) it may result in synergistic antimicrobial effects

(E) it allows a decrease in dose that may reduce toxicity

341. A 35-year-old woman with AIDS presents with fever, chills, a productive cough, and profound dyspnea. Her history is notable for multiple admissions for *Pneumocystis carinii* pneumonia (PCP) over the previous 18 months. During her most recent episode of PCP her CD4 count was found to be 70. Her antiretroviral regimen includes zidovudine (AZT), zalcitabine (ddC), and saquinavir. She takes trimethoprim-sulfamethoxazole intermittently for PCP prophylaxis. On presentation, the temperature is 38.0°C (100.4°F), pulse is 110 and regular, blood pressure is 100/70, and respiratory rate is 30 and labored. Her exam is notable for diffuse wasting, oral leukoplakia, and coarse breath sounds bilaterally. Her laboratory values are notable for WBC 3.0 and LDH 850, and her ABG reveals pH 7.48, Pa_{CO_2} 18 mm Hg, and Pa_{O_2} 50 mm Hg. Her chest x-ray is notable for diffuse bilateral interstitial infiltrates. The patient is admitted to the ICU with a presumptive diagnosis of PCP and is intubated and mechanically ventilated for acute hypoxemic respiratory failure. Which of the following statements about this patient's condition is true?

(A) With the use of combination antiretroviral therapy and the advent of protease inhibitors, the incidence of PCP is declining so that it is no longer the leading cause of ICU admission in patients with AIDS

(B) Bronchoscopy with BAL and transbronchial biopsy should be performed immediately to confirm the diagnosis of PCP

(C) The combination of diffuse interstitial infiltrates and grossly elevated LDH in patients with AIDS is essentially diagnostic of PCP, and further investigation is not warranted

(D) Treatment with trimethoprim-sulfamethoxazole (TMP-SMX) should be withheld until after diagnostic bronchoscopy has been performed

(E) Despite early institution of appropriate antibiotic and corticosteroid therapy, mortality from PCP-related acute respiratory failure approaches 50 percent

342. A 70-year-old man presents 8 months after the placement of a Dacron graft for an abdominal aortic aneurysm and complains of coffee-ground emesis and decreased urinary output. On examination he smells of alcohol and has a low-grade fever, hypotension, and abdominal tenderness. Laboratory values include a hematocrit of 20 percent and a white blood cell count of 21,000/mm^3 with a shift to the left. Nasogastric aspirate is clear but guaiac-positive. The most likely diagnosis is

(A) urosepsis
(B) hemorrhage from a duodenal ulcer
(C) hepatic abscess
(D) aortoduodenal fistula
(E) variceal hemorrhage

Questions 343–344.

A 28-year-old man is involved in a motor vehicle accident and suffers rib and femur fractures, left-sided pulmonary contusion, splenic rupture, and a closed head injury. He undergoes emergency splenectomy and stabilization of his femur. CT of the head shows a cerebral contusion with no hemorrhage or skull fracture. On the fourth hospital day he becomes febrile to 39.5°C (103.1°F) and hypotensive (90/40), and his white blood cell count rises to 25,000. He remains obtunded and mechanically ventilated.

343. The LEAST appropriate next step is to

(A) culture urine, sputum, and blood
(B) replace all intravascular catheters
(C) withhold empirical antimicrobial therapy pending the results of further tests
(D) perform diagnostic thoracentesis for a left-sided pleural effusion
(E) obtain another CT scan of the head

344. Four days later he remains febrile with no source identified. He is comatose and jaundiced. The white blood cell count is 30,000 with a marked left shift. The serum glucose has risen to 280, the creatinine is 3.2, and the bilirubin is 12.5. Serum albumin is 2.5, SGPT is 110, alkaline phosphatase is 160, and prothrombin time is normal. The most likely cause of jaundice is

(A) sepsis-related cholestasis
(B) choledocholithiasis
(C) viral hepatitis
(D) ascending cholangitis
(E) periampullary edema from pancreatitis

345. An increased risk of primary bacteremia and pyogenic infections is seen in patients with defects in humoral immunity. All the following conditions are associated with humoral immunodeficiency EXCEPT

(A) Job syndrome (hyper-IgE syndrome)
(B) multiple myeloma
(C) chronic lymphocytic leukemia
(D) protein-losing enteropathy
(E) common variable hypogammaglobulinemia

346. A 55-year-old man received a hemicolectomy for a ruptured diverticular abscess 5 days ago. He was extubated postoperatively without difficulty and was placed on broad-spectrum antibiotics. Over the past 2 days he has had recurrent fevers, abdominal pain, and distention. Today he became hypotensive and tachycardic. After 2-L fluid resuscitation, physical examination reveals a temperature of 40.5°C (104.9°F) orally, pulse 135, blood pressure 90/palpable, and respiratory rate 30. The abdomen is diffusely tender and distended. An arterial blood gas on supplemental oxygen taken before fluid resuscitation showed pH 7.29, Pa$_{CO_2}$ 28 mm Hg, and Pa$_{O_2}$ 110 mm Hg. The anion gap is 19, and the arterial lactate level is 6 mg/dL. After fluid resuscitation, the patient has good mentation and a urine output of 30 mL/h. A repeat blood gas reveals pH 7.15, Pa$_{CO_2}$ 26 mm Hg, and Pa$_{O_2}$ 65 mm Hg. The anion gap is now 26 with an arterial lactate level of 14 mg/dL. The patient is to be prepared for reexploration of the abdomen. The most effective way to control the patient's lactic acidosis is to

(A) increase supplemental oxygen until Pa$_{O_2}$ rises substantially
(B) administer three ampules of sodium bicarbonate
(C) administer six ampules of sodium bicarbonate
(D) intubate and mechanically ventilate with sedation (and muscle relaxation if necessary) to assume the work of breathing
(E) begin administering norepinephrine at 2 μg/kg/min

347. The most common presentation of infection with cytomegalovirus (CMV) in patients with a solid organ transplant is

(A) pneumonitis
(B) hepatitis
(C) pancolitis with gastrointestinal hemorrhage
(D) retinitis
(E) neutropenia and fever

348. All the following clinical data portend a poor prognosis in patients with pneumococcal pneumonia EXCEPT

(A) age greater than 70 years
(B) multilobar involvement on chest x-ray
(C) neutropenia
(D) pleural effusion
(E) hypoxemia

Questions 349–350.

349. A 64-year-old man with a history of alcoholism is found unconscious at home and is brought to the emergency room by his granddaughter. The patient had complained of left ear pain throughout the previous week, which he had treated with a home remedy of "sweet oil" instilled in the affected ear. Over the 48 hours before presentation he had been notably confused and lethargic. In the ER his temperature was 37.5°C (99°F), pulse 120, blood pressure 90/40, and respiratory rate 20. He was unresponsive to deep pain on exam but moved all his extremities. His left tympanic membrane was opaque and bulging, with purulent material noted in the external canal. His funduscopic exam was normal, and he had left periauricular and anterior cervical lymphadenopathy. The neck was supple, and the Kernig and Brudzinski signs were absent. Examination of his lungs revealed evidence of right lower lung field consolidation, and he had a III/VI crescendo-decrescendo systolic murmur on auscultation of his precordium. His WBC count was 25,000 with 35 percent band forms, and his chest x-ray confirmed a right lower lobe airspace infiltrate with air bronchograms. CT of the head revealed diffuse cerebral atrophy, and a lumbar puncture was notable for a CSF glucose of 40 mg/dL, CSF protein of 110 mg/dL, and CSF leukocyte count of 1200 cells/mL with 70 percent neutrophils. Gram stain of the CSF revealed gram-positive diplococci. All the following statements regarding this patient's illness are true EXCEPT

(A) the organism identified in this patient's CSF is the most common cause of bacterial meningitis in patients over 40 years of age
(B) alcoholics are predisposed to developing meningitis of this nature
(C) additional foci of infection, such as otitis media and pneumonia, are seen in approximately 30 percent of patients with this form of meningitis
(D) the use of a rapid CSF diagnostic test such as latex agglutination assays may aid in the diagnosis of this condition
(E) the absence of fever and signs of meningeal irritation are relatively uncommon in an elderly patient with bacterial meningitis

350. A correct statement regarding therapy in this patient is

(A) initial treatment with penicillin G is appropriate given the gram-stain results
(B) a third-generation cephalosporin should be administered because of the risk of drug resistance with this organism
(C) corticosteroids have been shown to reduce mortality in adults with bacterial meningitis
(D) 7 days of antibiotic therapy should be adequate to treat this infection effectively
(E) empiric antibiotic therapy should be withheld until the lumbar puncture is performed

351. The most significant complication of an appropriately treated retropharyngeal space infection is

(A) carotid artery perforation
(B) laryngeal edema and airway obstruction
(C) abscess rupture and aspiration
(D) basilar meningitis
(E) acute necrotizing mediastinitis

352. The agent most often responsible for acute epiglottitis in adults is

(A) influenza virus
(B) *Haemophilus influenzae*
(C) *Streptococcus pneumoniae*
(D) *Staphylococcus aureus*
(E) *Mycoplasma pneumoniae*

353. The development of necrotizing fasciitis usually is preceded by

(A) minor trauma
(B) major abdominal or thoracic surgery
(C) obstetric complications
(D) vascular injury secondary to major vascular surgery or traumatic central line placement
(E) inappropriately treated local cellulitis

354. Factors that increase the risk of urinary tract infections in the intensive care unit include all the following EXCEPT

(A) urinary tract instrumentation
(B) the use of broad-spectrum antimicrobial agents
(C) systemic infection and bacteremia
(D) elevated urine osmolarity and acidic urine pH
(E) glycosuria

355. The diagnosis of tetanus is confirmed by which of the following?

(A) Blood cultures positive for *Clostridium tetani*
(B) Tissue cultures positive for *Clostridium tetani*
(C) Elevated serum creatine phosphokinase
(D) Clinical manifestations of diffuse muscle rigidity with a history compatible with *Clostridium tetani* exposure
(E) Positive tensilon test

356. True statements regarding Rocky Mountain spotted fever (RMSF) include all the following EXCEPT

(A) the infectious agent is a rickettsial organism, *Rickettsia rickettsii*
(B) pathogenesis involves invasion of vascular endothelial cells by the infecting organism
(C) diffuse vasculitis and increased vascular permeability result from a toxin-mediated process
(D) a clinical hallmark of RMSF is the diffuse macular, maculopapular rash that most often involves the extremities, including the palms and soles
(E) treatment of RMSF includes specific antibiotic therapy with doxycycline in addition to supportive therapy for potential organ system dysfunction

357. A 52-year-old female 50-pack-year smoker with a history of bronchiectasis presents with hemoptysis of approximately 250 mL over the last 12 hours. She is a resident of northern Wisconsin and was evaluated for an infiltrate of the right upper lobe 6 months ago and treated with ampicillin. Her purified protein derivative (PPD) skin test reacted to 6 mm of induration at that time. Sputum culture did grow *Mycobacterium avium-intracellulare*. Her physician instructed her that this might not be a true infection and wanted to perform a follow-up chest x-ray and sputum culture in 1 to 2 months. However, the patient failed to follow up. Other past medical history is notable only for a transfusion given 25 years ago in association with a cesarean section. Her chest x-ray now shows a 3-cm cavitary lesion in the apical segment of the right upper lobe and surrounding fibronodular-type infiltrate. Sputum smear reveals numerous acid-fast bacilli. Which of the following statements is correct regarding this patient's condition?

(A) This condition meets the Centers for Disease Control (CDC) criteria for the acquired immunodeficiency syndrome (AIDS)
(B) *Mycobacterium avium-intracellulare* is not associated with this particular presentation
(C) Surgical therapy is considered in this disease only when there is life-threatening hemoptysis that exceeds 600 mL over 24 hours
(D) The organism likely to be responsible shows a high degree of drug resistance in vitro
(E) Isoniazid (INH) and rifampin would be the chemotherapeutic regimen of choice

358. Manifestations of severe falciparum malaria include all the following EXCEPT

(A) metabolic alkalosis
(B) pulmonary edema
(C) hypoglycemia
(D) hemoglobinuria
(E) splenic rupture

359. All the following statements regarding toxic-shock syndrome are true EXCEPT

(A) risk factors include surgical or traumatic damage to skin, deep tissue infection with *S. aureus,* and insertion of a foreign body
(B) the syndrome is caused by circulating *S. aureus* toxin, not circulating bacteria
(C) erythroderma generally spares mucous membranes
(D) hypocalcemia and hypophosphatemia are common
(E) it may result in CSF pleocytosis

DIRECTIONS: Each question below contains four suggested responses of which **one or more** is correct. Select

A	if	**1, 2, and 3**	are correct
B	if	**1 and 3**	are correct
C	if	**2 and 4**	are correct
D	if	**4**	is correct
E	if	**1, 2, 3, and 4**	are correct

360. A 60-year-old man with COPD is intubated for respiratory failure. On day 5, he fails extubation and a new infiltrate is noted on chest x-ray. Important findings to corroborate the empirical diagnosis of new bacterial pneumonia include

(1) increased white blood cells and bacteria in sputum
(2) increased alveolar-arterial (A-a) gradient
(3) leukocytosis
(4) positive sputum culture

361. True statements concerning infection in neutropenic hosts include

(1) the usual signs and symptoms of infection may be absent
(2) anaerobes are an important cause of infection
(3) mortality is high with *Pseudomonas* infection
(4) gram-negative bacilli usually enter into the blood via the urinary tract

362. Conditions that may result in a hemodynamic profile akin to that of sepsis with a high output include

(1) arteriovenous fistula
(2) advanced liver failure
(3) infusion of interleukin-2 (IL-2)
(4) Paget's disease of bone

363. Early bronchoscopic transbronchial biopsy may be useful in the diagnosis of which of the following pneumonias seen in the population of immunocompromised patients?

(1) *Mycobacterium tuberculosis*
(2) Cytomegalovirus (CMV)
(3) *Pneumocystis carinii*
(4) *Pseudomonas aeruginosa*

364. A 23-year-old homosexual man is known to be HIV-seropositive, and his CD4 lymphocyte count is now 210/mm^3. He presents with 2 days of shortness of breath and cough but no sputum production. His chest x-ray shows diffuse patchy infiltrates. His lung examination reveals diffuse crackles. No other abnormalities are seen on careful skin examination. Infections likely to cause this presentation include

(1) *Pneumocystis carinii* pneumonia
(2) toxoplasmosis
(3) cryptococcosis
(4) herpes simplex pneumonia

365. A 24-year-old intravenous drug abuser was treated for *Pneumocystis carinii* pneumonia in another state 1 year ago. The patient now presents with lethargy, confusion, and weakness of the right upper extremity. CT of the head reveals a single mass lesion in the left cortex. Infections that commonly present in this fashion include

(1) toxoplasmosis
(2) CMV infection
(3) tuberculosis
(4) infection with varicella-zoster virus

366. Indications for cardiac valve replacement in patients with infective endocarditis include

(1) severe heart failure refractory to medical therapy
(2) fungal etiology
(3) mycotic aneurysms
(4) tricuspid valve endocarditis in intravenous drug users

367. A 33-year-old hemophiliac who is known to be HIV-positive with a history of *Pneumocystis carinii* pneumonia 3 months ago now presents with a severe headache, fever to 39.4°C (103°F), and neck pain. Physical examination discloses meningismus and photophobia, with no other neurologic abnormalities. CSF analysis reveals a normal glucose, an upper-normal level of protein, and 1 WBC/mm^3 with 98 percent lymphocytes. True statements concerning this patient's condition include

(1) the low number of WBCs and the normal glucose and protein essentially rule out the possibility of cryptococcal meningitis
(2) this could be a presentation of aseptic meningitis secondary to the HIV virus itself
(3) this is a common presentation for the progressive multifocal leukoencephalopathy of AIDS
(4) this could be consistent with CNS lymphoma, a disease well described in AIDS patients

368. Correct statements regarding herpes encephalomyelitis include

(1) profound memory loss can be a presenting symptom
(2) treatment with acyclovir is usually free of significant side effects and is approved for use during late pregnancy
(3) EEG can show signs localized to the temporal lobe
(4) CSF analysis is often hemorrhagic

Questions 369–371.

A 44-year-old man is admitted to the ICU with severe pneumonia. He notes that he has recently returned from a 10-day hunting trip to Tennessee. He noted the onset of fevers, myalgias, and headache 4 days before admission while returning home. A chest x-ray done at that time revealed a patchy infiltrate of the left lower lobe. He was treated with cephalexin, and though he was compliant with the antibiotic prescription, he failed to improve. He noted worsening dyspnea and presented to the emergency room. His physical examination is remarkable for marked distress and confusion. He is febrile, tachycardic, and tachypneic as well as mildly hypotensive. Chest examination reveals evidence of consolidation of both bases. Cardiac examination reveals flat neck veins and normal heart sounds. The abdomen is unremarkable. The admitting chest x-ray reveals dense ground-glass infiltrates in both lower lung fields. Laboratory data reveal a mild elevation in the white blood cell count; blood gases reveal hypoxemia.

369. The initial microbiologic differential diagnosis of the patient's presentation should include infection with

(1) *Rickettsia rickettsii*
(2) *Francisella tularensis*
(3) *Blastomyces dermatitidis*
(4) *Coccidioides immitis*

370. The patient is intubated for respiratory failure. The appropriate empirical antimicrobial therapy should include

(1) amphotericin B
(2) streptomycin
(3) doxycycline
(4) cefazolin

371. After intubation, a sputum sample was stained with 10% KOH and revealed yeast with broad-based buds. Likely sites of dissemination include

(1) skin
(2) kidney
(3) bone
(4) heart

372. A 37-year-old HIV-positive intravenous drug abuser presents with dizziness and fatigue. She has orthostatic changes in blood pressure and pulse but has no fever and her chest x-ray is within normal limits. Laboratory examination reveals hyperkalemia with a normal BUN and creatinine. A morning cortisol level is very low. True statements concerning this patient's presentation and evaluation include

(1) a corticotropin stimulation test would be helpful in establishing the diagnosis
(2) CMV may cause a lesion that leads to this condition
(3) mycobacterial disease in normal hosts and AIDS patients can be causative of this condition
(4) this patient most likely will go on to develop renal failure

373. A 70-year-old Mexican man is in the United States visiting for the first time and is brought to the emergency room by his family for complaints of headache and confusion. He is febrile to 38.3°C (101°F) with mild neck stiffness. The remainder of the evaluation is remarkable only for poor cognitive function without any focal neurologic deficits. His chest x-ray redemonstrates a left lower lobe infiltrate, unchanged from previous films. He has calcified hilar nodes on the left side as well. Lumbar puncture and CSF analysis are performed and reveal WBCs of 50/mm³ (85 percent lymphocytes and 10 percent neutrophils), a mildly elevated protein, and a normal glucose. Correct statements include which of the following?

(1) This presentation is inconsistent with an aseptic meningitis
(2) In the elderly, tuberculous meningitis is usually from a primary infection
(3) This presentation is inconsistent with fungal meningitis
(4) Empirical antituberculous therapy would be reasonable even in the face of a negative CSF Gram stain for acid-fast bacilli

374. True statements regarding sinusitis in a critically ill patient include which of the following?

(1) The diagnosis is readily made by physical examination
(2) Sinusitis is a relatively common cause of occult fevers in a nasally intubated patient
(3) Antibiotics directed at *Streptococcus pneumoniae* are usually effective
(4) Complications include subdural empyema, brain abscess, and sepsis

375. Complications of acute pyelonephritis include

(1) focal bacterial nephritis
(2) renal abscess
(3) perinephric abscess
(4) pyonephrosis

376. The initial management of a severe case of tetanus should focus on

(1) control of the airway and ventilation
(2) passive immunotherapy of intoxication by tetanospasmin
(3) antibiotics and consideration of further evaluation of the site of infection
(4) sedation with benzodiazepines

377. The hantavirus pulmonary syndrome (HPS) is characterized by

(1) prominent anemia secondary to pulmonary hemorrhage
(2) a mortality rate that approaches 50 percent
(3) successful therapy with intravenous amantadine
(4) pathogenesis significant for capillary leak resulting from endothelial dysfunction without permanent endothelial damage

378. A 30-year-old former native of India returns there for a short visit. One month after returning to the United States, he presents complaining of fever, chills, headache, and diarrhea. On examination he is confused and has retinal hemorrhages on funduscopic examination, dysconjugate gaze, and tender hepatosplenomegaly. Laboratory values reveal a severe anemia, elevated BUN and creatinine, and elevated liver function tests. Appropriate management would include

(1) prophylaxis against seizure with phenobarbital
(2) mannitol
(3) frequent serum glucose measurements
(4) dexamethasone

379. Potential therapies for viral hemorrhagic fevers (VHF) include

(1) amantadine
(2) ganciclovir
(3) acyclovir
(4) ribavirin

380. A 28-year-old woman is admitted to the intensive care unit with disorientation, hypotension, and fever. She was entirely well and completed walking the Appalachian Trail 1 week ago, finishing the trip in Georgia. Three days after her return home, she noted fever and headache. Two days later, nausea, vomiting, and mild abdominal pain developed. Today her family noted that she was confused and had a new rash and brought her to the hospital. Her last menstrual period was 3 weeks ago and she is not using tampons. On examination she is febrile to 40°C (104°F) orally, with a pulse of 120, respiratory rate of 28, and blood pressure of 90/40 after fluids. Her examination is unremarkable except for delirium without meningeal signs and a macular rash most prominent on the extremities and including the palms of the hands. There is no desquamation. A lumbar puncture is unremarkable. True statements concerning this problem and its management include

(1) the skin lesion described is erythema chronicum migrans (ECM)
(2) initial antibiotic therapy should include chloramphenicol or a tetracycline
(3) the start of therapy should await confirmation of the diagnosis by serologic testing for indirect immunofluorescent antibody
(4) rapid diagnosis can be made in some patients by skin biopsy

381. With regard to percutaneous abscess drainage, correct statements include which of the following?

(1) Success rates of 80 to 90 percent are typical
(2) It is a procedure that should be reserved only for an unstable patient who is unable to undergo a surgical incision and drainage
(3) Failure is often due to fistulae and premature withdrawal of the catheter
(4) The site requires more nursing care and is more prone to infection than is an open drainage site

DIRECTIONS: Each group of questions below consists of lettered headings followed by a set of numbered items. For each numbered item select the **one** lettered heading with which it is **most** closely associated. Each lettered heading may be used **once, more than once, or not at all.**

Questions 382–385.

Match each side effect with the antibiotic with which it is most likely to be associated.

(A) Ganciclovir
(B) Vancomycin
(C) Gentamicin
(D) Imipenem
(E) Piperacillin

382. Seizures

383. Neutropenia

384. Platelet defect

385. Nephrotoxicity

Questions 386–389.

Match each immunocompromised state below with the infectious agent with which it is most commonly associated.

(A) *Pseudomonas aeruginosa*
(B) *Streptococcus pneumoniae*
(C) *Mycobacterium avium* complex
(D) Cytomegalovirus
(E) *Mycoplasma pneumoniae*

386. Cyclosporine therapy for liver transplantation

387. Marrow ablative chemotherapy

388. Multiple myeloma

389. Acquired immunodeficiency syndrome (CD4 < 100)

Questions 390–392.

Choose the most appropriate empiric antibiotic regimen for each patient.

(A) Vancomycin and a third-generation cephalosporin
(B) Ampicillin and a third-generation cephalosporin
(C) Third-generation cephalosporin alone
(D) Clindamycin and cefuroxime
(E) Metronidazole, nafcillin, and a third-generation cephalosporin

390. A 32-year-old patient who has had a cadaveric renal transplant presents to the emergency room with meningismus and fever. A CSF Gram stain reveals 12 polymorphonuclear white blood cells and a single gram-positive rod.

391. A 55-year-old woman is followed for Wegener's granulomatosis. She has had fevers associated with sinusitis in the past. She remains on cyclophosphamide and prednisone therapy and presents with 2 days of fever and a hemiparesis of new onset. Head CT is delayed because of emergent trauma evaluations now in progress.

392. A trauma patient who has had a craniotomy for evacuation of an acute subdural hematoma develops lethargy and fever. An infused CT scan of the head is remarkable only for postsurgical changes. CSF examination reveals WBCs of 20/mm^3, 85 percent polymorphonuclear cells, elevated protein, and a glucose of 30 mg/dL with a serum value of 120 mg/dL.

Questions 393–399.

Match each description with the appropriate organism.

(A) *Vibrio cholerae*
(B) *Shigella dysenteriae*
(C) *Clostridium perfringens*
(D) *Salmonella typhi*
(E) *Clostridium difficile*
(F) None of the above

393. No red or white blood cells are seen on stool examination

394. This organism is part of the normal gastrointestinal flora

395. Enteritis may be associated with hemolytic-uremic syndrome

396. Enteritis may be associated with blanching erythematous macules or papules on the shoulders, thorax, or abdomen

397. Enteritis is associated with over 50 percent mortality

398. Doxycycline is considered the therapy of choice

399. Bone marrow biopsy is the most sensitive diagnostic test

Questions 400–402.

Match each patient with the most likely infectious organism.

(A) *Klebsiella pneumoniae*
(B) *Staphylococcus aureus*
(C) *Pseudomonas aeruginosa*
(D) *Haemophilus influenzae*
(E) *Streptococcus pneumoniae*

400. A 21-year-old woman with dyspnea, a hoarse voice, and stridor

401. A 47-year-old alcoholic with a necrotizing pneumonia

402. A 65-year-old ventilator-dependent man with hemoptysis and cavitary lung lesions on chest x-ray

DIRECTIONS: Each group of questions below consists of four lettered headings followed by a set of numbered items. For each numbered item select

A	if the item is associated with	(A) **only**	
B	if the item is associated with	(B) **only**	
C	if the item is associated with	**both** (A) and (B)	
D	if the item is associated with	**neither** (A) nor (B)	

Each lettered heading may be used **once, more than once, or not at all.**

Questions 403–404.

(A) Intravenous ganciclovir
(B) Intravenous acyclovir
(C) Both
(D) Neither

403. A 43-year-old homosexual man is HIV-positive and is on prophylaxis for *Pneumocystis carinii* pneumonia. He complains of increasing blurring of vision. Ophthalmologic examination reveals retinitis.

404. A 28-year-old patient with AIDS complains of painful, blistering lesions that started in one patch on one side of her thorax. The pain has increased, and she now states that these lesions cover most of her back and buttocks on the one side.

Questions 405–407.

(A) Cavernous sinus thrombosis
(B) Orbital cellulitis
(C) Both
(D) Neither

405. Fifth-nerve palsy

406. Periorbital edema

407. Bilateral involvement

Questions 408–409.

(A) Empiric intravenous amphotericin B
(B) Empiric antituberculous therapy
(C) Both
(D) Neither

408. A 55-year-old man was treated for bilateral upper lobe tuberculosis 15 years ago. He was left with cystic parenchymal changes in both upper lobes and mild obstruction on pulmonary function testing. He has felt well since then and has had stable weight, no fever or night sweats, and no pulmonary symptoms. He now presents with the sudden onset of hemoptysis of approximately 400 mL. Chest x-rays reveal cystic disease that is stable since previous studies; however, an intracavitary mass is noted in the right upper lobe. CT of the thorax demonstrates the intracavitary mass with a crescent of air between the mass and the wall of the cavity.

409. A 60-year-old woman with a history of a positive PPD, diabetes, and renal insufficiency is brought in by her family for malaise and poor appetite of approximately 2 weeks' duration. She has a low-grade fever in the emergency room, and chest x-ray reveals small nodular opacities throughout both lung fields. Blood gas reveals a mild respiratory alkalosis.

Questions 410–412.

(A) Myonecrosis (gas gangrene)
(B) Necrotizing fasciitis
(C) Both
(D) Neither

410. Normal overlying skin rules out the diagnosis

411. The setting of minor trauma or recent surgery is typical

412. Crepitation may be seen on examination

INFECTIOUS DISORDERS IN THE CRITICALLY ILL

ANSWERS

339. The answer is C. *(Chapter 40)* Nosocomial infections occur twice as often in patients in intensive care units as they do in patients in general medical and surgical wards in part because of the greater number of invasive procedures and indwelling catheters found in these patients. The highest rates occur in the surgical intensive care unit, where one-third of the patients are affected; the lowest rates occur in the coronary care unit. As a result of drug resistance transmitted by plasmids, infections with organisms with unusual resistance patterns occur at an increased frequency in patients in intensive care units.

340. The answer is C. *(Chapter 40)* Combination antimicrobial therapy has several beneficial effects, including improved outcome in polymicrobial sepsis as a result of broad-spectrum activity, the prevention of drug resistance, synergistic antimicrobial activity against a particular organism, and a reduction in drug dosage that may reduce drug-induced toxicity. Detrimental effects of antibiotic combinations include the possibility of synergistic toxicities and antagonistic activities, which are most important in situations in which host defenses are compromised. The combination of an inhibiting drug and a lethal drug often results in drug antagonism, as lethal drugs often require actively growing bacteria to have their maximal effect. In normal hosts, enough suppression of bacterial growth may occur to result in a cure; however, this may not be the case in patients with impaired host defenses.

341. The answer is E. *(Chapter 44)* Acute respiratory failure secondary to PCP remains the most common indication for ICU admission in patients with AIDS. Despite aggressive therapy with antibiotics and corticosteroids, mortality approaches 50 percent in patients with PCP-associated respiratory failure. The advent of new prophylactic regimens may prolong survival; however, these regimens have not been shown to reduce the incidence of PCP-induced respiratory failure significantly. The diagnosis of PCP is best achieved with bronchoscopy and BAL. The sensitivity of BAL for the diagnosis of PCP is approximately 95 percent. Given the diagnostic reliability of BAL and the inherent risks of transbronchial biopsy, biopsy (including open-lung biopsy) should be reserved for patients with a high suspicion for PCP and negative BAL. Routine laboratory evaluations may aid in the diagnosis of PCP but should not be used for a definitive diagnosis. The appearance on chest radiograms is quite variable in patients with PCP, ranging from a normal chest x-ray to focal infiltrates with air bronchograms to a diffuse interstitial pattern. The presence of an elevated LDH, while common in PCP, is not specific for this diagnosis. Finally, empiric therapy for PCP should be administered immediately upon suspicion of PCP. Delays in therapy are related to increases in mortality and do not significantly improve the yield of BAL.

342. The answer is D. *(Chapter 45)* The patient has signs and symptoms of both infection and upper gastrointestinal bleeding. Fever and increased WBCs in a patient with a synthetic graft warrant consideration of the graft as a source of the infection. Infection of an intraabdominal graft may present with fever, abdominal tenderness, and ureteral obstruction or hydronephrosis. An aortoduodenal fistula may develop between an infected aortic graft and the duodenum and present with hematemesis or circulatory collapse. Urosepsis and hepatic abscess usually do not result in upper gastrointestinal bleeding, and duodenal ulcers and variceal hemorrhage usually do not present with infection.

343. **The answer is C.** *(Chapter 41)* This patient is likely to be septic. Potential sources include the lungs, urine, sinuses, abdomen, wounds, and intravascular catheters. Broad culturing is indicated as a guide to antimicrobial therapy. However, given the high likelihood of serious infection (based on hemodynamic manifestations and a high white blood cell count) and the additional risk of being newly asplenic, it is a serious error to withhold empiric antibiotics. Lines should be changed and their tips should be cultured. While CT of the head might not be necessary, it could reveal sinusitis related to the endotracheal (and nasogastric) tube and might therefore contribute to management.

344. **The answer is A.** *(Chapter 41)* Nonobstructive cholestasis is a common accompaniment of sepsis. The cause is uncertain, but the phenomenon can be reproduced in animals with endotoxin infusion. A similar cholestasis is seen in humans who are treated with interleukin-2. While gallstones, pancreatitis, viral hepatitis, cholangitis, and operative injury to the biliary system are possible, they are less likely in this patient.

345. **The answer is A.** *(Chapter 41)* Job syndrome (hyper-IgE syndrome) is an inherited disorder characterized by abnormal neutrophil and monocyte chemotaxis. An increased incidence of serious infection is related to altered neutrophil chemotaxis and function rather than being a result of altered immunoglobulin function. Each of the other conditions is associated with hypogammaglobulinemia and an increased risk of infection, especially with *Pneumococcus* and *Haemophilus influenzae.*

346. **The answer is D.** *(Chapter 42)* The patient is in septic shock, with an intraabdominal source most likely. Assumption of the work of breathing in this setting is likely to reduce lactate production by the respiratory muscles and is the most efficacious means of controlling the acidosis acutely, particularly in view of the imminent reexploration of the abdomen. The fall in arterial Pa_{O_2} may well be related to the onset of low-pressure pulmonary edema consequent to volume resuscitation. Nonetheless, increasing the arterial oxygen tension is not likely to substantially alter oxygen delivery to peripheral tissues. Bicarbonate administration may raise serum pH but will increase Pa_{CO_2} or require a greater minute ventilation to maintain a constant Pa_{CO_2} and may actually increase lactate production. High doses of catecholamines may worsen splanchnic perfusion and are not warranted in view of the acceptable blood pressure and evidence of adequate renal and central nervous system perfusion.

347. **The answer is E.** *(Chapter 43)* CMV infection may manifest itself by all the listed conditions; however, neutropenia and fever without other clinical manifestations are probably the most common.

348. **The answer is D.** *(Chapter 47)* The mortality from pneumococcal pneumonia is in excess of 25 percent in patients over age 70. Multilobar involvement and hypoxemia are indicators of extensive disease. Neutropenia also carries a poor prognosis in that it suggests that overwhelming infection has suppressed bone marrow function or that underlying nutritional deficiencies may prevent an adequate bone marrow response. The development of pleural effusion in patients with pneumococcal pneumonia does require evaluation for the development of empyema, but it is common and does not suggest a poorer prognosis.

349. **The answer is E.** *(Chapter 48)* The clinical and laboratory data suggest a diagnosis of pneumococcal meningitis. Pneumococcal meningitis is the most common cause of bacterial meningitis in adults over age 40 and frequently is associated with distant foci of pneumococcal infection such as otitis media, sinusitis, endocarditis, and pneumonia. Severe pneumococcal infection is seen more frequently in patients with predisposing

conditions such as splenectomy, multiple myeloma, and alcoholism. Latex agglutination testing of the CSF should be considered in all patients suspected of having bacterial meningitis. Bacterial meningitis in the elderly is often difficult to diagnose, as these patients may present without fever, meningismus, or focal neurologic changes. Altered mental status may be the only presenting sign, and thus meningitis should be considered in all elderly patients with unexplained changes in mental status.

350.　The answer is B.　*(Chapter 48)*　Although many pneumococcal isolates may be sensitive to penicillin, the incidence of penicillin-resistant pneumococcus is rising rapidly. Elderly patients with severe pneumococcal infection should be treated with a third-generation cephalosporin pending the results of sensitivity testing. While corticosteroids have been shown to improve survival in children with *H. influenzae* type b meningitis, the widespread use of steroids in adults has not been validated. Patients with severe bacterial meningitis should be treated with a minimum of 10 to 14 days of IV antibiotics as indicated by the severity of illness and the response to antibiotic therapy. While antibiotic therapy may sterilize the CSF of patients with meningitis, empirical antibiotic therapy should be administered immediately, given the dangers of delayed therapy.

351.　The answer is E.　*(Chapter 50)*　Involvement of the carotid artery or meninges from the retropharyngeal space is rare. Laryngeal edema is obviously of concern and requires prompt evaluation and therapy but is readily dealt with by intubation or tracheostomy. Abscess rupture is also of significant concern because of the risk of aspiration of pus; however, prompt surgical drainage should prevent this problem. Necrotizing mediastinitis often presents as a catastrophic complication, such as pericardial tamponade. It carries a high mortality (approximately 25 percent), even with appropriate surgical and antimicrobial therapy.

352.　The answer is B.　*(Chapter 50)*　*Haemophilus influenzae* is recovered from blood in the majority of children with acute epiglottitis. It is also the most common organism among adults, although culture diagnosis is less common. *Streptococcus pneumoniae* and *Staphylococcus aureus* have also been reported to cause epiglottitis. The influenza virus and *Mycoplasma pneumoniae* are causes of laryngotracheobronchitis.

353.　The answer is A.　*(Chapter 51)*　Necrotizing fasciitis is a relatively uncommon but severe infection involving the subcutaneous tissue and deep fascia. The infection is characterized by extensive epidermal undermining, with sparing of the overlying skin until late in the course of infection. Approximately 80 percent of reported cases are preceded by minor trauma, with operative wounds and decubitus ulcers accounting for the remaining cases.

354.　The answer is D.　*(Chapter 52)*　The development of UTIs is a common sequela of critical illness. The use of bladder catheterization in the ICU increases the risk of UTI by 5 percent with each day the catheter is in place. Widespread antibiotic use diminishes the presence of protective host flora, leading to an increased risk of UTI. Increases in bacteremia and systemic infection significantly increase the risk of UTI development via hematogenous routes. Finally, glycosuria resulting from hyperglycemic conditions and the complications of critical illness encourage the growth of bacteria in the urinary tract. Increased urine osmolarity and decreased urine pH may be seen in the intensive care setting; however, these conditions diminish the growth of bacteria in the urine and consequently diminish the incidence of UTIs.

355.　The answer is D.　*(Chapter 55)*　The diagnosis of tetanus is made on clinical grounds alone. Evidence of diffuse muscle rigidity in light of a history of potential *C. tetani* exposure is sufficient to initiate therapy for tetanus. The use of cultures to diagnose tetanus is unnecessary and may potentially delay therapy. Tissue cultures are positive in less than 50 percent of cases and rarely are positive in blood cultures because of the non-invasive nature of the infection. While CPK levels may be elevated in tetanus, this finding is neither sensitive nor specific for this disease. The tensilon test is useful in diagnosing myasthenia gravis, not tetanus.

356.   The answer is C.   *(Chapter 41)*   Rocky Mountain spotted fever is the most prevalent rickettsial infection in the United States. It is caused by the transmission of *Rickettsia rickettsii* through the bite of the dog tick, *Dermacentor variabilis.* Pathogenesis involves rickettsial invasion of the vascular endothelial cells, leading to a vasculitis with increased vascular permeability involving a multiorgan distribution. The presence of a diffuse macular or maculopapular rash is a hallmark of RMSF. The rash usually occurs within 3 to 6 days of the onset of illness and primarily involves the extremities, including the palms of the hands and the soles of the feet. Manifestations of *R. rickettsii* invasion do not involve toxin-mediated injury.

357.   The answer is D.   *(Chapter 47)*   *Mycobacterium avium-intracellulare* is associated with progressive parenchymal disease in nonimmunosuppressed hosts. Surgical therapy is considered in these patients when the disease is localized—independent of whether there is massive hemoptysis. In vitro testing discloses multiple drug resistance. Therapy is almost always initiated with three or more drugs.

358.   The answer is A.   *(Chapter 54)*   Falciparum malaria is potentially life-threatening. Severe disease is associated with coma, anemia, renal and hepatic dysfunction, pulmonary edema, hypoglycemia, shock, seizures, lactic acidosis, hemoglobinuria, and splenic rupture. Metabolic alkalosis is not characteristic of malarial infections.

359.   The answer is C.   *(Chapter 41)*   Toxic-shock syndrome is caused by circulating *S. aureus* toxin. The onset may be fulminant even when the site of infection does not appear inflamed. Clinical manifestations include fever, headache, nausea, vomiting, myalgias, diarrhea, generalized erythroderma of skin and mucous membranes, conjunctival injections, tachycardia, and shock. Hypocalcemia and hypophosphatemia are particularly common.

360.   The answer is A (1, 2, 3).   *(Chapter 40)*   New pulmonary infiltrates are common in patients on the ventilator and should not automatically be attributed to pneumonia unless the following criteria are met: new fever, increased white blood cells and bacteria on Gram stain of a deep sputum specimen (< 10 epithelial cells per high-power field), increased A-a gradient, and leukocytosis. Patients on the ventilator usually are colonized with multiple organisms, making sputum cultures of minimal value in the treatment of nosocomial bacterial pneumonia.

361.   The answer is B (1, 3).   *(Chapter 40)*   Neutropenic patients are at increased risk of bacterial infection. While they usually develop fever, typical signs and symptoms of infection may be absent. The mortality is high in patients with *Pseudomonas aeruginosa,* especially when appropriate antibiotic therapy is not begun within 4 hours. Anaerobes are rarely of concern in patients with neutropenia. The gastrointestinal tract is the usual point of entry into the blood for gram-negative bacilli.

362.   The answer is E (all).   *(Chapter 42)*   All the conditions listed are characterized by a hemodynamic profile of high flow, low systemic vascular resistance, and, in the extreme, evidence of hypoperfusion. Arteriovenous fistula and Paget's disease are felt to represent instances of increased flow through arteriovenous anastomoses. Hemodynamic changes in advanced liver disease and after the infusion of IL-2 may have pathogenic mechanisms similar to the interaction between microbe and host cytokine that characterizes septic shock.

363. **The answer is A (1, 2, 3).** *(Chapter 43)* Transbronchial biopsy may be useful in the diagnosis of pneumonia caused by *M. tuberculosis,* CMV, and *Pneumocystis.* Bronchoscopy may be useful in the diagnosis of pneumonia caused by *Pseudomonas* only if quantitative cultures of lavage fluid or protected brush specimens are done. Biopsy alone is rarely diagnostic of the specific organism causing bacterial pneumonia.

364. **The answer is B (1, 3).** *(Chapter 44)* *Pneumocystis carinii* pneumonia is the most common cause of respiratory failure in AIDS patients and presents with a diffuse pulmonary infiltrate, though disseminated fungal infections and tuberculosis also may present this way. Toxoplasmosis does not cause this presentation, although it is a well-known pathogen in AIDS patients. Herpes simplex infection almost always presents with skin or mucous membrane disease before a diffuse pneumonia is present.

365. **The answer is B (1, 3).** *(Chapter 44)* Focal CNS lesions of this type are commonly caused by toxoplasmosis and tuberculosis in patients with AIDS. CMV, herpes simplex virus, and varicella-zoster virus commonly cause diffuse encephalitis.

366. **The answer is A (1, 2, 3).** *(Chapter 45)* Successful treatment of patients with infective endocarditis is greatly influenced by the pathogenicity of the infecting organism, the location of the infecting valve, and the presence or absence of complications. Determining when valve replacement is indicated is essential to successful management of endocarditis. The presence of severe heart failure that is refractory to aggressive medical management is an indication for urgent valve replacement. Additional indications for valve replacement include the identification of organisms that are relatively refractory to antimicrobial therapy and the presence of catastrophic embolic phenomena. Fungal endocarditis remains an indication for valve replacement because of the relative difficulty of clearing fungal organisms with antifungal agents alone. Mycotic aneurysms increase the likelihood of severe CNS hemorrhage and/or infection and thus require urgent attention. The risk of recurrent prosthetic valve infection in patients with tricuspid valve endocarditis resulting from intravenous drug use argues against routine valve replacement.

367. **The answer is C (2, 4).** *(Chapter 44)* It is important to realize that cryptococcal meningitis can present with a nearly normal CSF analysis and therefore that CSF cryptococcal antigen and India ink smear are important studies to rule out the presence of cryptococcus. HIV and HSV have been reported to cause aseptic meningitis, and CNS lymphoma can present with a normal CSF analysis even in the presence of meningeal involvement.

368. **The answer is E (all).** *(Chapter 49)* Herpes encephalomyelitis classically involves the temporal lobes with associated memory loss and is a hemorrhagic encephalomyelitis. Acyclovir is the drug of choice, and the only side effects reported with any regularity are neuropsychiatric abnormalities.

369. **The answer is A (1, 2, 3).** *(Chapter 47)* The differential diagnosis of a febrile illness contracted after outdoor activity is broad and includes the routine causes of febrile illness. In addition, consideration has to be given to infections that require exposure to a vector such as a tick and to unusual fungal infections. Infection with *R. rickettsii* and *F. tularensis* occurs after exposure to infected ticks, although *F. tularensis* also may be contracted from infected animals. *B. dermatitidis* infection probably requires inhalation of infected soil, although its mode of transmission is not clear. *C. immitis* also may present as an overwhelming illness in certain immunocompromised groups; however, it is not endemic to the area in which this patient had traveled but rather to the southwestern United States.

370. **The answer is A (1, 2, 3).** *(Chapter 47)* The antibiotic of choice for tularemia is streptomycin. Amphotericin B is the drug of choice for overwhelming blastomycosis. Therapy for Rocky Mountain spotted fever should include doxycycline or chloramphenicol. There is little role for cefazolin in this setting.

371.   **The answer is B (1, 3).** *(Chapter 47)*   Disseminated blastomycosis most commonly affects the skin and bone. Other areas of involvement include the meninges and the prostate.

372.   **The answer is A (1, 2, 3).** *(Chapter 44)*   This patient has a presentation and laboratory evaluation consistent with adrenal insufficiency. Adrenalitis has been reported with CMV and mycobacterial diseases in AIDS patients, and tuberculosis is a cause of adrenal insufficiency even in normal hosts. There is no association of adrenal insufficiency with renal failure in AIDS.

373.   **The answer is D (4).** *(Chapter 48)*   This presentation is consistent with aseptic, bacterial, tuberculous, or fungal meningitis. In this instance, empirical treatment for bacterial and tuberculous meningitis is reasonable. Acid-fast bacilli usually are not seen in tuberculous meningitis. The chest x-ray findings and the high prevalence of tuberculous in the patient's country strongly support the initiation of antituberculous therapy. Tuberculous meningitis can be primary in immunosuppressed patients and young children but usually arises from reactivation of a parameningeal focus or another site in adults.

374.   **The answer is C (2, 4).** *(Chapter 50)*   Sinusitis may complicate critical illness, particularly in patients with nasal intubations (for nasotracheal or nasogastric tubes). It is usually clinically silent, and the diagnosis frequently requires plain films or CT of the sinuses. The infection is usually polymicrobial, and antibiotics are directed at both gram-positive and gram-negative organisms. The sequelae of untreated infection include intracranial extension and sepsis.

375.   **The answer is E (all).** *(Chapter 52)*   A patient with acute pyelonephritis should improve within 72 hours of appropriate antimicrobial therapy. If the patient fails to improve or deteriorates, it is likely that a complication such as acute focal bacterial nephritis (a renal mass resulting from focal parenchymal infection without pus), renal abscess, perinephric abscess (pus collection between the kidney and Gerota's fascia), or pyonephrosis (pus in the collecting system with obstruction) has occurred.

376.   **The answer is E (all).** *(Chapter 55)*   Tetanus is caused by intoxication with tetanospasmin, the neurotoxin produced by *Clostridium tetani*. The bacteria are obligate anaerobes that thrive in devitalized tissue. *C. tetani* is extremely sensitive to penicillin, and this agent should be given to all patients with tetanus (metronidazole may be used in patients allergic to penicillin). Furthermore, a careful search for dead tissue should be made if the source of the infection is not obvious. Tetanospasmin is released into the tissues when autolysis of the bacteria occurs. It is then taken up by motor neurons and transported to the central nervous system. Before its uptake by the motor neuron, tetanospasmin may be neutralized by specific antibodies (tetanus immune globulin). Once it is taken up by the motor neuron, the toxin is no longer available for neutralization. Therefore, early administration of tetanus immune globulin is key to reducing the degree of intoxication. Once it is in the central nervous system, tetanospasmin acts to block the actions of inhibitory neurons on motor neurons. This results in the protracted spasms characteristic of the disease. Benzodiazepines, through their interactions with the γ-aminobutyric acid receptor complex, act to inhibit motor neuron activity and so reduce the spasms. Protracted spasms of the diaphragm and chest wall may impair ventilation, and spasm of the laryngeal muscles may cause upper airway obstruction. Furthermore, therapy with benzodiazepines for muscle spasm may cause central nervous system respiratory depression. Any patient with tetanus should be followed in the intensive care unit for evidence of inadequate ventilation. In patients with protracted spasms or sedation-related hypoventilation, elective endotracheal intubation should be performed. Because of the risk of laryngeal muscle spasm, physicians capable of performing a cricothyroidotomy or tracheostomy should be in attendance during the intubation.

377. The answer is C (2, 4). *(Chapter 56)*   Hantaviruses are natural parasites that have been implicated in the pathogenesis of viral hemorrhagic fevers. The hantavirus pulmonary syndrome (HPS) is characterized by a predominance of fever, shock, and pulmonary symptoms primarily from pulmonary edema. The pathologic lesions seen in HPS are most compatible with endothelial dysfunction leading to capillary leak. Permanent endothelial damage is not seen in HPS; thus, recovery in survivors is generally rapid and occurs without persistent sequelae. Despite the transient nature of the endothelial changes, the mortality rate of HPS approaches 50 percent. Anemia is not a common finding in HPS. In fact, an elevated hematocrit is generally seen owing to the high incidence of capillary leak with resultant hemoconcentration. Ribavirin is the recommended therapy for HPS, although data documenting its efficacy are lacking.

378. The answer is B (1, 3). *(Chapter 54)*   The patient has malaria, with evidence of cerebral involvement, from infection with *Plasmodium falciparum*. This diagnosis should be considered in any febrile patient with a history of travel to an endemic area. Most patients present with symptoms within 1 month of leaving the endemic area and may complain of fever, chills, headache, lethargy, backache, myalgias, vomiting, and diarrhea. Physical examination may reveal anemia, jaundice, and tender hepatosplenomegaly. Renal and hepatic dysfunction, hypoglycemia, and pulmonary edema are all complications of falciparum malaria. Cerebral malaria presents with impaired consciousness progressing to coma, convulsions, dysconjugate gaze, and extensor posturing. Retinal hemorrhages indicate impending coma. The diagnosis is made by observation of parasites in the blood smear. Management consists of appropriate chemotherapy and supportive care, which includes monitoring for hypoglycemia and treatment of hyperpyrexia. In patients with cerebral malaria, prophylaxis against seizures with phenobarbital is recommended; however, dexamethasone and mannitol have not been shown to be of proven benefit.

379. The answer is D (4). *(Chapter 56)*   At present, the only effective antiviral agent identified is ribavirin. Amantadine, acyclovir, and ganciclovir have not been shown to be clinically effective.

380. The answer is C (2, 4). *(Chapter 41)*   The case description is typical of Rocky Mountain spotted fever, a rickettsial illness transmitted by ticks. Most cases are not encountered in the American west but in the southeast, including North Carolina and Georgia. The initial febrile illness may be followed by an aggressive vasculitic phase with multiorgan failure. Appropriate antibiotic therapy consists of either chloramphenicol or a long-acting tetracycline such as doxycycline. Therapy should be started promptly and not delayed until serologic testing has been performed. Biopsy of skin lesions with staining of the tissue with an immunofluorescent antibody specific for the spotted-fever group of rickettsiae can provide a rapid diagnosis when the test is positive. Erythema chronicum migrans is a rash typical of another tick-borne illness, Lyme disease.

381. The answer is B (1, 3). *(Chapter 97)*   Percutaneous abscess drainage is a significant advance for effective drainage of abscess fluid, with a high reported success rate. Nursing care tends to be less involved than that required after open drainage procedures. Failure is often due to failure to recognize fistulae, noncommunicating adjacent fluid collections, and premature withdrawal of the catheter before definitive drainage has been documented.

382–385. The answers are 382-D, 383-A, 384-E, 385-C. *(Chapter 40)*   Imipenem is a β-lactam antibiotic with a wide range of antimicrobial activity. Mild renal failure and elevated liver enzymes are reported side effects, but of greatest concern is the association of this drug with seizures. Most often seizures occur in patients with renal failure or preexisting seizure disorders.

   The major clinical indication for ganciclovir is in the treatment of cytomegalovirus infections. Its primary toxic effects involve rapidly proliferating tissues such as the bone marrow, gonads, and gastrointestinal tract. The most common and significant side effects seen with ganciclovir therapy are bone marrow suppression and neutropenia.

Piperacillin is an antipseudomonal penicillin that can cause a qualitative platelet defect and impaired hemostasis. Piperacillin blocks ADP-stimulated platelet aggregation.

The aminoglycosides, including gentamicin, are the antibiotics most often associated with renal failure in clinical practice. The nephrotoxicity is dose-related and more often occurs in the elderly and those with volume contraction, preexisting renal disease, or concurrent administration of other nephrotoxic drugs. Vancomycin may contribute to existing renal dysfunction but is a relatively uncommon direct cause of renal failure.

386–389.   The answers are 386-D, 387-A, 388-B, 389-C.   *(Chapter 43)*   The immunosuppressive effects of cyclosporine are seen primarily in the inhibition of cytotoxic T lymphocytes. While the beneficial effects of T-cell suppression include preventing rejection of solid organ transplants, the harmful side effects of immunosuppression include increased susceptibility to devastating viral infections. Cytomegalovirus is of particular concern in a transplant recipient who is receiving cyclosporine.

Marrow ablative chemotherapy can result in profound, prolonged neutropenia. Severe neutropenia is associated with a substantial increase in life-threatening bacterial infections. In particular, gram-negative bacteremia including *Pseudomonas aeruginosa* is of primary concern in a febrile neutropenic patient.

Patients with multiple myeloma may develop hypogammaglobulinemia, which predisposes them to infection with encapsulated organisms, including *S. pneumoniae* and *H. influenzae.*

Infection with the human immunodeficiency virus (HIV) leading to the acquired immunodeficiency syndrome (AIDS) produces a spectrum of immune defects. Patients with AIDS are predisposed to bacterial, fungal, protozoal, and mycobacterial infections. Increasingly, infections with mycobacterial organisms have been associated with diminished CD4 lymphocyte counts. While *M. tuberculosis* is found with increased frequency in HIV patients at most stages of disease, *M. avium* complex is seen predominantly with CD4 counts less than 100.

390–392.   The answers are 390-B, 391-E, 392-A.   *(Chapter 48)*   The Gram stain in the transplant patient is suggestive of *Listeria monocytogenes.* Ampicillin and penicillin G are active against *Listeria,* and one should be included in the empirical therapy. Third-generation cephalosporins do not have activity against *Listeria* but would have activity against gram-negative organisms. The antibiotic coverage can be narrowed later according to culture results.

The 55-year-old woman has a history suggestive of brain abscess. Such abscesses are often polymicrobial and include anaerobic organisms. Clindamycin has significant activity against anaerobes but does not penetrate brain abscesses well.

The evaluation of the trauma patient suggests postneurosurgical meningitis. Staphylococci and gram-negative organisms need to be covered empirically, and the regimen can be adjusted according to culture results.

393–399.   The answers are 393-A, 394-E, 395-B, 396-D, 397-C, 398-A, 399-D.   *(Chapter 53)* The organisms that cause noninflammatory diarrhea—which include *Vibrio cholerae,* enterotoxigenic *E. coli, Aeromonas hydrophilia,* rotavirus, and the Norwalk agent—do not disrupt the intestinal epithelium and therefore are not associated with red or white blood cells on stool examination. Doxycycline is the antibiotic of choice for patients with cholera.

Pseudomembranous colitis results from the suppression of the normal colonic bacterial flora by antibiotics and results in overgrowth of *Clostridium difficile* which is part of the normal gastrointestinal flora. Except for vancomycin, virtually all antibiotics can cause this disease, the most common being clindamycin, ampicillin, and the cephalosporins.

Patients with severe colitis caused by *Shigella dysenteriae* 1 or *E. coli* 0157:H7 have developed hemolytic-uremic syndrome. Treatment of uncomplicated dysentery with trimethoprim-sulfamethoxazole and treatment of ampicillin-resistant infections with ampicillin have been associated with this complication. Although fatalities have been reported from this complication, the majority of these patients have reversible renal failure and recover completely.

Patients with enteric fever from *Salmonella typhi* have abdominal pain in 50 percent of cases; diarrhea occurs in about one-third. The diarrhea consists of either stools or semisolid stools described as "pea soup." Melena occurs less commonly. Rose spots occur in more than half of light-skinned persons but often are not visible in dark-skinned patients. They fade quickly after a few days of treatment. The preferred method of diagnosis is isolation of *S. typhi* from a blood culture. The blood culture is positive in most patients during the first 2 weeks of illness. Urine and stool cultures are positive less frequently but should be taken to increase the diagnostic yield. The bone marrow culture is the most sensitive test—positive in nearly 90 percent of cases.

Necrotizing enteritis is an acute and often fatal complication of infectious diarrhea and is due most commonly to *C. perfringens*. It usually occurs in children in developing countries. Regardless of whether medical or surgical treatment is employed, mortality exceeds 50 percent.

400–402.   The answers are 400-D, 401-A, 402-B.   *(Chapter 47)*   The woman in question has acute epiglottitis, most commonly caused by *Haemophilus influenza*.

Klebsiella pneumoniae often colonizes the oropharynx of alcoholics. The organism is aspirated and may cause a severe necrotizing pneumonia.

Chronic ventilator-dependent patients are predisposed to colonization and infection with *Staphylococcus aureus*. Furthermore, evidence of cavitary chest lesions and hemoptysis should raise suspicion of a necrotizing pneumonia caused by *S. aureus*.

403–404.   The answers are 403-A, 404-B.   *(Chapter 44)*   The findings in the 43-year-old man are highly suggestive of CMV retinitis, which can lead to blindness. Ganciclovir is indicated for CMV retinitis. Its administration is limited mainly by bone marrow suppression. CMV can also cause encephalitis, enterocolitis, and pneumonitis in these patients.

405–407.   The answers are 405-A, 406-C, 407-A.   *(Chapter 45)*   Cavernous sinus thrombosis results from direct spread of bacteria from a contiguous source of infection such as facial cellulitis, middle-ear infection, or peritonsillar abscess. Patients usually present with external ophthalmoplegia, decreased sensation around the eye, periorbital edema, and chemosis. It can be hard to distinguish this from orbital cellulitis initially. Clues to cavernous sinus thrombosis include fifth-nerve palsy, bilateral involvement, a fixed and dilated pupil, and meningitis.

408–409.   The answers are 408-D, 409-B.   *(Chapter 47)*   The man's presentation is classic for an intracavitary mycetoma or aspergilloma. Patients with chronic cystic disease are at risk for the development of this condition. This infection is not invasive per se, and intravenous amphotericin B is not helpful. Bronchial artery embolization can be considered, and if hemoptysis is massive, many recommend surgery, although many postoperative complications are reported in this patient group. Recurrent tuberculosis is a very remote possibility.

This elderly woman presents with nonspecific symptoms but with risk factors and a chest x-ray that are suggestive of miliary tuberculosis. Empirical antituberculous therapy and the initiation of diagnostic studies are warranted. Fungal disease can occasionally present in this manner, but therapy should be withheld until diagnostic studies have been performed or until the patient deteriorates despite therapy for miliary tuberculosis.

410–412.   The answers are 410-D, 411-C, 412-C.   *(Chapter 51)*   Both of these deep infections may occur with minimal or no skin manifestations. They typically occur in the setting of trauma and may result in crepitation. In necrotizing fasciitis, infection spreads rapidly along fascial planes and extensively undermines apparently normal skin. Eventually, however, thrombotic venous occlusion leads to widespread skin necrosis.

The clinical appearance of myonecrosis may be similar, with the distinction made during operative exploration. Bacterial myonecrosis is characterized by a "cooked" appearance of the muscle. Antibiotic therapy and immediate surgical intervention are crucial in both conditions.

NEUROPSYCHIATRIC DISORDERS IN THE CRITICALLY ILL

QUESTIONS

DIRECTIONS: Each question below contains four or five suggested responses. Select the **one best** response to each question.

413. A 52-year-old alcoholic is admitted to the ICU after an episode of hematemesis. On admission he is alert and oriented, but within 2 hours he becomes progressively confused and disoriented. He is observed getting out of bed and walking to the bedside sink with an ataxic gait. After he is placed on the bed, physical examination reveals a heart rate of 120 beats per minute, blood pressure of 180/100 mm Hg, and a respiratory rate of 22 breaths per minute. The patient is diaphoretic. Cardiac, lung, and abdominal examinations are unremarkable. Neurologic examination reveals ophthalmoplegia but no other focal findings. You should emergently

(A) give the patient 1 mg midazolam (Versed) intravenously
(B) give the patient 2 mg haloperidol intravenously
(C) give the patient thiamine
(D) put the patient in four-point restraints

414. In addition to calcium channel blockers, therapy for vasospasm after a subarachnoid hemorrhage should include

(A) diuresis
(B) nitroprusside
(C) hypervolemic/hypertensive therapy
(D) angiotensin-converting enzyme inhibitors

415. The most sensitive indicator of a subarachnoid hemorrhage is

(A) clinical history
(B) neurologic exam
(C) infused head CT
(D) lumbar puncture

416. In the ICU, Doppler studies of carotid arteries are not useful in differentiating cardioembolic from atherosclerotic causes of brain infarction because

(A) of the high incidence of asymptomatic atherosclerosis and the inconsistent relationship between the degree of atherosclerotic disease and consequent brain infarction
(B) the technology is not available in the ICU
(C) of high false-negative rates
(D) of low false-positive rates

417. A 38-year-old man with an unremarkable past medical history presents after the acute onset of severe headache and coma. The most probable cause of this patient's neurologic event is

(A) embolic stroke
(B) intracerebral hemorrhage
(C) seizure
(D) subarachnoid hemorrhage

418. The following statements regarding tissue plasminogen activator (t-PA) for acute ischemic stroke are true EXCEPT

(A) treatment with t-PA improved clinical outcome at 3 months compared with placebo
(B) an increased incidence of intracerebral hemorrhage was observed in patients receiving t-PA
(C) benefits of therapy may be seen when t-PA is given within 24 hours of the onset of symptoms
(D) patients receiving t-PA showed no improvement compared with those receiving placebo during the first 24 hours

419. The prognosis of a patient with status epilepticus is most influenced by

(A) duration of seizures
(B) age of the patient
(C) development of respiratory failure
(D) etiology of the seizures

420. Which of the following statements about status epilepticus is true?

(A) Initial evaluation should focus on the airway, breathing, and circulation
(B) Midazolam is the benzodiazepine of choice because of its relatively short half-life
(C) An EEG demonstrating seizure activity should be obtained before initiating anticonvulsant therapy with phenytoin or phenobarbital
(D) Barbiturate coma should be considered in patients with status epilepticus approaching 4 hours' duration

421. Mechanical ventilation would be indicated in a patient with myasthenia gravis

(A) when peak expiratory force is less than 60 percent of predicted
(B) when vital capacity is less than 10 mL/kg
(C) only when Pa_{CO_2} is elevated
(D) prophylactically with the administration of aminoglycosides

422. True statements regarding sleep deprivation include

(A) it is an expected and uncontrollable by-product of the critical care environment
(B) it is a minor stress in comparison to the patient's underlying critical illness
(C) it has both psychological and physiologic effects
(D) it can be treated with sedative drugs
(E) it gives the patient time to integrate the experience of critical illness

423. According to the President's Commission for the Study of Ethical Problems in Medicine and Biomedical and Behavioral Research, the criteria for death include

(A) brain stem function absent regardless of the presence of cerebral function
(B) cerebral function absent regardless of the presence of brain stem function
(C) irreversible cessation of circulatory and respiratory function
(D) cessation of cerebral and brain stem function whether or not the cause of coma is known
(E) absence of cerebral and respiratory functions

424. All the following statements concerning intracranial pressure (ICP) are true EXCEPT

(A) under normal conditions, ICP has little influence on cerebral blood flow
(B) under normal conditions, central venous pressure has little influence on cerebral blood flow
(C) significant obstruction to CSF flow will not have an effect on ICP for weeks because of the low rate of CSF turnover
(D) the Cushing's response of bradycardia and hypertension in association with elevated ICP usually is seen only in the setting of catastrophic brain injury
(E) "plateau waves" (large, transient increases in ICP) have been associated with vasodilation on angiography and are seen in both normal patients and those with CNS disease

425. A 58-year-old woman with a prior history of an ischemic stroke developed acute bacterial endocarditis related to an intravenous catheter infection with subsequent respiratory failure and septic shock that required intubation and mechanical ventilation. Antibiotic therapy with imipenem and fluids have improved her septic shock and respiratory status; however, the patient remained unarousable. An infused CT of the head revealed an old ischemic stroke involving the right temporal lobe but no new abnormalities. A lumbar puncture showed only a mild increase in protein. The most appropriate approach to the patient would now include

(A) observation and broadening of antibiotic coverage while awaiting CSF culture results
(B) follow-up CT in 48 to 72 hours to rule out a new infarct as the problem
(C) an electroencephalogram (EEG)
(D) magnetic resonance imaging (MRI) of the brain to rule out lesions not disclosed on CT
(E) none of the above

426. Cerebral vasospasm associated with subarachnoid hemorrhage (SAH)

(A) is maximal at 24 to 48 hours after an injury
(B) cannot be demonstrated angiographically
(C) may be ameliorated by the aggressive administration of intravenous fluids
(D) is apparently independent of the presence of blood in the subarachnoid space
(E) does not affect the long-term neurologic outcome

427. Prognosis in nontraumatic coma

(A) is extremely poor when renal failure is associated with coma

(B) is better for structural lesions than for hepatic encephalopathy

(C) is extremely poor in patients with coincident shock

(D) is just as poor in drug overdose as in other causes

(E) is such that a majority of patients go on to an independent existence

428. Regarding CNS dysfunction with the sepsis syndrome, which of the following is true?

(A) Most episodes of neurologic dysfunction are related to direct infectious involvement of the CNS

(B) The response of cerebral blood flow to Pa_{CO_2} seems to be preserved

(C) Owing to protective alterations in autoregulation, perfusion abnormalities have not been implicated

(D) Studies of metabolic changes have failed to disclose any alterations in amino acid or neurotransmitter concentrations

(E) CNS dysfunction in the sepsis syndrome is uncommon

429. A 32-year-old woman is seen 2 days after a small-bowel resection for Crohn's disease. Her previous central venous line was used for chronic total parenteral nutrition but was withdrawn because of infusion problems and possible infection. A new subclavian line was put in 3 hours ago, but no medications or other solutions have been infused pending final approval of placement from the surgeon, who is currently involved in an emergency surgery. The patient becomes precipitously diaphoretic and markedly agitated with a temperature of 37°C (98.6°F), a pulse of 110 beats per minute, and blood pressure of 140/90. The most plausible explanation for this patient's behavioral change is

(A) paradoxical thromboembolus to the CNS from removal of a long-standing central venous catheter

(B) hypoglycemia

(C) bacteremia of new onset

(D) air embolus

(E) hypoperfusion from a tension pneumothorax

430. The most important consideration regarding "ICU psychosis" is that

(A) it is often manifest at night, when nursing is less available

(B) it still requires a patient to be closely monitored in the ICU after all other problems have been resolved

(C) it is primarily a diagnosis of exclusion of other organic encephalopathies

(D) it is more common in those with previous CNS dysfunction

(E) it often requires psychiatric consultation to be managed effectively

431. All the following statements regarding autoregulation of cerebral blood flow are true EXCEPT

(A) mean systemic blood pressures below 50 to 60 mm Hg are associated with linear decreases in blood flow with pressure

(B) elevations in blood pressure have little effect on cerebral blood flow

(C) chronic hypertension can result in decreases in blood flow at values of blood pressure usually associated with normal flow

(D) acidosis and head trauma affect the blood pressure limits of autoregulation

432. Which of the following would be predicted to have the greatest potential for CNS injury?

(A) Anemia to hemoglobin of 5 g/dL with normal blood flow

(B) Anemia to hemoglobin of 5 g/dL with a Pa_{O_2} of 35 mm Hg and increased blood flow

(C) Anemia to hemoglobin of 5 g/dL and a Pa_{CO_2} of 25 mm Hg with a Pa_{O_2} of 60 mm Hg

(D) Hemoglobin of 20 g/dL with a Pa_{O_2} of 56 mm Hg

(E) Cessation of flow for 3 minutes with prior hemoglobin of 13 g/dL and a Pa_{O_2} of 150 mm Hg

DIRECTIONS: Each question below contains four suggested responses of which **one or more** is correct. Select

A	if	**1, 2, and 3**	are correct
B	if	**1 and 3**	are correct
C	if	**2 and 4**	are correct
D	if	**4**	is correct
E	if	**1, 2, 3, and 4**	are correct

433.   Patients at increased risk for developing delirium include those who have

(1)   severe burn injury
(2)   HIV-spectrum disorders
(3)   cardiotomy
(4)   age > 60 years

434.   True statements regarding cerebral hemorrhage include

(1)   hemorrhages into the basal ganglia and cerebellum are the most common type of intracerebral hemorrhage
(2)   amyloid angiopathy usually leads to hemorrhage in the subcortical hemispheric white matter
(3)   intracranial aneurysms may rupture into the brain as well as the subarachnoid space
(4)   intracerebral hemorrhages caused by amyloid angiopathy occur most commonly in middle age

435.   In patients with atherothrombotic cerebral infarction,

(1)   cerebral edema is the major cause of late (after 1 week) mortality
(2)   corticosteroids improve mortality
(3)   reduction of intracranial pressure by mannitol has a long-term benefit
(4)   glycerol has not provided consistent improvements in morbidity and mortality

436.   Clinical complications of a ruptured intracranial aneurysm include

(1)   rebleeding
(2)   vasospasm
(3)   hydrocephalus
(4)   hypovolemic shock

437.   Therapies that improve the outcome of ruptured intracerebral aneurysms include

(1)   prophylactic treatment of vasospasm
(2)   emergent clipping
(3)   drainage of hydrocephalus
(4)   early blood transfusions

438.   In which of the following clinical situations should prompt treatment of an elevated blood pressure be strongly considered?

(1)   Acute intracerebral hemorrhage
(2)   Papilledema with a focal neurologic defect
(3)   Acute subarachnoid hemorrhage
(4)   Myocardial ischemia in the setting of an acute brain infarct

439.   Emergency neurosurgical interventions should be strongly considered in which of the following clinical situations?

(1)   Acute ischemic strokes
(2)   All cerebellar hematomas
(3)   Deep hematomas arising from the basal ganglia
(4)   Subarachnoid hemorrhages

440.   Among the therapies listed below, which should be employed routinely in the treatment of acute stroke?

(1)   Intravenous heparin for an acutely progressing stroke
(2)   Mannitol/hyperventilation/corticosteroids for cerebral edema
(3)   Establishment of mild hypoosmolarity
(4)   Early ambulation

441.   Potential consequences of status epilepticus include

(1)   pulmonary edema
(2)   renal failure
(3)   respiratory failure
(4)   hypoglycemia

442.   Quadriplegics with high cervical injuries who inspire only with the accessory muscles experience which of the following?

(1)   Abdominal paradoxical motion with inspiration
(2)   Worsened hypercapnia and hypoxemia when breathing spontaneously in the supine position compared with the (supported) upright position
(3)   Hypoxemia as a result of hypoventilation and microatelectasis
(4)   Inward motion of the upper and middle rib cage during inspiration

443. Therapy for botulism would include

(1) mechanical ventilation
(2) high-dose penicillin
(3) trivalent antitoxin against neurotoxins A, B, and E
(4) gastric lavage and enemas

444. True statements about coma and a persistent vegetative state include

(1) early CT of the brain is the most valuable test to diagnose the structural causes of coma
(2) overall mortality from coma in the intensive care unit is approximately 50 percent
(3) the majority of cases of coma result from metabolic disturbances or drug ingestion
(4) a persistent vegetative state refers to patients with persistent coma at 2 weeks

445. Which of the following clinical conditions would preclude the declaration of death by clinical assessment of irreversible cessation of cerebral function?

(1) Hypothermia
(2) Two isoelectric electroencephalograms taken 4 hours apart
(3) Recent ingestion of barbiturates
(4) Ongoing sepsis

446. True statements concerning the ongoing assessment of CNS function in the critically ill include

(1) further CNS investigation is appropriately initiated on the basis of collateral history obtained from nursing and respiratory therapy
(2) a change in CNS function in a critically ill person often is first heralded by a change in the level of consciousness
(3) serial neurologic examinations are an important part of the daily assessment of neurologic status in critically ill patients
(4) given a high incidence of CNS dysfunction in patients with more than one organ failure, metabolic brain failure should be assumed and examinations of the CNS (e.g., lumbar puncture, brain CT) should be withheld

447. Hepatic encephalopathy has been associated with which of the following?

(1) Hyperreflexia on neurologic examination
(2) Cerebral edema
(3) Coexistent hypoglycemia
(4) A uniformly irreversible and progressive deterioration

448. Criteria for establishing the clinical diagnosis of brain death include

(1) absence of all brain stem reflexes
(2) apnea during a period that significantly raises Pa_{CO_2}
(3) drug overdose ruled out
(4) decerebrate posturing with physical stimulation

449. With regard to cerebral blood flow and energy sources for the brain, true statements include which of the following?

(1) Pa_{O_2} does not have an appreciable effect on blood flow
(2) The fall in cerebral blood flow with an abrupt decrease in Pa_{CO_2} can be maintained for a few days to weeks
(3) Cerebral blood flow and cerebral metabolic rate of oxygen consumption are linked only over the range of normal oxygen consumption values
(4) The reserves of glucose and glycogen are small in the brain and can be exhausted in a matter of minutes under conditions of aerobic metabolism

450. Rheologic manipulations of blood have been clearly shown to improve CNS dysfunction

(1) in hyperviscosity syndromes associated with an elevation in serum protein
(2) in recovery from a global hypoxic insult such as a hypotensive episode
(3) in polycythemia
(4) within 48 hours of a focal ischemic stroke

451. Brain injury during ischemia has been postulated to be mediated by which of the following?

(1) Massive influx of calcium into the cell
(2) Altered sodium and calcium flux mediated by excitatory neurotransmitters
(3) Prolonged postischemic hypoperfusion
(4) Hyperemic perfusion state once flow is restored

DIRECTIONS: The group of questions below consists of lettered headings followed by a set of numbered items. For each numbered item select the **one** lettered heading with which it is **most** closely associated. Each lettered heading may be used o**nce, more than once, or not at all.**

Questions 452–454.

Match each clinical situation with the appropriate pupillary findings.

(A) Small, reactive
(B) Large, nonreactive
(C) Pinpoint, reactive
(D) Unilateral, large nonreactive
(E) Midsized, reactive

452. Opiate overdose

453. Hepatic encephalopathy

454. Uncal herniation

DIRECTIONS: Each group of questions below consists of four lettered headings followed by a set of numbered items. For each numbered item select

A   if the item is associated with   (A) **only**
B   if the item is associated with   (B) **only**
C   if the item is associated with   **both** (A) and (B)
D   if the item is associated with   **neither** (A) nor (B)

Each lettered heading may be used **once, more than once, or not at all.**

Questions 455–458.

(A)   Diazepam

(B)   Phenytoin

(C)   Both

(D)   Neither

455.   Will often cause central nervous system depression in therapeutic concentrations

456.   Will have a rapid onset of action

457.   May cause hypotension

458.   May cause cardiac arrhythmias

NEUROPSYCHIATRIC DISORDERS IN THE CRITICALLY ILL

ANSWERS

413. **The answer is C.** *(Chapter 57)* The patient presents with the classical symptoms of Wernicke's encephalopathy and must be given thiamine. Benzodiazepines can then be used to control his alcoholic withdrawal.

414. **The answer is C.** *(Chapter 58)* Prophylactic augmentation of circulating blood volume and mean arterial pressure is associated with about a 10 percent incidence of postoperative morbidity related to vasospasm. This represents about a 50 percent reduction from vasospasm-related morbidity in previous decades. Hypervolemic/hypertensive therapy is delivered by administering saline or colloids to achieve a pulmonary wedge pressure of 15 to 18 mm Hg. Vasoactive agents such as dopamine and phenylephrine also are used to increase mean blood pressure.

415. **The answer is D.** *(Chapter 58)* Lumbar puncture is the most sensitive test for the detection of a subarachnoid hemorrhage. The clinical history and examination often assist in the initial assessment of a patient with a neurologic disorder; however, essential findings are often absent or difficult to interpret. An infused head CT is useful in the detection and localization of intracranial pathology, but it may miss the diagnosis in 10 to 20 percent of cases.

416. **The answer is A.** *(Chapter 58)* Because of the high incidence of asymptomatic atherosclerosis and the inconsistent relationship between the degree of atherosclerotic disease and consequent brain infarction, examination of carotid or vertebral arteries by Doppler or ultrasound has little value in differentiating cardioembolic from atherosclerotic causes of brain infarction.

417. **The answer is D.** *(Chapter 58)* Cerebrovascular disease usually produces the sudden onset of focal brain dysfunction. The primary exception is pure subarachnoid hemorrhage with symptoms restricted to the sudden onset of severe headache, with or without loss of consciousness.

418. **The answer is C.** *(Chapter 58)* Despite an increased incidence of intracerebral hemorrhage, patients receiving t-PA within 3 hours of the onset of symptoms of acute ischemic stroke showed an improved clinical outcome at 3 months. Benefits of t-PA therapy were not evident within the first 24 hours of treatment. Benefit of t-PA therapy has not been demonstrated in patients receiving treatment more than 3 hours after the onset of symptoms.

419. **The answer is D.** *(Chapter 59)* Currently, with appropriate therapy, mortality results from the condition that precipitates status epilepticus rather than from the repeated seizures. In one series, all patients with a prior history of seizures and no acute neurologic event survived. All deaths in this series were attributable to the underlying disease.

420. **The answer is A.** *(Chapter 59)* The initial evaluation of a patient with status epilepticus should focus on the need for airway maintenance, mechanical ventilation, and hemodynamic support. Benzodiazepines enter the brain quickly and have a rapid onset of anticonvulsant activity. Long-acting benzodiazepines such as lorazepam are preferred because of the increased incidence of seizure recurrence with short-acting agents. While EEG may be a helpful tool in further characterizing seizure activity, therapy should not be withheld while one is awaiting EEG results. Furthermore, epileptic seizures are paroxysmal events. The absence of seizure activity on EEG should not preclude appropriate therapy. Within 60 minutes of continuous seizure activity, the brain begins to suffer irreversible damage. Barbiturate coma should be considered within this period of time.

421. **The answer is B.** *(Chapter 60)* The vital capacity can be measured at the bedside, and respiratory failure is often heralded when vital capacity decreases below 10 mL/kg. An elevation of Pa_{CO_2} is a late sign of impending respiratory failure, and mechanical ventilation should be considered before the onset of hypercapnia. Peak expiratory force assesses respiratory muscle strength, but mechanical ventilation would not be instituted at a level of 60 percent of predicted. Aminoglycosides may worsen myasthenia, but not predictably. The patient should be closely monitored, not "prophylactically" mechanically ventilated.

422. **The answer is C.** *(Chapters 2, 10)* Sleep deprivation is cited by patients as being a common and major stressor during their stays in critical care units. It has numerous psychological (anxiety, irritability, paranoia, delusions) and physiologic (hyperactivity, decreased tissue healing, cardiac dysrhythmias) effects that jeopardize the patient's well-being. Its incidence can be lessened by careful attention to decreasing noise levels, monitoring, and treatment intervention at night. Sedatives often interfere with, rather than promote, sleep.

423. **The answer is C.** *(Chapter 61)* Death is defined by the President's Commission as either irreversible cessation of circulatory and respiratory function or irreversible cessation of the entire brain. Both cerebral and brain stem function must be absent. The cause of coma must be established and must explain the loss of brain function, there must not be a possibility of recovery, and the absence of brain function must persist for an appropriate period.

424. **The answer is C.** *(Chapter 89)* CSF fluid turns over four to six times daily, and significant obstruction of CSF flow can result in acute elevations in intracranial pressure with acute CNS symptoms. The normal intracranial pressure (10 mm Hg) and normal central venous pressure (5 to 10 mm Hg) usually have little influence on cerebral blood flow. Plateau waves can influence cerebral blood flow and have been seen in association with CNS disease and during REM sleep in normal persons.

425. **The answer is C.** *(Chapter 59)* This patient has suffered a previous stroke and is receiving imipenem. Both of these circumstances can predispose to seizures. Subclinical seizures that are causing apparent unresponsiveness would be important to identify. Bacterial meningitis is unlikely with an unremarkable lumbar puncture and the improvement in the patient's septic shock. Further imaging of the brain would be unlikely to reveal a cause for her mental status and would not be the best next step in the evaluation.

426. **The answer is C.** *(Chapter 58)* Aggressive intravenous fluid therapy may improve cerebral perfusion by hyperperfusion, which apparently dilates the vasospastic cerebral artery. Crystalloid typically is given in the range of 150 to 200 mL/h. The vasospasm is usually maximal at 1 week, has been related to the presence of blood in the subarachnoid space, and is angiographically present in the majority of patients with SAH, of whom a third will become symptomatic. Vasospasm after SAH is associated with a worsening neurologic outcome.

427.   The answer is C.   *(Chapter 61)*   With regard to nontraumatic coma, prognostication is unfortunately in a rudimentary stage of development. Renal failure and hepatic failure in association with coma often have potentially reversible metabolic causes and are associated with better prognoses. Unfortunately, most patients do not recover from nontraumatic coma to lead an independent existence, and when shock is associated with coma, a very poor prognosis has been demonstrated (95 percent mortality in some studies).

428.   The answer is B.   *(Chapter 41)*   The response of cerebral blood flow to Pa_{CO_2} is preserved in sepsis, leading to concern that sepsis-related hyperventilation may cause decreases in cerebral blood flow with adverse consequences. Neurologic dysfunction is very common in sepsis, although direct infectious etiologies are not felt to be common. Abnormalities in amino acid metabolism have been found and implicated as potential contributors.

429.   The answer is B.   *(Chapter 57)*   Hypoglycemia is most plausible given that the continuous source of calories has been discontinued. Signs of sympathetic discharge support this diagnosis. Agitation is not an uncommon presentation of hypoglycemia, and this readily correctable cause of neurologic dysfunction must be acted on in such a setting.

430.   The answer is C.   *(Chapter 57)*   Although the other responses may be true, the symptoms of ICU psychosis overlap considerably with those of other organic encephalopathies, and this requires that other possibilities be clearly ruled out first. Assuming that abnormal perceptions or behavior are due to the ICU environment may result in missing important metabolic, structural, or infectious processes during a window of opportunity for correction. Many measures may be undertaken for a patient with altered mental status from the experience of critical illness, including minimizing polypharmacy, restoring sleep-wake cycles, allaying fears, and controlling pain.

431.   The answer is B.   *(Chapter 58)*   Elevations in blood flow do occur with increases in pressure above 125 to 150 mm Hg in normal persons. Chronic hypertension, acidosis, hemorrhagic shock, and head trauma can affect both the upper and the lower limits of autoregulation.

432.   The answer is E.   *(Chapter 58)*   Whereas all the other possibilities result in marginal decreases in oxygen delivery, cessation of flow is the least tolerated insult. Oxygen stores and brain electrical activity can diminish in a matter of seconds after circulatory arrest.

433.   The answer is E (all).   *(Chapter 57)*   Patients at high risk to develop delirium include children, illicit drug users, the elderly, and patients with HIV/AIDS, postcardiotomy, organic brain disease, and severe burns.

434.   The answer is A (1, 2, 3).   *(Chapter 58)*   Hemorrhages into the basal ganglia and cerebellum often occur in a middle-aged patient with long-standing hypertension and are not the most common type of intracerebral hemorrhage. Arteriovenous malfunctions must be considered in younger patients. Intracerebral hemorrhages caused by amyloid angiopathy become important from the seventh decade on. Other rare causes of intracerebral hemorrhage are thrombocytopenia, DIC, and hemophilia.

435.   The answer is D (4).   *(Chapter 58)*   Cerebral edema is the major cause of early mortality after cerebral infarction. No effective treatment is available. Corticosteroids and glycerol have not provided consistent improvements in morbidity and mortality. Mannitol and hyperventilation temporarily reduce intracranial pressure but have no long-term benefit.

436.   The answer is A (1, 2, 3).   *(Chapter 58)*   The common complications of ruptured intracranial aneurysm are rebleeding, delayed ischemia or vasospasm, and hydrocephalus, which all can cause further brain damage. Volume within the cranium is insufficient for bleeding to cause hypovolemia.

437. The answer is A (1, 2, 3). *(Chapter 58)* Improved results over the last decade strongly suggest that emergent clipping in patients with a subarachnoid hemorrhage, coupled with acute ventricular drainage for hydrocephalus and prophylactic treatment for vasospasm, is associated with an improved outcome.

438. The answer is C (2, 4). *(Chapter 58)* Optimal treatment of the hypertension that accompanies acute cerebrovascular disease is somewhat uncertain. There are no known hazards to the brain from the spontaneous transient elevation in systemic blood pressure that accompanies strokes. For subarachnoid hemorrhage, increasing the mean arterial pressure is actually one of the therapies used to prevent vasospasm. The benefits of lowering blood pressure in the setting of intracerebral hemorrhage are less clear. Rebleeding occurs rarely, and its relationship to early arterial hypertension is unknown. However, unlike the questionable benefit of hypertensive therapy in the setting of acute cerebrovascular disease, there is no level to which blood pressure can be reduced that does not carry the risk of further neurologic deterioration. Thus, clear indications for prompt control of elevated blood pressure in the setting of acute cerebrovascular disease occur only when neurologic deficits are secondary to the hypertension itself (malignant hypertension) and when systemic hypertension is causing damage to other organs (myocardial ischemia, dissecting aortic aneurysm). When treated, the elevated blood pressure should be lowered carefully and judiciously with constant monitoring of neurologic status.

439. The answer is D (4). *(Chapter 58)* Since carotid endarterectomy is associated with high morbidity and mortality and because the prevailing evidence suggests that most hemispheric infarctions are due to distal embolization, an improvement in outcome from emergent surgery is unlikely. For intracerebral hematomas, the primary goal of surgery is to alleviate the effects of the hematoma's acting as an intracranial mass lesion, not to reverse the effects of local tissue destruction. Thus, surgery plays no role in treating small hemorrhages. The value of surgery is best proved for cerebellar hemorrhages that *result in brain stem compression.* However, many patients with cerebellar hematomas do well without surgical intervention or simply with ventricular drainage for hydrocephalus. Patients with superficial hematomas arising from the basal ganglia and signs of increased intracranial pressure may show improvement after surgical evacuation. Emergent clipping in patients with a subarachnoid hemorrhage, coupled with acute ventricular drainage for hydrocephalus and prophylactic treatment for vasospasm, is associated with an improved outcome.

440. The answer is D (4). *(Chapter 58)* Recent studies have demonstrated no benefit of anticoagulation with heparin in patients with a transient ischemic attack or a partial stable stroke. Although several controlled trials have demonstrated a benefit of long-term oral anticoagulation in patients whose initial presentation was progressing stroke, more recent evidence from uncontrolled trials of heparin in acute progressing stroke has demonstrated that further progression usually occurs in spite of early anticoagulation. Since this issue is unresolved and because of the risk of converting a bland to a hemorrhagic infarct, intravenous heparin for an acutely progressing stroke cannot be recommended as a routine therapy.

Although cerebral edema is the major cause of early mortality after cerebral infarction, no effective treatment is available. Because of the potential side effects and because there has been no documented long-term benefit, corticosteroids, glycerol, mannitol, and hyperventilation should not be used routinely to treat cerebral edema that complicates acute stroke. However, these manipulations may be of short-term value in, for example, a patient with brain stem compression from edematous cerebellar infarct in whom craniotomy and removal of the edematous tissue may be of benefit.

Since hypoosmolarity can exacerbate brain edema, it should be avoided. Prolonged bed rest carries an increased risk of iliofemoral venous thrombosis, pulmonary embolism, and pneumonia. Thus, since there is no clinical evidence or pathophysiologic reason to support routinely restricting patients with acute stroke to bed, ambulation should be instituted as soon as possible.

441. **The answer is E (all).** *(Chapter 59)*   There are numerous systemic effects of repeated generalized tonic-clonic seizures or status epilepticus. They include tachycardia, bradycardia from increased vagal tone, cardiac arrhythmias, hyperpyrexia, excessive sweating, respiratory failure after a series of seizures, noncardiac pulmonary edema, rhabdomyolysis leading to renal failure, respiratory and metabolic acidosis, hypoxemia, hyperkalemia, hypoglycemia, and hyponatremia.

442. **The answer is A (1, 2, 3).** *(Chapter 60)*   Owing to the dysfunction of the diaphragms (innervated by the phrenic nerves), diminished vital capacity with resultant abnormalities of gas exchange is common in patients with high cervical cord injuries. Abdominal paradox results when the denervated diaphragm is influenced by negative thoracic pressure and gravity's effect on the abdominal contents. Inward motion of the chest cage results from a lower cervical injury with residual diaphragm function.

443. **The answer is E (all).** *(Chapter 60)*   Gastric lavage and enemas can eliminate unabsorbed neurotoxin from the gut while penicillin and antitoxin are being administered. Mechanical ventilation is required in about one-third of these patients, and most survive.

444. **The answer is B (1, 3).** *(Chapter 61)*   Coma is defined as a state of "unarousable psychologic unresponsiveness in which the subject lies with eyes closed." Assessment of the structural causes of coma is best performed by brain CT. Metabolic abnormalities and toxic ingestions account for the majority of cases of coma. Despite the overwhelming morbidity associated with coma, overall mortality remains stable at 15 percent. The persistent vegetative state describes the presence of coma, usually as a result of ischemic/hypoxic brain injury, for at least 4 weeks.

445. **The answer is B (1, 3).** *(Chapter 61)*   Hypothermia and barbiturate overdose may both cause reversible cessation of brain function. Therefore, their presence precludes the clinical diagnosis of irreversible cessation of brain function. In patients with iatrogenic barbiturate coma in whom there is a suspicion of death, cerebral viability may be assessed by ancillary studies such as measurement of cerebral blood flow. An electroencephalogram may confirm or exclude the diagnosis of irreversible cessation of brain function (for instance, in a patient who mistakenly received a dose of muscle relaxant) but is not necessary for the diagnosis. Ongoing sepsis similarly does not influence the diagnosis of cessation of brain function.

446. **The answer is A (1, 2, 3).** *(Chapter 57)*   Personnel can unfortunately accept CNS dysfunction as the norm in the ICU because of its high incidence, but this does not preclude the need for ongoing, thorough evaluation and physical examination, which can be especially valuable for determining focal defects of evidence of infection that requires further testing. An impairment in the level of consciousness is the most commonly noted early finding in critically ill persons. Nurses and other caregivers can provide invaluable information for identifying new findings.

447. **The answer is A (1, 2, 3).** *(Chapter 57)*   Hepatic encephalopathy can be induced by reversible processes, such as infection, and can present with a spectrum of neurologic abnormalities that can include general hyperreflexia. Cerebral edema can be a complication, though it is more common in acute, fulminant liver failure. Severe liver dysfunction is a common cause of hypoglycemia.

448. **The answer is A (1, 2, 3).** *(Chapter 61)* Irreversible cessation of brain function is best judged by an experienced observer. Conditions such as shock, hypothermia, and drug effects must be excluded. Absence of cerebral and brain stem reflexes is required, and thus seizure activity and posturing (decerebrate or decorticate) are inconsistent with a diagnosis of brain death. Reflexes purely of the spinal cord do not preclude this diagnosis.

449. **The answer is D (4).** *(Chapter 58)* The brain is in constant need of oxygen and glucose delivery because of the small reserve of these substrates. Blood flow to the brain is significantly linked to oxygen consumption over a wide range. Both Pa_{CO_2} and Pa_{O_2} influence cerebral blood flow, but the decrease in blood flow associated with an abrupt fall in Pa_{CO_2} is of relatively short duration (24 to 72 hours), during which time blood flow returns to baseline despite the persistence of hypocapnia.

450. **The answer is B (1, 3).** *(Chapter 58)* Plasmapheresis in severe hyperproteinemic states and phlebotomy with hemodilution in polycythemia have been shown to improve CNS function. There is conflicting evidence for the efficacy of hemodilution or other rheologic manipulations after ischemic brain injury.

451. **The answer is A (1, 2, 3).** *(Chapter 58)* Postischemic injury has been associated with flux of calcium into the neuron. Excitatory neurotransmitters have been postulated to contribute to metabolic derangements that can further potentiate cell injury. Upon restoration of flow, a hyperemic phase followed by a hypoperfusion phase (which can last for hours to days) has been noted. Only the hypoperfusion phase has been seen as clearly deleterious.

452–454. **The answers are 452-C, 453-A, 454-D.** *(Chapter 61)* Opiates cause pinpoint-sized pupils that are reactive to light (although this may be hard to demonstrate).

Metabolic encephalopathies typically leave the sympathetic and parasympathetic inputs to the ciliary muscles intact until the near-terminal stage. This can be an important diagnostic tool in a patient with other brain stem dysfunction.

Compression of third-nerve fibers by a herniating temporal lobe may impair sympathetic ciliary innervation before the development of an ophthalmoplegia.

455–458. **The answers are 455-A, 456-A, 457-C, 458-B.** *(Chapter 59)* The advantage of diazepam in treating seizures is its rapid onset of activity resulting from quick distribution to the CNS. Disadvantages are its tendency to depress respiration and consciousness, its tendency to cause occasional hypotension, and its short CNS half-life, which limits its effectiveness to less than a half hour. The initial drug of choice for treating status epilepticus should be phenytoin. Its main advantages are its effectiveness in controlling seizures, relatively long half-life, and lack of significant CNS depression. Disadvantages include its tendency to cause hypotension and cardiac arrhythmias, the time required to give a full loading dose, and its relative ineffectiveness in suppressing focal epileptic activity.

HEMATOLOGIC AND ONCOLOGIC DISORDERS IN THE CRITICALLY ILL

QUESTIONS

DIRECTIONS: Each question below contains four or five suggested responses. Select the **one best** response to each question.

459. All the following statements are true regarding thrombocythemia in excess of 1 million platelets per cubic millimeter EXCEPT

(A) patients with this finding are at risk for hemorrhagic complications that can be predicted by a prolonged bleeding time
(B) patients with this finding are at risk for thrombotic events
(C) splenectomy is generally necessary for definitive management
(D) markedly increased megakaryocytes can be seen on bone marrow examination
(E) platelet levels can be quickly and safely reduced with platelet pheresis

460. The pentad of findings that characterizes thrombotic thrombocytopenic purpura (TTP) includes all the following EXCEPT

(A) fever
(B) microangiopathic hemolytic anemia
(C) renal dysfunction
(D) abnormal liver function profile

461. A 20-year-old woman was admitted with thrombocytopenia and seizures. A clinical diagnosis of thrombotic thrombocytopenic purpura was made, and she was treated with therapeutic plasmapheresis with plasma exchanges. The following arterial blood gas values (room air) were obtained before her fifth plasma exchange therapy: pH 7.54, Pa_{CO_2} 49 mm Hg, and Pa_{O_2} 83 mm Hg. The following additional values were also obtained: Na^+ 146 mEq/L, K^+ 3.6 mEq/L, Cl^- 89 mEq/L, CO_2 42 mEq/L, BUN 12 mg/dL, and creatinine 1.0 mg/dL. What is the etiology of her alkalosis?

(A) Volume contraction
(B) Hypokalemia
(C) Citrate toxicity
(D) Respiratory acidosis

462. Which of the following should be included in the differential diagnosis of dyspnea in a patient with a malignancy?

(A) Pulmonary embolism
(B) Radiation pneumonitis
(C) Constrictive pericarditis
(D) Superior vena cava syndrome
(E) All of the above

Questions 463–464.

A 62-year-old man with acute myelogenous leukemia is admitted to the ICU for a hemoglobin of 9.0 g/dL and a white blood cell count of 190×10^9 cells/L with 95 percent blasts. He is somnolent but not difficult to arouse and describes mild dyspnea. On examination, he is afebrile with a normal pulse and blood pressure. His breathing is unlabored at 22 breaths per minute. His lungs have diffuse fine crackles throughout both lung fields, and his lips and fingernails are pink. Pulse oximetry reveals an Sp_{O_2} of 97 percent. An arterial blood gas is obtained with the following results: pH 7.32, Pa_{CO_2} 32 mm Hg, and Pa_{O_2} 38 mm Hg.

463. Which of the following options is the correct intervention for the diminished Pa_{O_2}?

(A) Proceed to intubate the patient for acute hypoxemic respiratory failure
(B) Send a carboxyhemoglobin level
(C) Rerun the original blood-gas sample on a co-oximeter
(D) Place a second blood-gas sample on ice and send it immediately to the laboratory for rapid analysis

464. Appropriate management of this patient's condition should include

(A) immediate high-dose chemotherapy aimed at cytoreduction

(B) transfusion of two units of packed red blood cells to improve the oxygen-carrying capacity

(C) anticoagulation to prevent further complications of leukostasis

(D) placement of a Quinton catheter followed by emergent leukophoresis

465. An 18-year-old woman was admitted to the hospital for induction therapy for acute lymphocytic leukemia with high-dose cytarabine (ara-C) and daunorubicin. One day after the completion of her therapy she complained of diffuse abdominal pain. On physical examination her blood pressure was 110/70 mm Hg, heart rate was 110 beats per minute, respiratory rate was 22 breaths per minute, and temperature was 38.9°C (102°F). Her cardiopulmonary examination was unremarkable except for her tachycardia. Her abdominal examination revealed absence of bowel sounds, mild distention, and diffuse tenderness without any rebound tenderness. She was moved to the intensive care unit for observation. Over the next 2 hours her abdominal tenderness became severe and localized to her lower right quadrant with rebound tenderness. Her hematocrit was 36 percent, WBC was 0.1×10^9 cells per liter, and arterial blood gas on room air was pH 7.33, Pa_{CO_2} 32 mm Hg, and Pa_{O_2} 110 mm Hg. At this point you should

(A) observe the patient closely

(B) perform exploratory laparotomy

(C) give steroids

(D) intubate the patient

466. Of the following tissues, the one LEAST sensitive to the acute effects of radiotherapy is

(A) skin

(B) nerve

(C) ileal mucosa

(D) lung

(E) bone marrow

467. A 40-year-old man received MOPP [mechlorethamine, vincristine (Oncovin), procarbazine, prednisone] chemotherapy and mantle irradiation in a dose of 40 Gy for Hodgkin disease. The last dose of mantle irradiation was completed 6 weeks ago. The patient now complains of new-onset dyspnea on exertion. Cough, fatigue, and low-grade fevers are also present. Physical examination is unremarkable. CT scans of the thorax and abdomen do not show any evidence of lymphoma but reveal perihilar infiltrates bilaterally, which are also seen on the chest radiograph. Arterial blood gas measurements reveal pH of 7.40, Pa_{CO_2} of 30 mm Hg, and a Pa_{O_2} of 55 mm Hg. Bronchoscopy with bronchoalveolar lavage is negative for mycobacterial, fungal, and opportunistic organisms. A transbronchial biopsy is nondiagnostic. A follow-up chest radiograph 1 week later reveals no progression but no resolution of the infiltrates. Therapeutic and diagnostic considerations would include

(A) avoidance of supplemental oxygen since this may worsen the patient's condition

(B) immediate tapering of the prednisone used as part of the patient's chemotherapy regimen

(C) informing the patient that this is a rapidly progressive pulmonary complication of treatment with a poor prognosis

(D) beginning cyclosporine

(E) anticipating that these infiltrates will remain localized to the described area

468. A 58-year-old man is admitted for evaluation of weakness and weight loss. He was well until 18 months ago, when he was found to have nasopharyngeal carcinoma. He was treated with 70 Gy (7000 rads) over 7 weeks with curative intent. After treatment, his tumor mass was no longer detectable and he felt well and returned to work. Beginning 4 months ago, he complained of anorexia and began to lose weight. ENT examination showed no evidence of local recurrence. A chest radiograph was normal. In the past 3 weeks he has noted progressive weakness, nausea, worsening anorexia and a 50 lb weight loss. Vague abdominal pain led to esophagogastroduodenoscopy and a barium enema, both of which were normal. CT of the abdomen revealed no abnormality, and the pancreas was well visualized. While getting out of bed to use the bathroom, the patient collapsed.

On examination he was cachectic and responded to voice. His blood pressure was 80/50, heart rate was 115, and respirations were 32. He was given 2 L of normal saline and transferred to the intensive care unit. Deterioration in mentation led to endotracheal intubation and mechanical ventilation. A rapid bedside glucose determination revealed a level of 45 mg/dL. Fifty milliliters of 50% dextrose was given without improvement. Laboratories confirmed that glucose level was 42 mg/dL, sodium 125, potassium 4.8, chloride 96, bicarbonate 16, BUN 52, and creatinine 2.1. The white blood cell count was 5500 with 35 percent neutrophils, 2 percent bands, 54 percent lymphocytes, and 9 percent eosinophils. The hematocrit was 38 percent, and the platelets were 320,000.

After an additional 3 L of saline, the blood pressure was 85/45 mm Hg. Dopamine was infused up to a dose of 10 μg/kg per minute with no improvement in blood pressure. The patient was now awake but lethargic. The next step in management should be

(A) begin an infusion of norepinephrine
(B) begin ceftriaxone for presumed meningitis
(C) administer dexamethasone 4 mg intravenously
(D) begin mebendazole 100 mg per naso-gastric tube
(E) place a pulmonary artery catheter

Questions 469–470.

A 54-year-old man with Burkitt's lymphoma who received chemotherapy 12 hours previously develops tetany. Laboratory data are notable for sodium 134, chloride 100, bicarbonate 13, potassium 7.0, blood urea nitrogen 30, creatinine 3.2, calcium 4.5, phosphate 12, magnesium 2.4, and uric acid 15.0.

469. What is the most likely cause of this patient's condition?

(A) Obstructive uropathy
(B) Uric acid nephropathy
(C) Tumor lysis syndrome
(D) Hypoparathyroidism

470. Further management of this patient should include all the following EXCEPT

(A) aggressive hydration
(B) allopurinol
(C) sodium polystyrene sulfonate (Kayexalate)
(D) acidification of urine

DIRECTIONS: Each question below contains four suggested responses of which **one or more** is correct. Select

A	if	**1, 2, and 3**	are correct
B	if	**1 and 3**	are correct
C	if	**2 and 4**	are correct
D	if	**4**	is correct
E	if	**1, 2, 3, and 4**	are correct

471. Medications associated with toxic neutropenia in the intensive care unit include

(1) chloramphenicol
(2) phenytoin
(3) cimetidine
(4) amiodarone

472. Disseminated intravascular coagulation (DIC) is suggested by

(1) elevated D-dimer levels
(2) microangiopathic hemolysis by smear
(3) hypofibrinogenemia
(4) prolonged clotting times

473. Correct statements regarding uremic bleeding include

(1) it is a thrombocytopathic process
(2) it can be corrected with intravenous desmopressin (DDAVP)
(3) it is characterized by an abnormal bleeding time
(4) it is not corrected by dialysis or corticosteroids

474. A 40-year-old man with sickle cell anemia presented to the emergency room with a sickle cell crisis. He was admitted to the floor and treated with analgesics, intravenous fluids, and supplemental oxygen. His hematocrit on admission was 26 percent with 15 percent reticulocytes. His WBC was 5×10^9 cells per liter, and his chest x-ray was normal. One day after admission he developed fever, severe chest pain, and shortness of breath and was transferred to the ICU. On arrival to the ICU, he became hypotensive and obtunded. Physical examination demonstrated a narrow pulse pressure, cold and clammy extremities, cyanosis, jugular venous distention, and a right ventricular heave. Chest x-ray demonstrated diffuse, bilateral alveolar infiltrates. His arterial blood gas on 100% mask was pH 7.30, Pa_{CO_2} 46 mm Hg, and Pa_{O_2} 45 mm Hg. Your management should include

(1) broad-spectrum antibiotics
(2) intubation and mechanical ventilation
(3) exchange transfusion
(4) methylprednisolone sodium succinate (Solu-Medrol)

475. Thrombocytopenia associated with decreased platelet survival time

(1) is seen in bleeding and sepsis
(2) may be associated with antiplatelet antibodies
(3) may require treatment with intravenous γ-globulin
(4) may be treated with platelet administration

476. A 48-year-old woman with small cell carcinoma of the lung metastatic to bone presents with a 3-day history of progressively increasing lethargy. Possible etiologies of this patient's changes in mental status include

(1) hypercalcemia
(2) syndrome of inappropriate antidiuretic hormone (SIADH)
(3) leptomeningeal carcinomatosis
(4) sepsis

477. True statements about alterations in host defenses in recipients of bone marrow transplants include which of the following?

(1) Circulating granulocytes generally recover within 3 weeks after marrow infusion
(2) IgM and IgG serum levels are normal at 1 year
(3) Serum and secretory IgA levels are low for longer than 1 year
(4) Chronic graft-versus-host disease (GVHD) does not confer any additional immunosuppression

478. True statements about spinal cord compression include which of the following?

(1) Pain localized to the spine or paravertebral area is present in less than 50 percent of these patients
(2) X-ray studies of the spine will demonstrate abnormalities of vertebral bodies in about two-thirds of patients with back pain
(3) Abnormalities on x-ray will correctly predict the presence or absence of epidural metastases in about 40 percent of these patients
(4) Patients who are paraplegic at diagnosis have less than a 10 percent chance of significant neurologic recovery and should not be treated

479. True statements regarding pericardial effusions in cancer patients include

(1) malignant pericardial effusions are an immediate or contributory cause of death in close to 90 percent of patients who are symptomatic
(2) mesothelioma is the most common primary pericardial malignancy
(3) lung and breast cancer are the two most common solid malignancies involving the pericardium
(4) close to half of all pericardial effusions are nonmalignant

480. Platelet transfusion may fail to significantly elevate the platelet count in patients with

(1) drug-related thrombocytopenia
(2) disseminated intravascular coagulation (DIC)
(3) thrombotic thrombocytopenic purpura
(4) dilutional thrombocytopenia

481. Plasmapheresis may be a useful therapy in

(1) myasthenia gravis
(2) Goodpasture syndrome
(3) thrombotic thrombocytopenic purpura (TTP)
(4) thyroid storm

DIRECTIONS: Each group of questions below consists of lettered headings followed by a set of numbered items. For each numbered item select the **one** lettered heading with which it is **most** closely associated. Each lettered heading may be used **once, more than once, or not at all.**

Questions 482–486.

Match each disease or procedure with the appropriate morphologic abnormality.

(A) Teardrop cells
(B) Schistocytes
(C) Target cells
(D) Howell-Jolly bodies
(E) Heinz bodies (special stain)

482. Glucose 6-phosphate dehydrogenase deficiency

483. Liver disease

484. Splenectomy

485. Myelodysplasia

486. Thrombotic thrombocytopenic purpura

Questions 487–490.

Match each effect with the appropriate agent.

(A) Vincristine and vinblastine
(B) Bleomycin
(C) Carmustine (BCNU)
(D) Methotrexate
(E) Cisplatin

487. Torsade de pointes associated with severe hypomagnesemia

488. Respiratory deterioration after intraoperative administration of oxygen in a concentration greater than 30%

489. Necrotizing leukoencephalopathy appearing months after therapy that included cranial irradiation

490. Paralytic ileus that can mimic an acute abdomen

DIRECTIONS: Each group of questions below consists of four lettered headings followed by a set of numbered items. For each numbered item select

A   if the item is associated with   **(A) only**
B   if the item is associated with   **(B) only**
C   if the item is associated with   **both** (A) and (B)
D   if the item is associated with   **neither** (A) nor (B)

Each lettered heading may be used **once, more than once, or not at all.**

Questions 491–494.

    (A) Acute graft-versus-host disease
    (B) Chronic graft-versus-host disease
    (C) Both
    (D) Neither

491. Mortality is most often associated with infection

492. Bronchiolitis obliterans

493. Noninfectious diarrhea

494. Occurs within 3 months of autologous bone marrow transplant

Questions 495–498.

    (A) Transfusion reaction causing intravascular hemolysis
    (B) Transfusion reaction causing extravascular hemolysis
    (C) Both
    (D) Neither

495. Can occur if the antibody that reacts with red cells is of the IgM or IgG type capable of activating complement through C9

496. May be rapid and may cause shock, DIC, back pain, and acute renal failure

497. Will usually require no specific therapy, though urinary output and hemoglobin should be followed

498. Can occur in acute and delayed hemolytic transfusion reactions

HEMATOLOGIC AND ONCOLOGIC DISORDERS IN THE CRITICALLY ILL

ANSWERS

459. The answer is C. *(Chapter 64)* Splenectomy should be avoided because it can result in marked platelet elevations and fatal vasoocclusive events.

460. The answer is D. *(Chapter 65)* The pentad of clinical findings in TTP is fever, microangiopathic hemolytic anemia, renal dysfunction, neurologic dysfunction, and thrombocytopenia.

461. The answer is C. *(Chapter 62)* This patient has a metabolic alkalosis resulting from citrate infusion. Citrate is used as an anticoagulant in the blood products during plasmapheresis and is converted to bicarbonate by the liver leading to metabolic alkalosis. Hypokalemia and volume contraction are other causes of metabolic alkalosis but are unlikely in this case.

462. The answer is E. *(Chapter 67)* Both chemotherapy and radiation therapy have pulmonary and cardiac toxicities that can result in dyspnea. Examples include radiation pneumonitis, congestive heart failure from adriamycin therapy, and radiation-induced constrictive pericarditis. Dyspnea is the most common symptom of superior vena cava syndrome. Pericardial tamponade and pulmonary embolism should always be considered and ruled out as causes of dyspnea in a patient with an underlying malignancy.

463. The answer is D. *(Chapter 66)* This patient's apparent hypoxemia is due to the high O_2 consumption of his white blood cells in the blood sample. Placement of the blood sample on ice will decrease the metabolism of the cells, and prompt measurement of the Pa_{O_2} will minimize the fall in Pa_{O_2}. This patient does not manifest signs of acute hypoxemic respiratory failure, and thus intubation is not indicated. Measurement of the carboxyhemoglobin level will be nonrevealing. Patients with carbon monoxide poisoning usually present with a normal Pa_{O_2} and a low oxyhemoglobin level. The use of co-oximetry will not correct the blood-gas analysis. The measurement of the initial blood gas accurately reflects the low Pa_{O_2} of the sample, resulting from blast cell consumption of oxygen.

464. The answer is D. *(Chapter 66)* Leukemic blast crisis, as represented in this case, constitutes an oncologic emergency. In addition to the metabolic derangements precipitated by the number of leukemic blasts, leukostasis involving multiple organs requires prompt attention. The goals of therapy involve reducing the tumor burden and decreasing serum viscosity. Leukophoresis is indicated in this condition for a rapid, although transient, reduction in the number of circulating blasts. While cytoreductive chemotherapy eventually will play an important role in the management of this patient, rapid destruction of this quantity of blasts probably will trigger massive metabolic derangements from tumor lysis syndrome. The use of leukophoresis before cytoreductive chemotherapy may decrease the tumor burden, resulting in less severe consequences of tumor lysis. Red blood cell transfusions should be avoided if at all possible because of the increase in serum viscosity associated with transfusions and the resulting increase in leukostasis. Anticoagulation with heparin will not prevent leukostasis, but will increase the risk of catastrophic bleeding.

465. **The answer is B.** *(Chapter 66)* This patient has agranulocytic enterocolitis, which is a complication of high-dose chemotherapy. Management consists of supportive care and antibiotics. However, patients with localizing signs or bowel perforation (if demonstrated by abdominal x-rays or other modalities) should have exploratory laparotomy. This patient was taken to the operating room, and an exploratory laparotomy was performed that revealed a ruptured appendix and peritonitis as well as diffuse bowel inflammation. Ascitic fluid cultures grew *Escherichia coli* and *Pseudomonas aeruginosa.* Steroids play no role in this condition, and the patient is not in respiratory failure and does not require intubation.

466. **The answer is B.** *(Chapter 69)* The majority of radiation effects are expressed at the time of cellular reproduction. The tissues most susceptible to the acute effects of radiotherapy are those which require continuous proliferation, such as skin, bone marrow, and gut mucosa. Nerve function does not require regular cellular renewal, and so this tissue is relatively resistant. Lung tissue is intermediate in sensitivity to radiation.

467. **The answer is E.** *(Chapter 69)* The working diagnosis for the described condition is radiation pneumonitis, given the presentation at 6 to 12 weeks after radiation, the limitation of the infiltrates to the radiation field, and the consistent symptoms. One may wish to pursue an open-lung biopsy to rule out lymphangitic spread of cancer definitively. Radiation pneumonitis has not been proved to be responsive to steroid therapy, though this may be tried in selected cases. Flares upon withdrawal of steroids have been well documented although poorly understood. Cyclosporine plays no role at present in the treatment of this disorder. While manifestations may occur outside the radiation field, particularly in patients who are also receiving chemotherapeutic agents, this is unusual.

468. **The answer is C.** *(Chapter 69)* This patient's chronic illness in the absence of metastatic disease, along with acute hypotension poorly responsive to fluids and vasoactive drugs, suggests a diagnosis of adrenal insufficiency. The presence of hyponatremia and eosinophilia makes the diagnosis highly likely. One of the complications of high-dose radiotherapy for nasopharyngeal carcinoma is pituitary failure, which can present as adrenal, thyroid, or gonadotropin insufficiency. Secondary adrenal insufficiency typically does not present with hypokalemia, since aldosterone production is not impaired. Treatment should begin immediately with dexamethasone (or hydrocortisone). The diagnosis can be confirmed if a random cortisol measurement is very low or by performing an ACTH stimulation test (as long as hydrocortisone has not been given). Norepinephrine is unlikely to raise the blood pressure adequately in adrenal insufficiency and does nothing to correct the fundamental problem. Mebendazole is an appropriate therapy for some parasitic infections, but the eosinophilia here is due to adrenal insufficiency. A pulmonary artery catheter might provide information useful in guiding fluid management; however, it will not treat the patient and is an unnecessary distraction in this critically ill patient.

469. **The answer is C.** *(Chapter 67)* Tumor lysis syndrome occurs after the treatment of certain malignancies that are exquisitely sensitive to the effects of chemotherapy. Burkitt lymphoma and leukemias are among the malignancies that are associated with this syndrome. Laboratory abnormalities include hyperuricemia, hyperkalemia, hyperphosphatemia, and lactic acidosis and result from rapid and massive killing of tumor cells, which release their intracellular contents into the bloodstream. Complications include tetany from hypocalcemia, cardiac arrhythmias from hypocalcemia and hyperkalemia, and renal failure from hyperuricemia.

470. **The answer is D.** *(Chapter 67)* To promote uricosuria, patients should be hydrated vigorously to ensure a urine output of at least 100 to 200 mL/h. The urine should be alkalinized. Allopurinol, which decreases the production of uric acid, should be administered. Hypocalcemia and hyperkalemia should be treated aggressively, potentially with hemodialysis.

471. **The answer is A (1, 2, 3).** *(Chapter 63)* Chloramphenicol, phenytoin, and cimetidine are all associated with toxic neutropenia. Amiodarone has multiple toxicities, including thrombocytopenia. Neutropenia, however, has not been attributed to the use of amiodarone.

472. **The answer is E (all).** *(Chapter 64)* All the listed factors are consistent with DIC. Elevated fibrin degradation products also would be expected.

473. **The answer is A (1, 2, 3).** *(Chapter 64)* Uremic bleeding is associated with platelet dysfunction and is corrected with desmopressin (DDAVP). The bleeding time is typically elevated. Dialysis, corticosteroids, and cryoprecipitate have been useful in certain patients.

474. **The answer is A (1, 2, 3).** *(Chapter 104)* This patient has acute chest syndrome, which presents with fever, chest pain, pulmonary infiltrates, and hypoxemia. Sludging in the hypoxic environment of the small pulmonary arterioles is the presumed cause of most cases of acute chest syndrome. Therapy should correct the hypoxemia and decrease the fraction of circulating hemoglobin that is sickle hemoglobin to minimize sludging. This patient was in respiratory failure and required intubation with mechanical ventilation. Broad-spectrum antibiotics should be used routinely, since infection may underlie the acute chest syndrome. Rarely can pneumonia be ruled out with confidence. Steroids play no role in the treatment of this condition.

475. **The answer is E (all).** *(Chapter 64)* Bleeding and sepsis can reduce platelet survival, and platelet transfusion can be used in these conditions for clinical bleeding. Idiopathic thrombocytopenic purpura (ITP) has been associated with the use of certain medications. Potential offending agents should be stopped, and intravenous γ-globulin may be administered for 3 to 5 days to enhance platelet survival. Many drug-related thrombocytopenias with diminished platelet survival are associated with antiplatelet antibodies.

476. **The answer is E (all).** *(Chapter 67)* The differential diagnosis of mental status changes in a patient with an underlying malignancy should include hypercalcemia, hyponatremia, uremia, sepsis, meningitis, leptomeningeal carcinomatosis, and brain metastases.

477. **The answer is A (1, 2, 3).** *(Chapter 68)* Patients with chronic GVHD have persistently decreased cell-mediated immunity and specific antibody responses. These alterations are due to the GVHD and are independent of immunosuppressive treatment.

478. **The answer is C (2, 4).** *(Chapter 67)* Pain localized to the spine or the paravertebral area is present in more than 90 percent of patients with compression of the spinal cord and is thus a very sensitive symptom. X-rays demonstrate destruction, collapse, or loss of pedicles in two-thirds of patients with back pain. These abnormalities will correctly predict the presence or absence of epidural metastases in over 80 percent of patients, but a myelogram, CT, or MRI is necessary to confirm the diagnosis. Patients who are ambulatory at diagnosis have a 65 to 80 percent chance of being ambulatory after therapy. Patients who are paraparetic at presentation have approximately a 50 percent chance of being ambulatory after treatment. For patients who are paraplegic at diagnosis, the morbidity of treatment outweighs the benefits.

479. **The answer is E (all).** *(Chapter 27)* Mesothelioma is a rare cause of pericardial effusion; however, it is the most common primary malignancy of the pericardium. Most malignant pericardial effusions represent disseminated malignancies, most often lung or breast cancer, leukemia, or lymphoma. Close to half of all pericardial effusions in cancer patients are nonmalignant in nature, related to previous radiation, chemotherapy, or infection. Others are sympathetic effusions.

480. **The answer is A (1, 2, 3).** *(Chapter 62)* Platelet transfusions usually are not effective in patients with rapid destruction (e.g., idiopathic thrombocytopenic purpura, drug-related thrombocytopenia) and may not be effective in patients with fever, sepsis, DIC, or platelet antibodies. Platelet transfusions are contraindicated in patients with thrombotic thrombocytopenic purpura and hemolytic-uremic syndrome. Dilutional thrombocytopenia, which usually is seen after a massive blood transfusion, can lead to difficulties with hemostasis and is readily treatable with platelet transfusion.

481. **The answer is E (all).** *(Chapter 62)* Plasmapheresis involves the removal of 1.5 L of plasma, which is then replaced with an albumin-salt solution. In addition to being useful in the disorders listed, plasmapheresis is considered useful in hyperviscosity syndromes, idiopathic, rapidly progressive glomerulonephritis, and rapidly progressive glomerulonephritis from vasculitis, overdose with certain drugs, and Guillain-Barré syndrome.

482–486. **The answers are 482-E, 483-C, 484-D, 485-A, 486-B.** *(Chapter 63)* Teardrop cells are seen in extramedullary hematopoesis, marrow replacement, iron deficiency, and myelodysplasia. Anemia in thrombotic thrombocytopenic purpura is due to microangiopathic hemolytic anemia with schistocytes. Target cells are seen in liver disease, iron deficiency, and hemoglobinopathies. Howell-Jolly bodies are seen with splenectomy, and Heinz bodies are characteristic of glucose 6-phosphate dehydrogenase deficiency.

487–490. **The answers are 487-E, 488-B, 489-D, 490-A.** *(Chapter 69)* Cisplatin is associated with renal toxicity that can include severe magnesium wasting. Bleomycin can cause severe pulmonary fibrosis, and it is generally recommended to limit supplemental oxygen to less than 30% to avoid the potentiation of injury. Methotrexate in association with cranial irradiation can cause multifocal leukoencephalopathy, which presents with confusion and long-tract signs. Vinblastine and vincristine cause autonomic and peripheral neuropathy. Severe autonomic neuropathy is thought to be the cause of ileus.

491–494. **The answers are 491-C, 492-B, 493-A, 494-D.** *(Chapter 68)* Graft-versus-host disease (GVHD) is a complication of bone marrow transplantation (BMT) that is characterized by an immunologic reaction between donor lymphocytes and "foreign" antigens present on host tissue. GVHD is categorized as acute or chronic on the basis of the time of presentation (before or after 3 months), organ involvement, and histology. Mortality in both acute and chronic GVHD is most affected by infectious complications. The development of histologic bronchiolitis obliterans is recognized in up to 10 percent of patients who receive allogeneic BMTs. Patients with acute GVHD may develop airflow obstruction; however, the histologic appearance differs from the classic obliterative bronchiditis seen in patients with chronic GVHD. Acute GVHD commonly affects the gastrointestinal tract, often producing copious bloody diarrhea. The pathogenesis is usually noninfectious inflammation of the GI tract, although infections such as CMV may be seen. Diarrhea in chronic GVHD is less common and usually represents an infectious pathogen. GVHD is rarely seen in autologous BMT given the lack of donor-recipient antigenic disparity.

495–498. **The answers are 495-A, 496-A, 497-A, 498-C.** *(Chapter 62)* Intravascular hemolysis occurs when IgM or IgG antibody binds complement through C9. It can be rapid, occurring after only a few milliliters of blood is transfused, and can lead to shock, acute renal failure, and DIC. Symptoms include fever and chills, headache, back pain, and chest pain. Treatment includes stopping the transfusion immediately and administering fluids and furosemide. Extravascular hemolysis occurs with IgG or IgM antibodies that do not bind complement. The reaction is usually not clinically severe, but fever and chills, hyperbilirubinemia, and anemia may occur.

RENAL AND METABOLIC DISORDERS IN THE CRITICALLY ILL

QUESTIONS

DIRECTIONS: Each question below contains four or five suggested responses. Select the **one best** response to each question.

499. All the following may contribute to myoglobinuric nephropathy EXCEPT

(A) uric acid precipitation
(B) ferrihemate tubular toxicity
(C) ischemia of the nephron resulting from vasoconstriction
(D) ureteral obstruction
(E) oxygen free radicals formed by iron derived from heme groups

500. A correct statement regarding rhabdomyolysis is

(A) muscle pain is a uniform complaint in an awake patient with rhabdomyolysis
(B) release of myoglobin into the urine causes urinary discoloration
(C) the influx of fluid into damaged muscle cells often leads to intravascular volume depletion
(D) the absence of myoglobinuria essentially rules out the diagnosis of rhabdomyolysis
(E) hypophosphatemia is a known complication of rhabdomyolysis that requires prompt attention

501. All the following drugs cause hyperkalemia EXCEPT

(A) heparin
(B) captopril
(C) theophylline
(D) propranolol
(E) ibuprofen

502. A 35-year-old woman with a history of sarcoidosis complicated by invasive aspergillosis is admitted with hemoptysis and undergoes resection of the left upper lobe. She had received amphotericin B for treatment of the aspergillosis and now describes a 3-month history of anosmia and polyuria. Postoperatively, she is noted to have polyuria (urine volume 4.5 L for 24 hours). Physical examination is notable for tachycardia and orthostatic hypotension. Laboratory data reveal a sodium of 162 and a serum osmolarity of 324. All the following statements are true EXCEPT

(A) the presence or absence of thirst would help distinguish the cause of the polyuria and hypernatremia
(B) fluid deprivation will help distinguish the cause of the polyuria and hypernatremia
(C) the administration of desmopressin (DDAVP) will distinguish the cause of the polyuria and hypernatremia
(D) replacement of free water should occur over 36 to 72 hours to avoid cerebral edema
(E) further pituitary evaluation probably is indicated

503. A 38-year-old woman with a history of hypothyroidism presents with a 7-day history of weakness, fatigue, anorexia, nausea, diarrhea, poor oral intake, and a low-grade fever. She also reports a 15-lb weight loss over the last 3 months. Blood pressure is 80/40 mm Hg, falling to 60/palpable when rising. Pulse is 115, and temperature 38.0°C (100.4°F). Except for dry mucous membranes, the remainder of the physical examination is unremarkable. Laboratory data include a white blood cell count of 11,000/mm^3 with no premature forms, hemoglobin 11.0 g/dL, sodium 125 mEq/L, potassium 5.1 mEq/L, blood urea nitrogen 50 mg/dL, and creatinine 2.1 mg/dL. The best next step in this patient's management would be

(A) treatment with vigorous intravenous hydration followed by careful observation of the response to therapy
(B) measurement of a random cortisol level followed by vigorous intravenous hydration and careful observation of the response to therapy
(C) performance of a rapid ACTH stimulation test followed by vigorous intravenous hydration and a careful observation of the response to therapy
(D) treatment with 4 mg intravenous dexamethasone and vigorous intravenous hydration followed by a rapid ACTH stimulation test and careful observation of the response to therapy

504. A 40-year-old woman with a history of chronic renal insufficiency presents with a blood pressure of 80/40 mm Hg and a heart rate of 130 beats per minute. The laboratory abnormality most suggestive of the diagnosis of adrenocortical insufficiency would be

(A) hyperkalemia
(B) hyponatremia
(C) hypoglycemia
(D) hypercalcemia
(E) anemia

505. Diabetic ketoacidosis results from insulin deficiency in concert with elevation of all the following EXCEPT

(A) epinephrine
(B) somatostatin
(C) growth hormone
(D) glucocorticoids
(E) glucagon

506. Which of the following principles is correct for the interpretation of arterial blood gas data?

(A) The magnitude of bicarbonate compensation is the same for the acute and chronic primary respiratory disorders
(B) Alveolar ventilation completely compensates for metabolic acid-base disturbances
(C) Bicarbonate is directly measured by most blood-gas machines
(D) Secondary compensation for a primary acid-base disturbance is never complete
(E) Muscle and kidney contribute equally in the compensation for respiratory acid-base disturbances

507. A 24-year-old man is found unconscious. The arterial blood gas analysis reveals a pH 7.24, Pa$_{CO_2}$ 60, and Pa$_{O_2}$ 70. The acid-base disorder is

(A) metabolic acidosis
(B) respiratory acidosis and metabolic alkalosis
(C) respiratory acidosis and metabolic acidosis
(D) acute respiratory acidosis
(E) respiratory alkalosis and metabolic alkalosis

Questions 508–509.

508. A 72-year-old man weighing 60 kg is brought to the intensive care unit with acute mental status changes. His serum Na is 168 mEq/L, blood pressure is 90/65 mm Hg, and heart rate is 120 beats per minute. He has poor skin turgor. The free water (liters) required to normalize serum sodium is approximately

(A) 3
(B) 4
(C) 5
(D) 6
(E) 7

509. In the patient described above, which of the following is true?

(A) Rapid normalization of the serum Na may lead to central pontine myelinolysis
(B) The initial fluid of choice to reverse the hyperosmolar state is intravenous 5% dextrose in water
(C) This condition puts him at risk for intracranial hemorrhage
(D) The free water deficit should be corrected to decrease the serum Na by 3 to 4 mEq/L per hour
(E) If corrected appropriately, mortality is less than 10 percent

DIRECTIONS: Each question below contains four suggested responses of which **one or more** is correct. Select

A   if   **1, 2, and 3**   are correct
B   if   **1 and 3**   are correct
C   if   **2 and 4**   are correct
D   if   **4**   is correct
E   if   **1, 2, 3, and 4**   are correct

Questions 510–511

A 57-year-old woman with long-standing COPD and diabetes mellitus has a pelvic mass detected on physical examination and confirmed by infused CT. Three days later, the patient develops fever, nausea, vomiting, and diarrhea. In the emergency room her BUN is 50 mg/dL, her creatinine is 3.6 mg/dL, and her potassium is 7.2 mmol/L. Urine output is 15 mL/h, and urine sodium is less than 10 mEq/L. ECG shows widening of the QRS complex with occasional ventricular ectopy.

510. Possible diagnoses include

(1) hypovolemia
(2) tumor lysis syndrome
(3) myocardial dysfunction
(4) acute tubular necrosis

511. Appropriate management in the first hour includes

(1) intravenous calcium
(2) hydration with 0.9% normal saline
(3) renal ultrasound
(4) lidocaine

512. Risk factors for contrast nephropathy include

(1) previous contrast nephropathy
(2) diabetes mellitus
(3) gout
(4) volume depletion

513. The use of continuous venovenous hemofiltration dialysis (CVVHD) may be preferable to conventional hemodialysis in which of the following settings?

(1) Severe peripheral vascular disease limiting available central venous access
(2) Heparin-induced platelet antibodies limiting the use of anticoagulation
(3) Life-threatening pulmonary edema caused by massive volume overload
(4) Cardiovascular instability that limits rapid ultrafiltration

514. Antibiotics that can be given to patients with acute renal failure without dosage adjustment include

(1) amphotericin B
(2) clindamycin
(3) erythromycin
(4) ciprofloxacin

515. Appropriate guidelines for fluid correction in hyponatremia include

(1) serum sodium should not increase > 20 to 25 mEq/L during the first 48 hours
(2) the maximum level of serum sodium during acute correction is 150 mEq/L
(3) hypernatremia should be avoided
(4) hypertonic saline (3%) should not be used

516. Lactic acidosis is likely to occur in which of the following clinical situations?

(1) Shock
(2) Cyanide intoxication
(3) Fulminant hepatic failure
(4) Isoniazid intoxication

517. A 24-year-old man was crushed in a construction accident. Evaluation in the emergency room revealed evidence of head trauma and multiple fractures. Evaluation of the head trauma with plain films of the skull and CT of the head revealed no fractures or intracranial fluid collections. The patient's fractures were externally stabilized. He was treated with aggressive volume resuscitation (300 mL/h) and received bicarbonate and mannitol. Urine volumes in excess of 150 mL/h were maintained for the first 72 hours to prevent the development of myoglobinuric renal failure. On the fourth hospital day fluids were restricted to maintenance, but polyuria persisted. Plasma sodium was 138 mEq/L. Further evaluation should include

(1) fluid deprivation
(2) discontinuation of mannitol
(3) measurement of urine osmolarity
(4) administration of desmopressin

518. Which of the following arguments may be made against the use of bicarbonate therapy in lactic acidosis?

(1) Bicarbonate infusion may worsen intracellular acidosis

(2) Bicarbonate administration may cause systemic vasodilation and hypotension

(3) Bicarbonate administration may decrease ionized calcium levels

(4) The reduction in hydrogen ion concentration gained by bicarbonate administration may be diminished if the lungs are unable to excrete the carbon dioxide produced

519. Which of the following statements may be made in support of bicarbonate therapy for lactic acidosis?

(1) Diminished contractility occurs in isolated cardiac muscle exposed to an acidic milieu

(2) Cardiac output improves in patients with lactic acidosis treated with sodium bicarbonate but not with a similar infusion of sodium chloride

(3) Decreased densities of beta-adrenergic receptors occur in cells exposed to an acidic milieu

(4) Treatment with bicarbonate results in decreased production of lactic acid

520. Complications of aggressive therapy for diabetic keto-acidosis include

(1) hyperchloremic metabolic acidosis

(2) hypocalcemia

(3) cerebral edema

(4) hypokalemia

521. A 75-year-old woman is brought to the emergency room unresponsive. Her examination is notable for a temperature of 34.0°C (93.2°F), pulse of 90 beats per minute, and blood pressure of 95/60 mm Hg. Her skin is dry and coarse with scaling of the knees and elbows. Her cardiac and lung exams are relatively normal. She is responsive to painful stimuli only, moving all four extremities. Her deep tendon reflexes are delayed. Laboratory evaluation reveals a white blood cell count of 18,000 cells/mm^3 with 25 percent bands, and her hematocrit is 26.4 percent. Urinalysis reveals > 20 WBC/hpf with many bacteria. The sodium is 124, potassium 6.8, BUN 68, and creatinine 4.5. ABG reveals a pH 7.25, Pa$_{CO_2}$ 55, and Pa$_{O_2}$ 60. The serum thyroxine level is 1.5 mg/dL, and the thyroid-stimulating hormone level is 7.0 mU/L. Initial management should include

(1) intravenous thyroxine (T$_4$)

(2) tri-iodothyroxine (T$_3$) per nasogastric tube

(3) intravenous hydrocortisone

(4) intubation and mechanical ventilation

522. A 67-year-old woman with a diagnosis of hyperthyroidism made 1 year earlier is admitted to the intensive care unit. Her initial thyrotoxicosis had been managed with propylthiouracil, which had been stopped because of evidence of hepatotoxicity and a skin rash. Thyroidectomy had been planned, but the patient was lost to follow-up. She now presents with a 2-month history of weight loss and diarrhea. Her family indicates that her behavior has become increasingly bizarre in the past 2 days. There is no history of drug use. On initial examination she is febrile to 39°C (102.2°F) orally, with a pulse of 158, blood pressure of 150/60, and respiratory rate of 28. She is tremulous. There is a goiter but no exophthalmos. Her neurologic examination shows no focal abnormality or meningeal signs, but she is confused and her behavior is inappropriate. Initial drug management should include

(1) intravenous hydrocortisone after a cortisol level is obtained

(2) intravenous sodium iodide

(3) oral iopanoic acid (Telepaque)

(4) intravenous propranolol

523. True statements about the rapid ACTH stimulation test include which of the following?

(1) A blunted or flat cortisol response can be due to primary or secondary adrenocortical insufficiency

(2) The test is only a screening procedure

(3) A normal response eliminates the possibility of primary adrenocortical insufficiency

(4) A normal response eliminates the possibility of secondary adrenocortical insufficiency

524. True statements about the physiologic stress response that occurs in critically ill patients include which of the following?

(1) It has been shown to occur in patients who are comatose

(2) It results in decreased release of renin and angiotension

(3) It results in increased release of ACTH

(4) It results in increased immunity and a decreased chance of infection

525. Causes of lactic acidosis include

(1) hypoxemia

(2) liver failure

(3) methanol

(4) extreme exercise

526. Causes of hypomagnesemia include

(1) gastrointestinal tract losses

(2) skin losses

(3) renal losses

(4) internal redistribution

DIRECTIONS: Each group of questions below consists of lettered headings followed by a set of numbered items. For each numbered item select the **one** lettered heading with which it is **most** closely associated. Each lettered heading may be used **once, more than once, or not at all.**

Questions 527–530.

Match each patient with the appropriate lettered set of blood-gas measurements.

	pH	Pa_{CO_2}	Pa_{O_2}	HCO_3
(A)	7.39	68	48	40
(B)	7.05	19	124	5
(C)	7.31	15	120	7
(D)	7.14	80	60	26
(E)	7.33	80	32	40

527.   A 22-year-old woman with diabetes mellitus

528.   A 33-year-old man with severe kyphoscoliosis and protracted vomiting from small bowel obstruction

529.   A 42-year-old woman who presents with paresis after eating last summer's home-grown tomatoes

530.   A 17-year-old boy with agitation, tinnitus, abdominal pain, and nausea after a drug overdose

Questions 531–534.

Match the factors below with the appropriate acid-base status.

(A) Metabolic acidosis (elevated anion gap)
(B) Metabolic acidosis (normal anion gap)
(C) Metabolic alkalosis (chloride-unresponsive)
(D) Metabolic alkalosis (chloride-responsive)

531.   Administration of acetazolamide

532.   Nasogastric suctioning

533.   Administration of corticosteroids

534.   Diarrhea

DIRECTIONS: Each group of questions below consists of four lettered headings followed by a set of numbered items. For each numbered item select

A   if the item is associated with   (A) **only**
B   if the item is associated with   (B) **only**
C   if the item is associated with   **both** (A) and (B)
D   if the item is associated with   **neither** (A) nor (B)

Each lettered heading may be used **once, more than once, or not at all.**

Questions 535–536.

  (A) Hypophosphatemia
  (B) Hyperphosphatemia
  (C) Both
  (D) Neither

535. Focal neurologic findings

536. Cardiomyopathy

Questions 537–540.

  (A) Autoimmune adrenalitis
  (B) Adrenal hemorrhage
  (C) Both
  (D) Neither

537. May be associated with gastrointestinal symptoms and signs

538. May be associated with a sudden fall in hematocrit

539. May present without the typical laboratory abnormalities of Addison disease

540. May be associated with vitiligo

Questions 541–543.

  (A) Hypomagnesemia
  (B) Hypermagnesemia
  (C) Both
  (D) Neither

541. Coma

542. Respiratory depression

543. Tetany

Questions 544–545.

  (A) Euthyroid sick syndrome
  (B) Primary hypothyroidism
  (C) Both
  (D) Neither

544. Elevated reverse T_3 concentration

545. Decreased T_4 concentration

Questions 546–548.

  (A) Alcoholic ketoacidosis
  (B) Diabetic ketoacidosis
  (C) Both
  (D) Neither

546. Extremely high ratio of β-hydroxybutyrate to acetoacetate exists

547. Hepatic synthesis of ketoacids exceeds peripheral utilization of them

548. Free fatty acids are very high, and insulin is barely detectable

Questions 549–551.

  (A) Hypomagnesemia
  (B) Hypocalcemia
  (C) Both
  (D) Neither

549. Will potentiate the toxic effects of digoxin

550. Can cause refractory hypokalemia

551. Can cause nephrogenic diabetes insipidus

Questions 552–553.

(A) Cerebral edema with herniation
(B) Central pontine myelinolysis
(C) Both
(D) Neither

552.   A 50-year-old alcoholic was found lethargic at his apartment. Neurologic evaluation revealed no focal abnormalities and only a minimal reaction to voice. Evaluation disclosed an initial serum sodium of 106 mEq/L. The patient is corrected rapidly with hypertonic saline to a serum sodium of 140 mEq/L over 12 hours. Four days later, he develops quadriparesis, a diminished level of consciousness, and cranial nerve abnormalities.

553.   A 42-year-old woman received chemotherapy for lymphoma. For 1 week she experienced diarrhea with 15 to 20 watery stools per day. The nursing staff noted that she had become somnolent, with a heart rate of 125 and blood pressure of 110/80 mm Hg with an orthostatic change of 25 mm Hg. Stat laboratory determinations reveal a serum sodium of 155 mEq/L.

RENAL AND METABOLIC DISORDERS IN THE CRITICALLY ILL

ANSWERS

499. The answer is D. *(Chapter 71)* Obstructive uropathy does not play a major role in the development of myoglobinuric renal failure at the macroscopic level. Potential mechanisms for the development of myoglobinuric nephropathy include tubular obstruction from urate crystals or pigment, direct cellular toxicity from myoglobin or ferrihemate, formation of oxygen free radicals by the heme groups of myoglobin, and ischemia secondary to decreased renal perfusion or local vasospasm.

500. The answer is C. *(Chapter 71)* Profound hypovolemia is a known complication of rhabdomyolysis that occasionally can progress to shock. The cause of hypovolemia is believed to be the influx of fluid into damaged skeletal muscle cells. The signs and symptoms of rhabdomyolysis, including muscle pain, weakness, and paresthesias, may assist in the diagnosis of this disorder but often are obscured or absent. Myoglobin visibly discolors urine at concentrations over 100 mg/L. Even in cases with severe muscle destruction, urine myoglobin rarely exceeds 25 mg/L. Myoglobinuria, when present, supports the diagnosis of rhabdomyolysis. It is not, however, uniformly present. Hyperphosphatemia is a known complication of rhabdomyolysis. Severe hypophosphatemia, by contrast, may predispose patients to the development of rhabdomyolysis.

501. The answer is C. *(Chapter 73)* Theophylline and β agonists are drugs that can cause hypokalemia. In addition to the other listed drugs, digitalis, succinylcholine, and α-methyldopa may cause hyperkalemia.

502. The answer is B. *(Chapter 73)* The patient has multiple possible causes of polyuria. These include neurogenic diabetes insipidus (DI) caused by sarcoidosis, nephrogenic DI resulting from sarcoidosis or amphotericin B, and secondary DI caused by resetting of the thirst osmostat (yet another potential complication of neurosarcoidosis). The development of hypernatremia excludes the diagnosis of secondary DI. Therefore, administration of DDAVP should be the next diagnostic step, although the presence of thirst would support the diagnosis of nephrogenic DI. Given the significant hypernatremia, replacement of free water is indicated and should proceed at a moderate pace to avoid the development of cerebral edema. If neurogenic DI is diagnosed, further pituitary evaluation is indicated.

503. The answer is D. *(Chapter 76)* In a young woman with a history of endocrine disease who presents with systemic symptoms, gastrointestinal complaints, hypotension, hyperkalemia, and hyponatremia, one should strongly consider the diagnosis of adrenocortical insufficiency secondary to autoimmune adrenalitis. Because adrenocortical insufficiency is fatal if untreated and because the side effects of 24 hours of glucocorticoids are minimal, one should treat with corticosteroids while awaiting the results of the rapid ACTH stimulation test. Dexamethasone should be the initial therapy because it does not interfere with the assay for cortisol. Since dexamethasone has no mineralocorticoid activity, hydrocortisone should be substituted immediately after diagnostic testing.

504.   The answer is C.   *(Chapter 76)*   Although hyperkalemia, hyponatremia, hypercalcemia, hypoglycemia, and anemia are found in patients with adrenocortical insufficiency, these laboratory abnormalities are neither sensitive nor specific markers of this disease. In the setting of hypotension, however, hypoglycemia should always raise the possibility of adrenocortical insufficiency. In a normal person, hypotension is associated with elevated levels of "stress hormones" such as cortisol and catecholamines, which should cause hyper- or at least normoglycemia.

505.   The answer is B.   *(Chapter 75)*   Diabetic ketoacidosis is a potentially life-threatening complication of insulin deficiency. Hyperglycemia and ketosis result from an imbalance of hormones characterized by diminished insulin and increased levels of catecholamines, glucagon, growth hormone, and glucocorticoids. Somatostatin is not directly associated with diabetic ketoacidosis but functions to down-regulate the production and release of both glucagon and growth hormone.

506.   The answer is D.   *(Chapter 74)*   The kidneys seek to compensate for primary respiratory disturbances, with the degree of compensation better in chronic disorders. Alveolar ventilation does not completely compensate for all the metabolic disturbance, often being in the range of 50 percent for metabolic acidosis. The secondary compensation for a primary acid-base derangement is never complete. Indeed, "complete compensation" indicates that another primary acid-base derangement is present.

507.   The answer is D.   *(Chapter 74)*   An acute rise in Pa_{CO_2} leads to a predictable fall in pH. For each rise of 10 mm Hg in Pa_{CO_2}, pH falls by 0.08 unit. Similarly, when there is an acute fall in Pa_{CO_2} of 10 mm Hg, pH rises by 0.08 units.

508.   The answer is E.   *(Chapter 73)*   The free water required to normalize serum sodium can be calculated from the following formula: free water deficit (L) = (Na − 140) / 140 × body weight (kg) × 0.6. In this example: [(168 − 140) / 140] × 6.0 × 0.6 ≅ 7.

509.   The answer is C.   *(Chapter 73)*   Acute hypernatremia may lead to neuronal shrinkage with physical separation of the brain from the meninges and a subdural or intraparenchymal hemorrhage. Central pontine myelinolysis is seen with rapid correction of hyponatremia. Initial volume resuscitation should be with crystalloid (0.9% NS) until the patient is approaching euvolemia. This may be combined with enteral tap water if the patient can tolerate enteral fluid administration. D_5W may exacerbate hyperosmolar states because of hyperglycemia resulting from peripheral insulin resistance. Serum Na levels should be decreased no greater than 1.5 to 2 mEq/L per hour. Symptomatic hypernatremia is associated with mortality greater than 40 percent in the elderly.

510.   The answer is A (1, 2, 3).   *(Chapter 70)*   A low urine sodium in the face of oliguric renal failure is most suggestive of prerenal azotemia. Decreased renal perfusion commonly result from either hypotension or myocardial dysfunction. Additional causes of oliguric renal failure with low U_{Na} include acute glomerulonephritis, early urinary obstruction, contrast nephropathy, interstitial nephritis, rhabdomyolysis, and uric acid nephropathy. The tumor lysis syndrome may cause oliguric renal failure by a variety of mechanisms, including formation of uric acid nephropathy. Acute tubular necrosis may cause oliguric renal failure but seldom is associated with a U_{Na} less than one.

511.   The answer is A (1, 2, 3).   *(Chapter 73)*   Hyperkalemia manifested by widening of the QRS complex on ECG demands prompt attention. Early intervention to stabilize the myocardial cell membrane with calcium administration is indicated in this patient. Glucose, insulin, and bicarbonate therapy also should be considered in an effort to shift potassium intracellularly. Finally, polystyrene sulfate may be employed to bind and remove potassium through the GI tract. Hemodialysis should be reserved for severe hyperkalemia and hyperkalemia that does not respond to the above interventions. Additional evaluation, including renal ultrasound, is indicated in this patient to rule out urinary obstruction.

Treatment of hypovolemia secondary to fever, diarrhea, and vomiting may be accomplished by hydration with 0.9% normal saline. Lidocaine is not indicated in the treatment of this patient.

512. **The answer is E (all).** *(Chapter 72)* In addition to the listed risk factors, preexisting renal failure, multiple contrast procedures, a high contrast dose, congestive heart failure, myeloma, and old age are risk factors for contrast nephropathy.

513. **The answer is D (4).** *(Chapter 72)* The primary indication for the use of continuous venovenous hemofiltration dialysis (CVVHD) instead of conventional hemodialysis is a patient with cardiovascular instability that demonstrates unacceptable hypotension during hemodialysis. CVVHD permits both ultrafiltration and dialysis at a relatively slow rate that limits cardiovascular complications such as significant hypotension. Like conventional hemodialysis, CVVHD requires large-bore central venous access and necessitates anticoagulation to prevent clotting of the dialysis filter. CVVHD does not provide a distinct advantage over hemodialysis in the rapid removal of volume in patients with life-threatening states of massive volume overload.

514. **The answer is A (1, 2, 3).** *(Chapter 72)* It is important to review the indications for and dosages of all drugs given to patients with renal failure. Among the listed antibiotics, only ciprofloxacin requires dosage adjustment in patients with renal failure. Other antibiotics that can be given without an alteration in dosage include nafcillin, rifampin, isoniazid, and chloramphenicol.

515. **The answer is B (1, 3).** *(Chapter 73)* Controversy exists about the appropriate rate of correction of hyponatremia because overly rapid correction may result in the rare but devastating syndrome of central pontine myelinolysis. Most experts agree that the serum sodium should not increase more than 20 to 25 mEq/L during the first 48 hours of therapy, regardless of its initial value. Hypernatremia should be avoided, and the maximum level of serum sodium should not exceed 130 mEq/L during acute correction. Hypertonic saline may be used safely if the above guidelines are followed.

516. **The answer is E (all).** *(Chapter 74)* Lactic acidosis is a common problem seen in the intensive care unit. It is most often due to tissue hypoperfusion, as seen in shock or local ischemia. It also may complicate intoxications in which oxygen delivery is impaired (carbon monoxide poisoning), intoxications in which oxidative phosphorylation is inhibited (cyanide poisoning), fulminant hepatic failure in which lactic acid metabolism is impaired, and ingestions of certain drugs, such as isoniazid and metformin.

517. **The answer is A (1, 2, 3).** *(Chapter 73)* The polyuria in this patient probably is due to excess administration of water. Other potential causes include solute diuresis resulting from administration of mannitol and loss of the medullary concentrating gradient after massive diuresis. The presence of hypertonic urine would support mannitol as the cause of the polyuria. Discontinuation of mannitol would confirm this suspicion. If the urine is hypotonic, either excess administration of water persists or the medullary concentrating gradient has been "washed out." Neurogenic diabetes insipidus is possible given the history of head trauma, but without any other manifestation of significant injury, it is unlikely. Fluid restriction would confirm the diagnosis of excess administration of water and would be therapeutic in reestablishing the medullary concentrating gradient.

518. **The answer is A (1, 2, 3).** *(Chapter 74)* Bicarbonate administration has several potential disadvantages. When bicarbonate combines with hydrogen ions, it produces carbon dioxide, which may diffuse into cells faster than does the bicarbonate. This intracellular excess of carbon dioxide may cause the generation of hydrogen ions. Also, when administered as a bolus, bicarbonate may cause systemic vasodilation and hypotension. This effect may be due to its osmotic effects. In patients who have received bicarbonate therapy, there is a significant fall in ionized calcium. This decrease in calcium may cause

decreased contractility as well as systemic vasodilation. Bicarbonate administration, while perhaps worsening intracellular acidosis, does not cause an extracellular respiratory acidosis per se. Any rehydration of carbon dioxide to carbonic acid in the extracellular space will only return the hydrogen ion concentration toward its original value. No additional hydrogen ions are formed.

519.   The answer is B (1, 3).   *(Chapter 74)*   Myocardial tissue exposed to an acidic milieu demonstrates decreased contractility, perhaps because of decreased availability of intracellular calcium. This decrease in contractility may be worsened by the decreased responsiveness to β-adrenergic agents mediated by a decrease in receptor density. Some patients treated with sodium bicarbonate do demonstrate an increase in cardiac output; however, in a controlled study the improvement in cardiac output was due to the volume response to bicarbonate infusion rather than to its effect on hydrogen ion concentration. Furthermore, treatment with bicarbonate has been demonstrated in animal models to increase the production of lactic acid.

520.   The answer is E (all).   *(Chapter 75)*   Careful monitoring of the patient's physical status, fluid intake, and electrolytes should prevent most complications of therapy for diabetic ketoacidosis. Hyperchloremic metabolic acidosis results from overaggressive rehydration with normal saline. Hypocalcemia can result from overaggressive replacement of phosphorus. Hypokalemia may be present initially, and potassium levels may fall with therapy. Cerebral edema, the most worrisome complication, is more common in children and can be fatal. Aggressive hydration, especially with hypotonic fluids, may contribute to this complication.

521.   The answer is E (all).   *(Chapter 77)*   This patient has classic myxedema coma, probably triggered by a urosepsis. Some questions may remain about the risk of thyroid replacement in an elderly patient with hypothyroidism; however, treatment of a patient with myxedema coma should not be delayed. T_4 and T_3 should be administered immediately. The addition of T_3 provides active hormone, which is essential given the delay in peripheral conversion of T_4 to T_3 in critical illness. The availability of intravenous T_3 is often limited, leading to the need for nasogastric administration. Steroid requirements for patients with myxedema coma often are reduced. However, 5 to 10 percent of these patients have associated primary hypoadrenalism. Supplemental corticosteroid should be administered until the function of the pituitary-adrenal axis is evaluated. This patient also has evidence of hypoventilatory respiratory failure, probably the result of profound hypothyroidism. Early intubation and mechanical ventilation should be considered in all patients with myxedema coma who present with cardiopulmonary instability.

522.   The answer is A (1, 2, 3).   *(Chapter 77)*   This patient is presenting in thyroid storm, as indicated by the fever, mental status changes, and hyperdynamic circulation. In view of a significant prior history of hepatotoxicity and possible allergy to propylthiouracil, this medication should not be used in her management. Iodine and oral cholecystographic agents can be used to block hormonal secretion, although extremely careful monitoring will be required since they will be administered without the usual antithyroid medications. Since some patients with thyroid storm are adrenally insufficient owing to high turnover of corticosteroids, exogenous steroids are advised initially. Propranolol is not recommended for thyroid storm, particularly in the elderly and patients with asthma or ventricular dysfunction.

523.   The answer is A (1, 2, 3).   *(Chapter 76)*   The rapid ACTH stimulation test is only a screening procedure, and the results should be verified by a more definitive test when the patient's condition stabilizes. Since this investigation tests the integrity of the entire hypothalamic-pituitary axis, an abnormal response can be due to either primary or secondary adrenocortical insufficiency. Although a normal response eliminates the possibility of primary disease, false-negative results have been reported in rare patients with secondary adrenocortical insufficiency and patients with early ACTH deficiency.

524. The answer is B (1, 3). *(Chapter 10)* Critical illness frequently triggers a physiologic stress response, and this has been shown to occur even in patients who are comatose. It also has been shown to result in sympathetic nervous system activation with release of catecholamines, increased corticotropic releasing factor with increased ACTH release, increased (not decreased) release of renin and angiotensin, and decreased immunity.

525. The answer is E (all). *(Chapter 74)* Excess lactic acid can result from overproduction or underconsumption. Failure of adequate oxygen delivery to individual tissues (e.g., bowel ischemia) or to all organs (e.g., hypoxemia, anemia, cardiogenic shock) results in overproduction of lactic acid. Similarly, lactic acidosis results when oxygen delivery is normal but insufficient for excessive activity (e.g., exercise, seizures). Other causes of lactic acidosis include failure of cellular oxygen utilization such as occurs with cyanide, carbon monoxide, salicylate, and methanol poisoning and underconsumption of lactate as occurs with liver failure.

526. The answer is E (all). *(Chapter 73)* The primary sources of magnesium loss include the gastrointestinal tract and the kidney. Rarely, magnesium is lost from the skin (e.g., with severe burns) or is redistributed internally (e.g., during treatment of diabetic ketoacidosis), resulting in hypomagnesemia.

527–530. The answers are 527-B, 528-A, 529-D, 530-C. *(Chapter 75)* Diabetic keto-acidosis usually results in a pure metabolic acidosis. Such an acidosis would be expected to decrease the Pa_{CO_2} by 1.0 to 1.5 mm Hg for each millimole change in the bicarbonate concentration.

Severe chest wall restriction may cause chronic alveolar hypoventilation and lead to the development of chronic respiratory acidosis. Chronic respiratory acidosis is characterized by an increase in the bicarbonate concentration of approximately 4 mmol for each rise of 10 mm Hg in the Pa_{CO_2}. In this instance, both the pH and the bicarbonate concentration are higher than expected for the level of Pa_{CO_2} elevation, suggesting the diagnosis of a mixed acid-base disorder, specifically, a metabolic acidosis superimposed on a chronic respiratory acidosis.

Botulism, intoxication with the neurotoxin produced by *Clostridium botulinum,* may cause the rapid onset of frank respiratory failure. Symptoms may include nausea and vomiting. Physical examination may be notable for orthostatic hypotension, ophthalmoplegia and ptosis, dilated pupils, and erythematous oropharynx and dry mouth. Weakness is descending in its progression, which may be rapid. Acute respiratory failure usually causes a pure respiratory acidosis, unless the associated hypoxemia causes tissue hypoxia, in which case a combined respiratory and metabolic acidosis ensues. In acute respiratory acidosis, the pH is expected to fall by approximately 0.08 unit for each increase of 10 mm Hg in the Pa_{CO_2}. The plasma bicarbonate may increase by 1 mmol/L for each increase of 10 mm Hg in the Pa_{CO_2}, somewhat ameliorating the increases in hydrogen ion concentration.

Salicylate intoxication may cause an acute metabolic acidosis. However, in younger patients it also may stimulate respiration and lead to a coincident respiratory alkalosis. In this instance, the decrease in Pa_{CO_2} is out of proportion to the fall in plasma bicarbonate, which suggests a mixed acid-base disorder, specifically, a combined metabolic acidosis and respiratory alkalosis.

531–534. The answers are 531-B, 532-D, 533-C, 534-B. *(Chapter 74)* Acetazolamide is a carbonic anhydrase inhibitor that results in bicarbonate wasting. Nasogastric suctioning and vomiting result in direct loss of hydrogen ions from the body and a "contraction alkalosis" through a renal mechanism (chloride and volume are lost in the gastric fluid, resulting in secondary hyperaldosteronism and consequent renal acidification). Similarly, corticosteroids directly stimulate distal nephron acidification through their mineralocorticoid effects. Diarrhea most often results in gastrointestinal bicarbonate loss and a normal anion gap metabolic acidosis.

535–536. The answers are 535-A, 536-A. *(Chapter 73)* The acute manifestations of phosphorus deficiency include central nervous system dysfunction (lethargy, altered mental status, focal neurologic findings), muscular weakness and rhabdomyolysis, hemolytic anemia, and defects in platelet and leukocyte function. A dilated cardiomyopathy, which responds only to phosphorus repletion, has been reported. The major clinical findings in cases of hyperphosphatemia include hypocalcemia and ectopic calcification, both resulting from the formation of calcium phosphate complexes.

537–540. The answers are 537-C, 538-B, 539-C, 540-A. *(Chapter 76)* Adrenocortical insufficiency of any etiology frequently is associated with gastrointestinal symptoms such as pain, anorexia, nausea, vomiting, and diarrhea. When abdominal signs occur, localizing signs are usually absent, though there may be tenderness and pain on deep palpation. The exception is adrenal hemorrhage, which can be associated with abdominal rigidity and rebound.

In the setting of trauma to the abdomen or thorax, recent surgery, severe medical illness, a history of thromboembolism, coagulopathy, or anticoagulant therapy, a sudden fall in hematocrit should immediately raise the possibility of adrenal hemorrhage.

The laboratory abnormalities associated with adrenocortical insufficiency—hyponatremia, hyperkalemia, prerenal azotemia, hypoglycemia, hypercalcemia, anemia, eosinophilia, and lymphocytosis—are neither specific nor sensitive markers for the disease, regardless of the etiology. However, the typical laboratory abnormalities are present less frequently when adrenocortical insufficiency occurs acutely, such as with adrenal hemorrhage and Waterhouse-Friedrichsen syndrome.

Autoimmune adrenalitis is associated with autoimmune disorders such as hypoparathyroidism, hypogonadism, hypo- and hyperthyroidism, diabetes mellitus, pernicious anemia, chronic active hepatitis, celiac disease, vitiligo, and alopecia in 40 to 70 percent of cases and may provide a clue to the diagnosis.

541–543. The answers are 541-C, 542-B, 543-A. *(Chapter 73)* The consequences of hypomagnesemia include coma, seizures, psychosis, and tetany. Hypermagnesemia can result in cardiac conduction abnormalities, respiratory depression, decreased deep tendon reflexes, hypotension, flaccid quadriplegia, and coma.

544–545. The answers are 544-A, 545-C. *(Chapter 77)* Nearly all critically ill patients have decreased serum levels of T_3, and 30 to 50 percent have low T_4 concentrations associated with normal or low serum TSH values. The reduction in T_3 levels results from a decrease in 5′-deiodinase activity that occurs in critical illness. This enzyme is responsible for the degradation of reverse T_3, explaining the increase in serum levels of reverse T_3 that occurs in critical illness. This syndrome has been termed the *euthyroid sick syndrome*. Patients with a T_4 value less than 3.0 μg/dL have a mortality of 68 to 84 percent, which is probably not improved by T_4 therapy. Primary hypothyroidism results from a failure of the thyroid gland to synthesize and secrete T_4. In this setting T_4 and T_3 are decreased, as is reverse T_3, while TSH is increased.

546–548. The answers are 546-A, 547-C, 548-C. *(Chapter 74)* Alcoholic ketoacidosis resembles diabetic ketoacidosis. Free fatty acid concentrations are very high, and insulin is barely detectable. Hepatic synthesis of ketoacids exceeds peripheral utilization of them, resulting in acidosis. In alcoholic ketoacidosis, synthesis of ketoacids results directly from alcohol metabolism and from free fatty acid breakdown. In contrast to diabetic ketoacidosis, the ratio of β-hydroxybutyrate to acetoacetate is very high in alcoholic ketoacidosis. This is a result of high NADH/NAD related to the metabolism of ethanol. Glucose typically is lower in patients with alcoholic ketoacidosis.

549–551. The answers are 549-A, 550-A, 551-D. *(Chapter 73)* Hypomagnesemia, hypercalcemia, and hypokalemia all potentiate the toxic effects of digoxin. Hypomagnesemia can cause refractory hypokalemia (by impairing renal absorption), refractory hypocalcemia (by impairing parathyroid hormone release), and hypophosphatemia. Nephrogenic diabetes insipidus may result from hypercalcemia.

552–553.   The answers are 552-B, 553-D.   *(Chapter 73)*   Destruction of the myelin sheaths in the central basis pontis with severe neurologic sequelae has been reported after rapid correction of severe hyponatremia. Alcoholics may be predisposed to this complication.

The dehydration and hypernatremia of the woman in the question may contribute to lethargy, but seizures or other permanent CNS damage is not likely with this degree of sodium imbalance.

GASTROINTESTINAL DISORDERS IN THE CRITICALLY ILL

QUESTIONS

DIRECTIONS: Each question below contains four or five suggested responses. Select the **one best** response to each question.

554. Which of the following statements regarding gastrointestinal bleeding is true?

(A) Morbidity and mortality from gastrointestinal bleeding do not depend on age
(B) Coexisting liver disease does not increase the risk of mortality
(C) There is no difference in outcome between patients who present to the hospital with gastrointestinal bleeding and patients who develop gastrointestinal bleeding in the hospital
(D) Patients with upper gastrointestinal bleeding who pass red stools have a worse outcome

555. The major cause of mortality in patients with fulminant hepatic failure is

(A) sepsis
(B) variceal hemorrhage
(C) acute hypoxemic respiratory failure
(D) cerebral edema
(E) the initial precipitant of fulminant hepatic failure

556. Toxic megacolon is most likely to complicate

(A) pseudomembranous enterocolitis
(B) Crohn colitis
(C) ischemic colitis
(D) ulcerative colitis

557. The most successful therapy in the management of fulminant hepatic failure is

(A) aggressive use of intracranial monitoring in the management of cerebral edema
(B) prophylactic antibiotics
(C) charcoal hemoperfusion
(D) orthotopic liver transplantation

558. Preexisting conditions or procedures that increase the risk of acute pancreatitis in critically ill patients include all the following EXCEPT

(A) radical neck dissection
(B) cardiac transplantation
(C) repair of an abdominal aortic aneurysm
(D) shock from any cause
(E) cardiopulmonary bypass

559. A true statement regarding hepatic failure from acetaminophen overdose is

(A) *N*-acetylcysteine (NAC) may be an effective antidote
(B) acetaminophen undergoes conjugation to sulfate and glucuronide metabolites in the liver, and this causes hepatic toxicity in large doses
(C) the dose of acetaminophen ingested and the time from ingestion to the institution of therapy are unreliable predictors of outcome
(D) NAC inactivates hepatotoxic acetaminophen metabolites

560. All the following statements regarding mesenteric ischemia are true EXCEPT

(A) mesenteric ischemia may result from venous thrombosis
(B) acute mesenteric ischemia presents with abdominal pain out of proportion to the findings on the physical examination
(C) in mesenteric ischemia peritoneal signs are a nonspecific finding
(D) all patients suspected of embolic or thrombotic occlusions should undergo urgent laparotomy

561. All the following statements regarding the contra-indications and adverse effects of esophagogastroduo-denoscopy (EGD) are true EXCEPT

(A) hemodynamic instability is the most common contraindication to safely performing EGD in a critically ill patient

(B) gastrointestinal obstruction at the small bowel level increases the risk of upper GI endoscopy

(C) suspicion of gastrointestinal perforation precludes EGD

(D) an endoscopy-induced mucosal tear at the gastro-esophageal junction usually is associated with self-limited bleeding, as in a non-instrument-induced Mallory-Weiss tear

(E) relatively few patients experience a change in Pa_{O_2} during endoscopy

562. Coagulation of bleeding sites during GI endoscopy

(A) has had an impact on mortality from GI bleeding

(B) is not recommended for a visible, unbleeding vessel because of the risk of perforation

(C) includes bipolar electrocoagulation, which has been associated with a decrease in transfusion requirements and the length of a hospital stay

(D) employs injection of hypertonic saline or ethanol only as temporizing measures before surgery

(E) is employed only after rebleeding occurs

563. Based on animal models, the strategy most likely to limit or prevent bacterial translocation across the intestinal mucosa and the systemic inflammatory response syndrome (SIRS) is

(A) broad-spectrum intravenous antibiotics

(B) decontamination of the gut with nonabsorbable oral antibiotics

(C) avoidance of antibiotics

(D) enteral feeding

(E) metoclopramide to limit bowel stasis

DIRECTIONS: Each question below contains four suggested responses of which **one or more** is correct. Select

A	if	**1, 2, and 3**	are correct
B	if	**1 and 3**	are correct
C	if	**2 and 4**	are correct
D	if	**4**	is correct
E	if	**1, 2, 3, and 4**	are correct

Questions 564–565.

A 35-year-old alcoholic man is admitted to the intensive care unit after he presented to the emergency room with two episodes of hematemesis. On admission to the intensive care unit, he is febrile with a blood pressure of 126/76 mm Hg with orthostatic changes, a heart rate of 110 beats per minute, and a respiratory rate of 20 breaths per minute. He has a 20-gauge intravenous line in his left hand.

564. At this point management should include

(1) transfusion of 2 units of unmatched packed red blood cells
(2) placement of a nasogastric tube
(3) peripheral vasopressin therapy
(4) placement of two large-bore intravenous lines

565. Two hours later, the blood pressure drops to 90/60 mm Hg and the heart rate becomes 130 beats per minute. The bedside nurse notes large quantities of melena. His blood tests obtained 1 hour ago become available and reveal hematocrit 34 percent, WBC 9.0×10^9 cells per liter, platelets 145×10^9 cells per liter, PT 15.8 seconds, and PTT 36 seconds. At this point you should

(1) place a pulmonary artery catheter to guide fluid therapy
(2) give 2 units of fresh frozen plasma
(3) perform emergent endoscopy
(4) give a 1-L fluid bolus

566. Which of the following may be useful in reducing intracranial pressure in fulminant hepatic failure?

(1) Hyperventilation
(2) Steroids
(3) Infusion of mannitol
(4) Elevation of the head

567. True statements regarding bleeding varices include which of the following?

(1) Compared with placebo, vasopressin has improved mortality
(2) Endoscopic variceal sclerotherapy lowers mortality from bleeding varices
(3) Compared with vasopressin alone, vasopressin plus nitroglycerin has improved mortality
(4) Blood transfusion requirements are reduced in patients who receive immediate endoscopic variceal sclerotherapy

568. Complications of acute pancreatitis include

(1) pancreatic necrosis
(2) adult respiratory distress syndrome (ARDS)
(3) pancreatic pseudocyst
(4) glomerulonephritis

569. A 38-year-old man with ulcerative colitis presents to the emergency room with fever, diarrhea, and abdominal pain. On examination the patient appears very ill with a heart rate of 132 beats per minute, a blood pressure of 110/50 mm Hg with orthostatic changes, and a respiratory rate of 22 breaths per minute. His abdominal x-ray demonstrates a 10-cm transverse colon. His room air blood gas shows pH 7.45, Pa_{CO_2} 32 mm Hg, and Pa_{O_2} 95 mm Hg. Indicated tests include

(1) emergency colonoscopy
(2) barium enema
(3) abdominal ultrasound
(4) an upright chest x-ray

570. In toxic megacolon, emergency surgery is indicated for

(1) a transverse colon 10 cm in diameter
(2) fever of 39.4°C (103°F), heart rate over 150, and diminished level of consciousness
(3) melena
(4) septic shock

571. Risk factors for mesenteric ischemia include

(1) polycythemia
(2) antithrombin III deficiency
(3) thrombocytosis
(4) malignancy

572. True statements regarding the use of early upper gastrointestinal endoscopy include which of the following?

(1) Proper use of endoscopy has reduced the mortality associated with acute upper GI bleeding
(2) With massive hematemesis from ongoing upper GI bleeding, a nasogastric tube and lavage are often sufficient and obviate the need for endotracheal intubation for airway protection during endoscopy
(3) A nasogastric lavage negative for blood effectively rules out the need for upper GI endoscopy in a critically ill patient
(4) A key reason for early endoscopy in a patient who experienced hypotension from upper GI bleeding is to establish the risk of rebleeding

573. Factors that may contribute to intestinal ischemia include

(1) the sympathetic outpouring related to circulatory shock
(2) underlying aortic atherosclerosis
(3) hypoperfusion around the time of cardiac arrest
(4) an infusion of dopamine at 2 μg/kg per minute

Questions 574–575.

574. A 57-year-old man suffers an acute myocardial infarction complicated by pulmonary edema necessitating mechanical ventilation. He is treated with afterload reduction, diuresis with furosemide, and continuous infusion of narcotic for analgesia. On the second hospital day, marked abdominal distention is noted. Potential salutary effects of nasogastric suction include

(1) a decreased risk of aspiration
(2) blunting of the intestinointestinal inhibitory reflex
(3) a rise in functional residual capacity (FRC)
(4) a reduction in left ventricular afterload

575. An abdominal film is requested and reveals a massively distended colon measuring 14 cm in greatest diameter. Appropriate next steps should include

(1) diagnostic peritoneal lavage to exclude peritonitis
(2) an assessment for diuretic-induced hypokalemia
(3) placement of a cecostomy tube
(4) administration of naloxone

DIRECTIONS: The group of questions below consists of lettered headings followed by a set of numbered items. For each numbered item select the **one** lettered heading with which it is **most** closely associated. Each lettered heading may be used **once, more than once, or not at all.**

Questions 576–577.

Match the clinical situations below with the appropriate procedure.

(A) Embolization
(B) Emergency surgery
(C) Angiography
(D) Nuclear medicine scan with technetium-labeled red blood cells
(E) Selective vasopressin infusion

576. A 70-year-old woman with known diverticular disease and maroon-colored stools over the last 3 days was found to be dizzy with a blood pressure of 100/60 mm Hg and a pulse rate of 100 beats per minute. She underwent angiography which was nondiagnostic and now continues to have guaiac-positive maroon-colored stools. Her blood pressure is 120/80 mm Hg with a pulse of 88 beats per minute.

577. A 74-year-old man with a myocardial infarction 1 month ago has taken ibuprofen for 1 year for arthritis in the right ankle. He presents to the emergency room with mixed maroon and bright red blood in his stool and with dizziness. An upper endoscopy for suspected gastric ulcer is difficult because of the large amount of blood present. A follow-up angiographic study reveals a single duodenal bleeding site. He passes multiple bloody stools and requires blood transfusion.

GASTROINTESTINAL DISORDERS IN THE CRITICALLY ILL

ANSWERS

554. The answer is D. *(Chapter 79)* Age is an important determinant of outcome with gastrointestinal bleeding. Mortality for patients older than 60 years is 30 percent higher than that for patients 60 years or less (13.4 versus 8.7 percent). Not surprisingly, underlying liver disease increases the risk of mortality from gastrointestinal bleeding. Patients who present to the hospital with gastrointestinal bleeding do better than do patients who develop gastrointestinal bleeding in the hospital. For upper gastrointestinal bleeding, the presence of black stool as opposed to brown stool does not carry a higher mortality or need for surgery. However, patients passing red stools who have upper gastrointestinal bleeding have a worse outcome. Patients with brown stool and clear nasogastric aspirate have a mortality of 8 percent, whereas patients with red blood in the stool and nasogastric aspirate have a mortality of 30 percent.

555. The answer is D. *(Chapter 80)* The majority of patients who die of fulminant hepatic failure are found to have cerebral edema at autopsy, and many of these patients have evidence of transtentorial herniation. Infection and sepsis are also quite common in these patients. Pulmonary edema may occur and is a significant complication but usually does not cause death. Gastrointestinal hemorrhage is also common but usually is related to gastritis or ulceration rather than to varices. Finally, the precipitant of fulminant hepatic failure is often unknown or is known with solely hepatic complications, such as acetaminophen overdose and viral hepatitis. Rarely, an overwhelming illness resulting in fulminant hepatic failure, such as heat stroke, may cause death through other mechanisms.

556. The answer is D. *(Chapter 78)* Toxic megacolon is usually a complication of ulcerative colitis but rarely supervenes in patients with pseudomembranous colitis, Crohn colitis, ischemic colitis, and infective colitis. Factors that may precipitate toxic megacolon include barium enema, opiates, anticholinergics, antidiarrheal agents, electrolyte derangements, and pregnancy.

557. The answer is D. *(Chapter 80)* Fulminant hepatic failure (FHF) is associated with mortality ranging from 50 to 90 percent, depending on the particular etiology. No medical intervention has been demonstrated to have a significant impact on survival in patients with FHF. Orthotopic liver transplanation in FHF has been associated with survival rates of 50 to 65 percent, significantly better than those of medical management.

558. The answer is A. *(Chapter 81)* An increasing number of illnesses in critically ill patients have been noted to precede the development of pancreatitis. After cardiac transplantation, pancreatitis is frequently reported and may be a result of cardiopulmonary bypass or the administration of heparin, cyclosporine A, or prednisone. Repair of an abdominal aortic aneurysm, especially after an acute rupture, may be associated with hypotension, microemboli, and vasoconstriction, which may produce hypoperfusion of the pancreas. Cardiopulmonary bypass is an independent risk factor and perhaps causes injury from microembolism, venous thrombosis, a low postoperative flow state, bleeding, hypothermia, or vasopressor use. Most of these risk factors are associated with hypoperfusion, and indeed shock from any cause increases the risk of pancreatitis. Major upper abdominal procedures, but not head and neck surgery, may be complicated by pancreatitis through direct dissection or another injury at surgery.

559.   **The answer is A.**   *(Chapter 99)*   Acetaminophen is largely conjugated in the liver to sulfate and glucuronide metabolites, which have no direct toxic effects. A minor metabolite of acetaminophen, *N*-acetyl-p-benzoquinonimine (NAPQI), is an electrophile with an affinity toward sulhydryl groups. It binds to cysteine groups on cellular proteins and glutathione, and this may adversely affect hepatocellular enzymes. The mechanism of action of *N*-acetylcysteine (NAC) is not fully understood, though it is metabolized to glutathione and may replace depleted glutathione stores, thus preventing hepatotoxicity. NAC does not inactivate NAPQI. Outcome in acetaminophen toxicity is inversely proportional to the dose of acetaminophen ingested and the time between ingestion and the institution of NAC therapy.

560.   **The answer is C.**   *(Chapter 82)*   In mesenteric ischemia, the presence of peritoneal signs suggests that intestinal infarction has already occurred.

561.   **The answer is E.**   *(Chapter 79)*   Most people experience a fall in Pa_{O_2} during upper endoscopy, and pulse oximetry monitoring is useful during this procedure in critically ill patients. It is important to hemodynamically stabilize the patient before endoscopy, especially with the knowledge that endoscopy itself has not been found to affect mortality in GI bleeding. Patients with significant obtundation or vomiting should have the airway secured before this procedure. Suspicion of a perforated viscus is a contraindication to this procedure. Bleeding from tears associated with EGD usually is self-limited.

562.   **The answer is C.**   *(Chapter 79)*   Thermal coagulation and electrocoagulation are now commonly applied to an actively bleeding vessel and a visible vessel that has about a 60 percent risk of rebleeding. The use of bipolar electrocoagulation has decreased the incidence of rebleeding, transfusion requirements, and length of stay but has not clearly affected mortality. Injection therapy is a good means of achieving hemostasis and can be permanent.

563.   **The answer is D.**   *(Chapter 78)*   Bacterial translocation represents failure of the normal function of the mucosal barrier of the gut. This functional loss is correlated with structural atrophy, a change seen within 24 hours of the onset of injury in experimental animals. Translocation across the gut mucosa may initiate the release of cytokines, and this cytokine cascade leads to systemic inflammation (SIRS). Both atrophy and translocation to mesenteric lymph nodes can be reduced substantially by means of prompt enteral feeding. Antibiotics do not reduce translocation. By raising gastric pH, antacids encourage colonization of the upper gastrointestinal tract with bacteria, a factor that has been implicated in nosocomial pneumonia. However, gastric colonization is not related to gut translocation. Metoclopramide has not been evaluated in this setting, but limiting stasis is unlikely to be beneficial unless there is a concomitant restoration of mucosal integrity.

564.   **The answer is C (2, 4).**   *(Chapter 79)*   Initial management of gastrointestinal bleeding is aimed at stabilizing the patient. This patient gives a history of hematemesis, and so placement of a nasogastric tube is indicated. At this point his vital signs are stable, but he still has a tachycardia. Two large-bore intravenous lines should be placed to facilitate rapid resuscitation. Unmatched blood transfusion is not indicated at this time. His source of bleeding is unknown, and so vasopressin therapy cannot be considered.

565.   **The answer is C (2, 4).**   *(Chapter 79)*   The patient is in hemorrhagic shock and needs fluid resuscitation. He should be given rapid fluid challenge and should be monitored for a response. At this point placement of a pulmonary artery catheter or endoscopy will detract from rapid resuscitation efforts. If he stabilizes with intravenous fluids, an emergent endoscopy can be performed safely to localize the site of bleeding. A pulmonary artery catheter should be placed if efforts to resuscitate him are not successful. His coagulopathy should be treated with fresh frozen plasma.

566. **The answer is B (1, 3).** *(Chapter 80)* In a controlled study evaluating the effects of dexamethasone therapy on intracranial pressure (ICP) in patients with fulminant hepatic failure, Edi and associates noted no difference in ICP between patients treated with the steroid and those not treated. Hyperventilation was demonstrated to reduce ICP, as was the infusion of mannitol. A subsequent study evaluated the effect of position on ICP in patients with fulminant hepatic failure and noted no difference in ICP with changes in elevation of the head.

567. **The answer is D (4).** *(Chapter 79)* Compared with placebo, vasopressin has not improved mortality and vasopressin plus nitroglycerin does not change mortality outcome compared with vasopressin alone. Neither portacaval shunt nor endoscopic variceal sclerotherapy (EVS) lowers mortality. Blood transfusion requirements are reduced in patients receiving immediate EVS. If active bleeding is present from a visible varix at the time of endoscopy, EVS can control bleeding in about 95 percent of patients, though rebleeding within 48 hours is likely (20 to 75 percent).

568. **The answer is A (1, 2, 3).** *(Chapter 81)* Local complications of necrotizing pancreatitis include pancreatic necrosis, pancreatic abscess, and pancreatic pseudocyst formation. Adult respiratory distress syndrome may accompany pancreatitis. Renal dysfunction is seen frequently in the setting of acute pancreatitis and is related to the hypoperfusion, hypotension, and volume loss associated with acute pancreatitis. No other specific renal injuries, such as glomerulonephritis, have been noted in patients with acute pancreatitis.

569. **The answer is D (4).** *(Chapter 78)* This patient has toxic megacolon, and barium enema and colonoscopy are contraindicated. Abdominal ultrasound and CT are usually not helpful in the management of such patients. An upright chest x-ray must be performed in search of free air below the diaphragm.

570. **The answer is C (2, 4).** *(Chapter 78)* Besides perforation, indications for emergency surgery include septic shock, imminent rupture of the transverse colon (12 cm or greater), and the presence of at least three of the following: temperature over 39.4°C (103°F), tachycardia over 150, positive blood cultures, and diminished level of consciousness.

571. **The answer is E (all).** *(Chapter 82)* Hypercoagulable states such as polycythemia, thrombocytosis, antithrombin III deficiency, and malignancy increase the risk of mesenteric venous thrombosis and thus of mesenteric ischemia.

572. **The answer is D (4).** *(Chapter 79)* Identifying a patient who is at risk for a significant recurrent bleed and is in need of early surgical intervention is an accepted criterion for early endoscopy in a patient who has had a recent severe upper GI bleeding event. Upper endoscopy has not been clearly associated with a decrease in mortality from GI bleeding. Nasogastric aspirates are reported to yield 14 percent false negatives and therefore would not rule out early endoscopy. A patient with massive hematemesis is at risk for aspiration. In these cases, a low threshold for endotracheal intubation and airway protection is suggested.

573. **The answer is A (1, 2, 3).** *(Chapter 82)* Intestinal ischemia results when oxygen delivery is insufficient to supply needs, especially of the metabolically active mucosa. The part of the bowel most vulnerable to ischemia is the midportion of the small bowel, since its supply is derived solely from the superior mesenteric artery (SMA). Contributors to decreased oxygen delivery include systemic factors such as hypoxemia, anemia, and decreased cardiac output as well as regional factors such as mesenteric vasoconstriction and atherosclerosis at the origin of the SMA. Low doses of dopamine do not have a detrimental impact on mesenteric blood flow and may even increase oxygen delivery.

574.   **The answer is A (1, 2, 3).**   *(Chapter 78)*   By reducing intraabdominal and intragastric pressure, nasogastric decompression lessens the chance of gastric regurgitation. Although the presence of a nasogastric tube causes incompetence of the gastroesophageal sphincter, this effect is outweighed by the benefit of reduced intragastric pressure. The intestino-intestinal inhibitory reflex describes the generalized, neurally mediated depression of bowel function that follows distention of any segment of bowel. By decompressing some of the proximal bowel, nasogastric suction diminishes some of the input to this reflex, leading to more rapid recovery of distant segments of bowel. FRC is the lung volume at which the inward recoil of the lungs balances the outward recoil of the chest wall. When the outward recoil of the chest is less (as it is in abdominal distention), FRC falls. By reducing abdominal pressure (and thereby aiding the outward recoil of the chest wall), nasogastric suction raises FRC. Nasogastric suction has no important effect on left ventricular afterload.

575.   **The answer is C (2, 4).**   *(Chapter 78)*   This patient has colonic pseudo-obstruction. Peritoneal lavage plays no role in the evaluation and risks perforation of the bowel. Reversible contributors to impaired gut motility should be sought, such as electrolyte disturbances (e.g., hypokalemia, hypomagnesemia), drug-induced atony (e.g., narcotics, clonidine), and hypothyroidism. Naloxone may result in dramatic improvement. If continued sedation is required, nonnarcotic alternatives should be employed. As the colonic diameter exceeds 12 cm, perforation becomes increasingly likely. If conservative measures do not lead to prompt improvement, colonoscopy is indicated to decompress the cecum. This procedure is successful about 70 percent of the time. Only if colonoscopy fails is operative intervention, such as cecostomy, indicated.

576–577.   **The answers are 576-D, 577-A**.   *(Chapter 79)*   The woman in the question presents with symptoms suggestive of diverticular hemorrhage, although other possibilities exist. Her bleeding site was not found on angiography, and she is now hemodynamically stable, which suggests a slower bleeding rate than would be expected to yield a positive repeat angiogram. Therefore, a nuclear medicine scan would be helpful in locating a bleeding site and directing further diagnostics.

Given a single identified bleeding site in a location with good collateral circulation in a patient with a contraindication to surgery (recent myocardial infarction), embolization has a significant chance of curtailing bleeding.

TRANSPLANTATION

QUESTIONS

DIRECTIONS: Each question below contains four or five suggested responses. Select the **one best** response to each question.

578. All the following may be complications of immunosuppression with cyclosporine EXCEPT

(A) seizures
(B) hypertension
(C) capillary leak syndrome
(D) hemolytic uremic syndrome
(E) elevated results of liver function tests

579. All the following statements regarding late complications of lung transplant are true EXCEPT

(A) infection remains the greatest threat to long-term survival
(B) late airway stenosis occurs in patients with both single and double lung transplants and can be managed nonsurgically by repeated dilations and endoluminal stenting
(C) while common in heart-lung transplants, bronchiolitis obliterans rarely is seen in isolated lung transplants
(D) *Pneumocystis carinii* pneumonia is a potential late infection that necessitates long-term prophylactic antibiotic therapy
(E) pulmonary function testing is useful in assessing the development of chronic rejection

580. The most common cause of hepatic allograft dysfunction after orthotopic liver transplantation is

(A) hepatic vein thrombosis
(B) hepatic artery thrombosis
(C) rejection
(D) ischemia of the graft
(E) CMV hepatitis

581. All the following statements regarding postoperative management of patients with heart-lung transplants are true EXCEPT

(A) excessive bleeding is one of the most dangerous early complications and is associated with increased mortality
(B) pooling of secretions below the tracheal anastomosis frequently precipitates severe coughing with catastrophic results
(C) patients receiving transplants for Eisenmenger complex may be at increased risk of bleeding because of large bronchopulmonary collaterals
(D) operative trauma to the vagus nerve may lead to gastric atony
(E) healing of the tracheal anastomosis in heart-lung transplants may be enhanced (compared with that in single- or double-lung transplants) by the collateral blood supply derived from the donor coronary and pulmonary arteries

582. A 45-year-old woman with end-stage liver disease undergoes an orthotopic liver transplantation. Twenty-four hours postoperatively she has hypoglycemia, coagulopathy, renal failure, and metabolic acidosis. Possible causes of her deterioration include all the following EXCEPT

(A) hepatic artery thrombosis
(B) sepsis
(C) primary nonfunction of the liver
(D) cyclosporine toxicity
(E) acute rejection

583. The most common cause of an increase in blood urea nitrogen (BUN) and creatinine after liver transplantation is

(A) cyclosporine toxicity
(B) hypovolemia
(C) sepsis
(D) hepatorenal syndrome
(E) aminoglycoside nephrotoxicity

DIRECTIONS: Each question below contains four suggested responses of which **one or more** is correct. Select

A	if	**1, 2, and 3**	are correct
B	if	**1 and 3**	are correct
C	if	**2 and 4**	are correct
D	if	**4**	is correct
E	if	**1, 2, 3, and 4**	are correct

584. True statements regarding patient selection for lung transplantation include which of the following?

(1) Cystic fibrosis is an absolute contraindication to transplantation because of the high risk of infection

(2) End-stage pulmonary fibrosis is treated effectively by single-lung transplantation

(3) Given the need for cardiopulmonary bypass in patients undergoing lung transplantation, candidates with lesions that may predispose to significant bleeding are eliminated from transplant consideration

(4) Heart-lung transplantation is the preferred procedure in patients with severe primary or secondary pulmonary hypertension

585. True statements concerning the implantation response after heart-lung transplantation include

(1) it is characterized by transient and reversible deterioration in lung compliance, gas exchange, and pulmonary vascular resistance

(2) it is characterized radiologically by interstitial edema

(3) it is most often seen in the first few post-operative days

(4) escalation of immunosuppressive drug regimens is highly recommended

586. True statements concerning the postoperative management of patients after heart transplantation include

(1) the most common cause of right ventricular dysfunction and tricuspid regurgitation in the postoperative period is infective endocarditis

(2) a denervated heart often requires chronotropic support with pacing or infusion of isoproterenol

(3) right ventricular biopsy should not be performed for at least 1 month postoperatively

(4) dual P waves are seen frequently on the posttransplant ECG

587. Pulmonary complications of liver transplantation include

(1) atelectasis

(2) metabolic alkalosis with compensatory respiratory acidosis

(3) pleural effusions

(4) lobar collapse

DIRECTIONS: The group of questions below consists of lettered headings followed by a set of numbered items. For each numbered item select the **one** lettered heading with which it is **most** closely associated. Each lettered heading may be used **once, more than once, or not at all.**

Questions 588–591.

Match each mechanism of action with the appropriate immunosuppressive agent.

(A) Cyclosporine
(B) Corticosteroids
(C) Azathioprine
(D) OKT3
(E) None of the above

588. Poorly understood reduction in interleukin-1 production

589. Nonspecific suppression of lymphocyte production

590. Inhibition of interleukin-2 production

591. Specific reduction in circulating T cells

TRANSPLANTATION

ANSWERS

578. The answer is C. *(Chapter 86)* The development of capillary leak is characteristically seen with the administration of OKT3, where large amounts of several cytokines are released. Pretreatment with steroids, histamine blockers, and acetaminophen attenuates the response, but pulmonary edema may occur in patients who are mildly volume-overloaded. Nephrotoxicity is the most common form of toxicity related to cyclosporine. Cyclosporine causes intense afferent arteriolar constriction, which in turn reduces glomerular perfusion and filtration. Hypertension is an important sequela of this glomerular hypoperfusion. Cyclosporine also may cause neurotoxicity ranging from neuropathy to seizures. It causes hepatic toxicity that usually consists of cholestasis with mild elevation of transaminases. Finally, cyclosporine rarely is associated with findings consistent with hemolytic uremic syndrome. Whether this is truly cyclosporine toxicity or a manifestation of host-graft interaction is not clear.

579. The answer is C. *(Chapter 86)* Late complications of lung transplantation remain a significant problem despite diagnostic and therapeutic advances. Bronchiolitis obliterans following transplantation was first reported in a series of heart-lung recipients. More recently, long-term follow-up of isolated lung transplant recipients showed an increased incidence in this population. Pulmonary infectious complications remain the leading cause of death in most published series of long-term lung transplant recipients. Airway stenosis, usually resulting from anastomotic ischemia, may be treated nonsurgically by dilation and stenting. *Pneumocystis carinii* pneumonia rarely is seen within 3 weeks of transplantation; however, it becomes a major pathogen thereafter. Antimicrobial prophylaxis is advised. Pulmonary function testing is a useful tool in the assessment of chronic rejection and bronchiolitis obliterans.

580. The answer is C. *(Chapter 86)* Poor hepatic function of a hepatic allograft after orthotopic liver transplantation can occur as a result of primary nonfunction of the graft, hepatic artery thrombosis, recurrent hepatic vein thrombosis in patients with Budd-Chiari syndrome, ischemia of the graft, and viral hepatitis, especially from CMV. The most common cause, however, is rejection.

581. The answer is B. *(Chapter 86)* The denervated heart-lung preparation actually demonstrates a diminished cough reflex to pooled secretions below the tracheal anastomosis, and postural drainage, suctioning, and breathing exercises are often necessary to aid expectoration.

582. The answer is D. *(Chapter 86)* Both liver failure and sepsis can result in hypoglycemia, coagulopathy, renal failure, and metabolic acidosis. Causes of hepatic failure include hepatic artery thrombosis (the most common vascular complication), primary nonfunction of the hepatic allograft, and acute rejection. Cyclosporine toxicity produces hypertension, tremulousness, hypertrichosis, and nephrotoxicity.

583. The answer is A. *(Chapter 86)* The most common cause of an increase in BUN and creatinine after transplantation is cyclosporine toxicity. Depletion of intravascular volume may occur owing to third-space losses and may contribute to the risk of cyclosporine-induced nephrotoxicity. Sepsis may contribute to persistent postoperative renal failure but is not the most common cause. Even patients with the hepatorenal syndrome have improvement in renal function if the new liver functions properly. Aminoglycosides should be used cautiously with careful monitoring of blood levels.

584. **The answer is C (2, 4).** *(Chapter 86)* At present, the main indication for single-lung transplantation is end-stage fibrosis. The classic indication for a heart-lung transplant remains pulmonary hypertension with cor pulmonale. Isolated single- or double-lung transplantation may be considered in patients with pulmonary hypertension who are believed to have reversible right heart failure. Cystic fibrosis is not an absolute contraindication to lung transplantation. Double-lung transplantation is the procedure of choice in this population given the risk of postoperative infection and gas-exchange abnormalities. The need for bypass is not universal during lung transplantation. Only 20 percent of single-lung transplants require cardiopulmonary bypass. Consequently, lesions that may predispose the patient to bleeding, such as lung biopsy sites, are no longer contraindications to transplantation.

585. **The answer is A (1, 2, 3).** *(Chapter 86)* The implantation response usually occurs within the first few postoperative days after heart-lung transplantation and is characterized by pulmonary edema and increased pulmonary vascular resistance. It has been ascribed to surgical trauma, denervation, lymphatic disruption, inadequate preservation, and other processes apart from rejection. When it occurs later than the first week, biopsy may be necessary to distinguish it from rejection. Treatment is supportive, and no adjustment in immunosuppression is necessary.

586. **The answer is C (2, 4).** *(Chapter 86)* Right ventricular dilation and dysfunction, along with tricuspid regurgitation, are common findings after cardiac transplantation and probably are related to the donor heart's adaptation to increased right ventricular afterload. The denervated heart often requires chronotropic stimulation. Right ventricular endomyocardial biopsy is crucial in following the patient for rejection and typically is done weekly during the first month, even if clear indications of rejection are absent. The recipient's atrial tissue as well as the donor heart may generate a P wave on the post-transplant ECG.

587. **The answer is E (all).** *(Chapter 86)* Respiratory problems are the most common complication of liver transplantation in the early postoperative period. These pulmonary complications include atelectasis, which can lead to lobar collapse, pleural effusion (usually right-sided), and metabolic alkalosis with compensatory respiratory acidosis as a result of nasogastric suction, diuretic and steroid therapy, and primary graft failure.

588–591. **The answers are 588-B, 589-C, 590-A, 591-D.** *(Chapter 86)* Corticosteroids are thought to block the production of interleukin-1 (IL-1) by macrophages through mechanisms that are not well defined. This reduction in IL-1 production results in less stimulation for expansion of clonal T-cell populations.

Azathioprine is an antimetabolite that inhibits the production of rapidly proliferating cell lines by blocking purine metabolism, thereby blocking DNA and RNA synthesis.

Cyclosporine exerts its immunosuppressive effect by interfering with the production of mRNA, which codes for the synthesis of interleukin-2 (IL-2). The lack of IL-2 again inhibits the propagation of clonal alloreactive T-cells.

OKT3 is a murine monoclonal antibody against CD3. This cell marker is specific for lymphocytes. The administration of OKT3 results in the disappearance of T cells from the circulation. T cells in lymph nodes appear to be less vulnerable.

TRAUMA

QUESTIONS

DIRECTIONS: Each question below contains four or five suggested responses. Select the **one best** response to each question.

592. Regarding acute head injury, which of the following statements is true?

(A) Anticonvulsants after head injury are indicated only in patients with demonstrable seizure activity
(B) The risk of CNS infection in patients with an open cranial injury is not affected by surgical debridement and restoration of dural integrity
(C) Systemic sepsis is an uncommon complication during recovery from an acute head injury
(D) Caloric requirements for patients with a head injury are similar to those required for patients with 20 to 40 percent body surface area burns
(E) Continuous intracranial pressure (ICP) monitoring should be reserved for patients with pressures greater than 20 cm H_2O

593. Which of the following statements regarding flail chest is correct?

(A) Mechanical fixation of the ribs is usually necessary
(B) Most patients with flail chest require mechanical ventilation
(C) Paradoxical movement of the chest wall is best seen when patients are ventilated with positive-pressure breaths
(D) Patients with flail chest who require mechanical ventilation should have a chest tube inserted on the involved side
(E) Discontinuation of mechanical ventilation depends on the disappearance of paradoxical movement

594. A 45-year-old alcoholic woman fell down a flight of stairs. In the emergency room, her blood pressure was 80/60 mm Hg and her pulse was 136 beats per minute. A supine chest x-ray showed left lower rib fractures and a left lower lobe infiltrate. The abdomen was diffusely tender with no guarding or rebound. A gastric aspirate was positive for trace blood. A fluid challenge was given with an increase in blood pressure to 105/70 mm Hg and a fall in pulse to 120 beats per minute. Which of the following would you do next?

(A) CT of the chest
(B) Upper GI endoscopy
(C) CT of the abdomen
(D) Ultrasound of the right upper quadrant and pancreas
(E) Upright chest x-ray

595. Which of the following statements regarding traumatic genitourinary injuries is true?

(A) Hematuria is absent in up to 40 percent of patients with genitourinary trauma
(B) Hematuria is the most important sign of genitourinary injury
(C) The routine use of IV pyelography is indicated in patients with abdominal trauma
(D) Microhematuria should be evaluated surgically regardless of the presence or absence of shock
(E) A majority of traumatic genitourinary injuries require early surgical intervention

596. A 23-year-old pedestrian is struck by an automobile, hitting his head on the pavement. Upon arrival he is minimally responsive to voice. His breathing is audible with occasional grunting. His vital signs reveal a blood pressure of 120/80 mm Hg with a pulse of 130 beats per minute. On examination he has an occipital hematoma, equal clear breath sounds bilaterally, and a regular heart rhythm. He has evidence of an open fracture of the left femur and is presumed to have a pelvic fracture. All distal pulses are present and equal, and there is no evidence of significant external hemorrhage. The skin is cool and appears pale. Blood is noted at the urethral meatus. Correct statements about the initial care of this patient include which of the following?

(A) Immediate orotracheal intubation should be the initial priority given the high risk of respiratory arrest

(B) Volume resuscitation should not exceed 2 L because of the risk of cerebral edema. A normal blood pressure indicates adequate perfusion at present

(C) Placement of a Foley catheter should be deferred

(D) After securing the airway, immediate reduction of the femur fracture should be performed because of the potential for limb ischemia and hemorrhage

(E) The development of hypotension, unresponsive to 2 L of crystalloid is an indication for immediate surgical exploration to rule out an abdominal or thoracic source of hemorrhage

597. Radiographic clues to the presence of an aortic rupture include all the following EXCEPT

(A) fracture of the first and second ribs
(B) deviation of the trachea to the left
(C) obliteration of the aortic knob
(D) a pleural cap
(E) obliteration of the aortic-pulmonary window

598. A 43-year-old man with blunt abdominal trauma exhibited marked deterioration in respiratory status with inflation of a pneumatic antishock suit. He should be considered as having which of the following?

(A) Tension pneumothorax
(B) Pulmonary embolus
(C) Splenic rupture
(D) Diaphragmatic rupture
(E) Aspiration pneumonia

599. Nutritional and metabolic support are important in multiple system organ failure (MSOF) to

(A) restore immune function
(B) decrease the hypermetabolic response
(C) attain nitrogen balance or at least minimize negative nitrogen balance
(D) allow substrate-limited metabolism
(E) decrease inflammatory mediators of MSOF

DIRECTIONS: Each question below contains four suggested responses of which **one or more** is correct. Select

A	if	**1, 2, and 3**	are correct
B	if	**1 and 3**	are correct
C	if	**2 and 4**	are correct
D	if	**4**	is correct
E	if	**1, 2, 3, and 4**	are correct

600. True statements regarding airway management in trauma patients include

(1) blind nasotracheal intubation in a patient with a suspected cervical spine injury is acceptable if the patient is conscious and breathing spontaneously

(2) in adults, a 14-gauge needle through the cricothyroid membrane establishes an adequate airway that can be used for a number of days

(3) a needle is preferred to an incision in the cricothyroid membrane of a child, as it minimizes damage to the cricoid cartilage, which is essential for upper airway stabilization

(4) most patients with multisystem trauma require endotracheal intubation

601. A 25-year-old man is pushed from a third-story balcony during a fight. Examination reveals that he is unconscious with multiple bruises on his face and head and has a fracture of the right humerus and both tibias. Appropriate initial management includes

(1) maintenance of a Pa_{O_2} and systolic blood pressure each > 100 mm Hg

(2) flexion and extension films of the cervical spine

(3) stabilization of cervical spine

(4) myelography

602. A patient with esophageal disruption may present with

(1) pneumothorax

(2) hemothorax

(3) mediastinal air

(4) a high-pH, high-amylase pleural effusion

603. For the purposes of trauma management, the neck is divided into three anatomic zones. True statements regarding these zones include which of the following?

(1) Zone I contains the esophagus, the thoracic duct, and the apex of the lung

(2) Penetrating injuries are most common in Zone II

(3) The base of the skull is contained in Zone III

(4) Vascular injury in penetrating neck wounds in Zone II is detected easily in clinical examination

604. A 69-year-old patient with chronic obstructive pulmonary disease (COPD) was admitted to the ICU in respiratory failure and was intubated after the third translaryngeal attempt. On his second day in the ICU, he developed fever, leukocytosis, and subcutaneous emphysema in the neck. Chest x-ray at that time did not demonstrate a pneumothorax or a new infiltrate. Indicated tests include

(1) endotracheal secretions for culture

(2) repeat chest x-ray in 2 hours

(3) soft tissue x-rays of the chest and neck

(4) Gastrografin swallow

605. In penetrating neck injury, airway compromise may result from

(1) compression and edema secondary to unrecognized expanding deep hematoma

(2) massive intraoral bleeding

(3) direct laryngotracheal injury

(4) secondary glottic edema from ongoing blood loss from a deep neck hematoma

606. Indications for immediate neck exploration after penetrating trauma include

(1) rapidly expanding hematoma

(2) uncontrolled bleeding

(3) shock

(4) airway obstruction

607. Peritoneal lavage is indicated in patients with abdominal trauma

(1) when a patient will be unavailable for repeated physical examinations because of surgical or radiologic investigation

(2) when findings from other injuries, such as rib fractures, confuse the evaluation of intra-abdominal structures

(3) when a patient's pain perception is abnormal (e.g., because of drug intoxication)

(4) when extraabdominal sources of hemorrhage are present that make it difficult to rule out simultaneous intraabdominal blood loss

608. In patients with blunt trauma to the liver,

(1) morbidity and mortality are higher than in patients with penetrating trauma

(2) CT and liver ultrasound clearly define the injury and may obviate the need for diagnostic peritoneal lavage in stable patients

(3) death usually results from associated injuries, particularly of the head and thorax

(4) hemorrhage from the damaged liver usually is contained within the capsule of the liver and rarely results in hemorrhagic shock

609. Appropriate management of pelvic fracture complicated by retroperitoneal hemorrhage includes

(1) high-dose corticosteroids to prevent fat embolism syndrome

(2) immediate exploration

(3) angiography in all patients

(4) external stabilization to avoid undue motion

610. In patients with penetrating trauma of the torso,

(1) a wound at the left nipple invariably will cause thoracic injury

(2) hemothorax draining 100 mL of blood per hour through a large-bore chest tube requires immediate surgical intervention

(3) tension pneumothorax relieved by inserting a needle may not require tube thoracostomy

(4) distended neck veins and hypotension could represent hemothorax or cardiac tamponade

611. In patients with acute cardiac tamponade,

(1) tamponade can occur from as little as 100 mL of fluid in the pericardial sac

(2) blood pressure is usually low with a normal pulse pressure

(3) aspiration of nonclotting blood during pericardiocentesis confirms a pericardial position of the needle

(4) successful pericardiocentesis (if done under sterile conditions and ECG guidance) saves the patient from having a formal thoracotomy

612. A 27-year-old man with blunt chest trauma presents with bilateral pneumothoraces and hemoptysis. A large, persistent air leak is noted after bilateral tube thoracostomies are performed. Correct statements include

(1) laceration of the right mainstem bronchus is the most likely injury

(2) additional chest tubes should be placed until the leak is corrected

(3) fiberoptic bronchoscopy is contraindicated

(4) thoracotomy is indicated

613. A traumatized patient is at particular risk of developing multiple system organ failure (MSOF) because of which of the following risk factors

(1) direct tissue injury

(2) intestinal ischemia

(3) prolonged shock

(4) inhibition of tumor necrosis factor-α

Questions 614–615.

A 16-year-old male is admitted to the intensive care unit after suffering an electrical injury while working on an amplifier for an electric guitar. On physical examination he is awake and alert, tachycardic, and mildly tachypneic. There are contact injuries on both hands. Further examination is notable for paresthesias of both hands and weakness in the distal upper extremities. The electrocardiogram demonstrates a global T-wave abnormality. Laboratory data are of note for mild hyperkalemia, hyperphosphatemia, and hypocalcemia. Urine is positive for ortho-toluidine reaction (positive urine dipstick for blood), but the microscopic examination is normal.

614. Further management at this juncture should include

(1) electrocardiographic monitoring
(2) careful debridement of the injured areas
(3) aggressive fluid resuscitation
(4) measurements of interosseous compartment pressure

615. The patient described above complains of shortness of breath and becomes progressively more tachypneic. Physical examination is unchanged except for inspiratory wheezing. Further immediate evaluation should include

(1) chest x-ray
(2) measurement of arterial blood gases
(3) sputum examination
(4) fiberoptic examination of the upper airway

616. True statements regarding compartment syndrome include

(1) if there is a distal pulse, compartment syndrome is not yet established
(2) the degree of postfasciotomy ischemia is directly correlated to the compartment pressure
(3) compartment pressures are generally lower than 30 to 40 mm Hg
(4) complications include myoglobinuria, acute renal failure, and muscular weakness

617. A 30-year-old construction worker was admitted 10 days ago for multiple fractures after a four-story fall. Her initial course was complicated by severe hemorrhagic shock and ARDS requiring nasotracheal intubation and mechanical ventilation. She was stabilized, and efforts to liberate her from the ventilator were initiated. A central venous catheter was placed, and parenteral feeding was initiated within 12 hours of admission. She now develops fever, worsening gas exchange, hypotension, low urine output, increased fluid requirements, elevated liver transaminases, and hyperglycemia. Possible causes of her deterioration include

(1) ventilator-associated pneumonia
(2) chronic sinusitis
(3) line sepsis involving the central venous catheter
(4) acute acalculus cholecystitis

DIRECTIONS: Each group of questions below consists of four lettered headings followed by a set of numbered items. For each numbered item select

A	if the item is associated with	(A) **only**
B	if the item is associated with	(B) **only**
C	if the item is associated with	**both** (A) and (B)
D	if the item is associated with	**neither** (A) nor (B)

Each lettered heading may be used **once, more than once, or not at all.**

Questions 618–619.

(A) Compartment syndrome
(B) Vascular ischemia
(C) Both
(D) Neither

618.   A 32-year-old construction worker with a crush injury to the right lower extremity and a displaced midshaft fracture of the femur

619.   A 64-year-old man who is hypotensive after a motor vehicle accident and who then has antishock garments applied and inflated for 4 hours

Questions 620–622.

(A) Spinal cord injury above T4
(B) Spinal cord injury above C5
(C) Both
(D) Neither

620.   Hypotension and bradycardia

621.   Ventilatory failure

622.   Autonomic dysreflexia

TRAUMA

ANSWERS

592. The answer is D. *(Chapter 89)*   Caloric requirements for patients with acute head trauma may increase by up to one and one-half to two times the normal requirements, approximating the caloric needs of burn patients. Aggressive treatment and prophylaxis of seizures after a head injury are warranted. The risk of CNS infection is reduced by surgical debridement and restoration of dural integrity in an open cranial injury. Systemic sepsis complicates recovery and should be diagnosed and treated aggressively. Early studies involving the management of head trauma revealed an improved outcome in patients undergoing ICP monitoring. In addition, approximately 50 percent of patients who die from head trauma succumb to uncontrollable ICP. Therefore, ICP monitoring should be considered for patients with severe head trauma regardless of initial ICP.

593. The answer is D. *(Chapter 91)*   Patients with flail chest often are managed without mechanical ventilation or mechanical fixation of the ribs when adequate analgesia is provided. When mechanical ventilation is required, prompt insertion of a chest tube on the injured side is indicated to prevent tension pneumothorax. Discontinuation of mechanical ventilation depends on the adequacy of gas exchange, not on whether the chest wall is stable. Paradoxical motion of the chest wall is best seen when patients breathe spontaneously and negative pleural pressures draw the involved area inward during inspiration.

594. The answer is C. *(Chapter 91)*   Splenic injury should be considered especially in patients who present with left upper quadrant pain or a left lower rib fracture. There may be associated shoulder pain on the left side. Patients with signs of massive intraperitoneal hemorrhage require immediate laparotomy. At laparotomy the goal is to control the hemorrhage with splenic salvage if possible. In stable patients CT or ultrasound can diagnose splenic injury.

595. The answer is B. *(Chapter 91)*   Hematuria may be absent in 5 to 10 percent of patients with genitourinary trauma; however, it remains the most important sign of injury. The use of routine IVP has recently been discouraged because of its relatively low yield and unacceptably high risk of complications. Surgical evaluation is indicated in patients with either gross hematuria or microhematuria with shock. Microhematuria without shock has not been shown to be associated with lesions that require surgical intervention. A majority of traumatic genitourinary injuries are considered minor and do not require initial surgical intervention.

596. The answer is C. *(Chapter 88)*   This patient is at risk for a cervical spine injury owing to the mechanism of injury. Therefore, stabilization of the spine should be done before attempts at intubation are made in this spontaneously breathing patient with probable variable airway obstruction secondary to the tongue. The patient does have signs of hypoperfusion despite a normal blood pressure; therefore, blood products will be warranted if the patient is unresponsive to the initial crystalloid. The most likely source of blood loss is the pelvis, and urinary tract catheterization should be deferred until a urethral injury is excluded. Surgical intervention aimed at identifying additional sources of injury and hemorrhage should not be pursued until further volume resuscitation is performed.

597.   The answer is B.   *(Chapter 91)*   Radiologic signs of aortic rupture include a widened mediastinum, fractures of the first and second ribs, obliteration of the aortic knob, a pleural cap, obliteration of the aortic-pulmonary window, and deviation of the trachea to the right.

598.   The answer is D.   *(Chapter 91)*   When there is diaphragmatic rupture, increasing intraabdominal pressure with an antishock suit can result in herniation of abdominal contents into the chest and cause respiratory deterioration. When this occurs, the antishock suit should be deflated promptly.

599.   The answer is C.   *(Chapter 17)*   Nutritional and metabolic support, preferably by the enteral route, is important to support the hypermetabolism and prevent the malnutrition seen in multiple system organ failure. The beneficial effects of nutrition have been found to correlate with the achievement of nitrogen balance. Nutritional support has not been shown to decrease inflammatory mediators or restore immune function. The goal of nutritional support is to prevent substrate-limited metabolism and support, rather than alter, the hypermetabolic state.

600.   The answer is B (1, 3).   *(Chapter 88)*   Ninety percent of trauma patients do not require endotracheal intubation. When indicated, blind nasotracheal intubation is acceptable in a conscious patient who is breathing. A 14-gauge needle is preferred if a cricothyroidotomy is to be performed on a child, but needle cricothyroidotomy in adults affords adequate ventilation only briefly before hypercapnia ensues.

601.   The answer is B (1, 3).   *(Chapter 90)*   Approximately 20 percent of patients with multiple trauma also have injuries to the spinal column. Cervical spine injury must be considered in any patient with significant injuries to the face or head, especially those unconscious from trauma. The initial management of a patient with a cervical spine injury includes resuscitative measures to ensure adequate oxygenation ($Pa_{O_2} > 100$ mm Hg) and circulation (BP $>$ 100 mm Hg) and stabilization of the cervical spine with a cervical collar. Initial x-rays include a lateral cervical spine film and an anteroposterior film of the chest and pelvis. Flexion and extension films of the cervical spine are indicated only after the lateral cervical spine film is negative and when a ligament injury is suspected; they should be performed only in an awake patient. A myelogram would not be done initially but only after plain films and CT were performed and usually only when an ischemic injury, dural defects, or avulsed nerve roots are suspected.

602.   The answer is A (1, 2, 3).   *(Chapter 91)*   Pleural effusions resulting from esophageal disruption typically have a very low pH (often near 6.9) and a high amylase. When present, these findings in the pleural fluid are strongly suggestive of esophageal disruption. Pneumothorax, hemothorax, and mediastinal air are helpful findings but are less specific.

603.   The answer is A (1, 2, 3).   *(Chapter 90)*   Zone I extends from the cricoid cartilage down to the level of the clavicle and represents the thoracic outlet, or the root of the neck. Included in this area are the proximal carotid, subclavian vessels, trachea, esophagus, thoracic duct, and apex of the lung. Zone II includes the area from the cricoid to the angle of the mandible and represents the mid-neck. Penetrating injuries are most common in this area and are easiest to evaluate. Zone III is the area between the angle of the mandible and the base of the skull. In any zone, penetrating neck wounds may harbor significant visceral and vascular injury with little or no clinical evidence.

604.   The answer is D (4).   *(Chapter 89)*   The patient has a perforation of the cervical esophagus or pyriform sinus, which has been reported to occur after translaryngeal intubation, diagnostic flexible endoscopy, or even passage of a nasogastric tube. This should be kept in mind in a patient who develops fever, leukocytosis, or subcutaneous emphysema in the neck after these procedures. Soft tissue x-rays of the chest and neck are useful in the absence of subcutaneous emphysema, since air within deep tissue planes may not be clinically palpable. If perforation is suspected, the diagnosis should be confirmed with a Gastrografin swallow, followed by a barium study if no leak is seen. Demonstration of a leak demands prompt intervention to control the soilage, restore continuity, and drain the resulting infection.

605.   The answer is E (all).   *(Chapter 90)*   All the conditions mentioned can lead to airway compromise in penetrating neck injury. Another complication of penetrating neck injuries is venous air embolism from a lacerated vein in a spontaneously breathing patient in the upright position. Although rare, it also may be the result of ill-advised wound exploration in the emergency room without preliminary intubation and positive-pressure ventilation.

606.   The answer is E (all).   *(Chapter 90)*   These patients should have their airways secured by intubation followed by rapid transfer to the operating suite. Even in the face of massive intraoral hemorrhage, oral intubation is usually possible. A cricothyroidotomy is the procedure of choice if oral intubation is not possible because of major structural deformity. Tracheostomy should be reserved for the few patients with direct injury to the larynx.

607.   The answer is E (all).   *(Chapter 91)*   All the listed conditions indicate peritoneal lavage. Contraindications include an existing indication for laparotomy, advanced pregnancy, previous abdominal operations with abdominal scars, morbid obesity, and coagulopathy.

608.   The answer is A (1, 2, 3).   *(Chapter 91)*   Blunt trauma to the liver carries a higher morbidity and mortality because of the irregular type of laceration and greater amount of tissue injury. Liver hemorrhage can result in hemorrhagic shock and is the usual indication for surgery. CT and ultrasound of the abdomen are useful to define the injury and may replace diagnostic peritoneal lavage.

609.   The answer is D (4).   *(Chapter 91)*   Retroperitoneal hemorrhage associated with pelvic fracture should be treated with immediate stabilization of the pelvis to prevent excessive motion of the pelvis and with transfusion. Exploration of the hematoma may result in massive, uncontrollable bleeding. When hemorrhage continues despite conservative therapy, angiography may identify the source of bleeding and allow for embolization of the bleeding artery. Fat embolism occurs most commonly from long-bone fractures, and though there is some evidence for the efficacy of steroids in preventing the fat embolism syndrome, steroids are not universally recommended because of the high rate of complications associated with their use, including the risk of infection and difficulty with wound healing.

610.   The answer is C (2, 4).   *(Chapter 91)*   Because of the configuration and variable location of the diaphragm and the uncertain trajectory of objects, wounds in the chest as high as the nipple can cause abdominal injury and wounds low in the abdomen can cause diaphragmatic and thoracic injury. Tension pneumothorax and massive hemothorax both require immediate intervention. When a needle or scalpel is used to treat tension pneumothorax, tube thoracostomy should follow. Tension pneumothorax, pericardial tamponade, and hemothorax can all cause hypotension with distended neck veins. Distended neck veins secondary to hemothorax occur when blood in the thorax causes mechanical obstruction to venous return.

611.   The answer is B (1, 3).   *(Chapter 91)*   Acute pericardial tamponade can occur from as little as 100 mL of fluid in the pericardial space. Similarly, removal of as little as 50 mL of fluid by pericardiocentesis may result in significant improvement. Patients with hemodynamically significant tamponade typically have a low blood pressure and a narrow pulse pressure indicating low stroke volume. Aspiration of nonclotting blood is a good indication that the needle is in the pericardial space, whereas blood that clots immediately should raise concerns of ventricular puncture. Both successful and unsuccessful pericardiocentesis should be followed by formal thoracotomy.

612.   The answer is D (4). *(Chapter 91)*   Hemoptysis coupled with a large, persistent air leak after blunt chest trauma suggests tracheobronchial laceration (most commonly of the left mainstem bronchus). After determining that the chest tubes are functioning properly, the patient should be placed on 100% oxygen. Fiberoptic bronchoscopy should be performed to localize the injury as long as it does not delay surgical intervention. Thoracotomy should be performed even if a lesion is not identified at bronchoscopy. Placement of an additional chest tube will not correct the underlying problem or the air leak and will only delay surgery.

613.   The answer is A (1, 2, 3). *(Chapter 17)*   Trauma patients are at an increased risk of developing MSOF because of the incidence of prolonged shock, direct tissue injury, intestinal ischemia, and altered cell-mediated immunity seen with trauma. A reduction in tumor necrosis factor-α is not seen in trauma victims.

614.   The answer is A (1, 2, 3). *(Chapter 93)*   Patients with electrical injury are at risk for multiple complications, including cardiac rhythm disturbances. Patients with ECG abnormalities, a history of loss of consciousness, or documented arrhythmia should be monitored for recurrent arrhythmias. Electrical injury produces extensive tissue damage that may not be readily apparent on the skin; therefore, all electrical wounds should be inspected and any nonviable tissue should be debrided. Because of extensive muscle damage, patients with an electrical injury frequently develop complications of rhabdomyolysis, including acute renal failure. The cornerstone of prevention of renal failure in rhabdomyolysis is fluid resuscitation. Finally, the monitoring of compartment pressure is extremely useful in determining which patients require fasciotomy before the onset of neurologic symptoms. Pressures in excess of 30 mm Hg indicate the need for fasciotomy. However, the pressures are reliable only in large muscle beds. Compartment pressures in the small compartments of the hand may not be accurate and should not dictate therapy.

615.   The answer is D (4). *(Chapter 93)*   The patient suffered an electrical injury whose course probably involved the upper airway, as evidenced by contact injuries on both hands. The electrical current passing through the upper airway might cause thermal injury to the airway, since the electrical resistance of the tissue generates heat. This injury might produce upper airway obstruction, which would be readily demonstrated by endoscopy. Chest x-ray and sputum examination would be unlikely to demonstrate any abnormality. Arterial blood gases probably would remain normal until the acute onset of respiratory failure.

616.   The answer is D (4). *(Chapter 92)*   In compartment syndrome, tissue hypoperfusion is the critical factor. The pulse distally may in fact be maintained in the face of impending or even established muscle and nerve necrosis. The degree of injury and ischemia after fasciotomy is correlated to the difference between mean arterial pressure and compartment pressure. Therefore, hypotension should be avoided. In compartment syndrome, compartment pressures are 30 to 40 mm Hg or higher. Complications of compartment syndrome include myoglobinuria, acute renal failure, infection of the fasciotomy site, loss of range of movement of the affected joint, and muscular weakness.

617.   The answer is E (all). *(Chapter 17)*   The patient has developed sepsis that may progress to MSOF. MSOF is a known, preventable complication of trauma. Ongoing efforts to identify and treat complicating infections are essential. The development of ventilator-associated pneumonia (VAP) is a serious complication in a critically ill patient. VAP usually develops after 72 hours of intubation and may progress to septic shock and MSOF. The use of central venous catheters serves as a potential source of sepsis. Nasotracheal intubation increases the risk of chronic sinusitis, and prolonged use of hyperalimentation increases the risk of developing acute acalculus cholecystitis.

618–619.   The answers are 618-C, 619-C.   *(Chapter 92)*   Crush injury predisposes to the development of compartment syndrome, and extremity fractures can lead to vascular disruption. If the vascular status is not improved by reduction and immobilization, angiography is warranted. Antishock garments used for 4 hours or more are known to be associated with complications of limb ischemia and compartment syndrome.

620–622.   The answers are 620-C, 621-B, 622-C.   *(Chapter 90)*   Patients in spinal shock from injuries above the level of T4 may manifest hypotension and bradycardia owing to loss of thoracic sympathetic outflow and unopposed vagal stimulation to the heart. Respiratory complications are greatest in patients with cervical cord injuries, especially when the patient has lost the intercostal and abdominal muscle function to initiate a cough. Phrenic nerve and hence diaphragmatic functions are affected in lesions above C5, thereby greatly increasing the risk of ventilatory failure. Patients with a spinal cord injury above T4 may manifest autonomic dysreflexia any time after recovery from spinal shock. This is usually a response to bladder or rectal distention or manipulation and presents with hyperhidrosis, headache, vasodilation above the neurologic level, and paroxysmal hypertension. Bradycardia may occur.

BURNS AND
ENVIRONMENTAL INJURY

QUESTIONS

DIRECTIONS: Each question below contains four or five suggested responses. Select the **one best** response to each question.

623. A patient with a deep burn of the abdomen, thorax, and face develops dyspnea with intraoral edema. The nose was not involved in the injury. Assuming that both oral and nasal routes are patent, intubation is best accomplished with a

(A) 6.5-mm endotracheal tube (ETT), passed orally
(B) 7.0-mm ETT, passed orally
(C) 7.5-mm ETT, passed orally
(D) 6.5-mm ETT, passed nasally
(E) 7.0-mm ETT, passed nasally

624. The most common organism involved in wound infection in the first week after a massive burn is

(A) β-hemolytic streptococcus
(B) α-hemolytic streptococcus
(C) *Pseudomonas aeruginosa*
(D) enterococcus
(E) *Staphylococcus aureus*

625. Well-documented causes of erythema multiforme (EM) include each of the following EXCEPT

(A) herpesvirus
(B) mycoplasma
(C) sarcoidosis
(D) sulfonamides
(E) phenytoin

626. Hyperventilation before breath-hold diving can cause blackout and drowning by

(A) increasing thoracic gas volume and predisposing to pulmonary barotrauma
(B) blocking the usual increase in cardiac output associated with diving
(C) decreasing the Pa_{CO_2} and thus diminishing the drive to breathe such that severe alveolar hypoxia and cerebral anoxia can ensue
(D) potentiating the bradycardic diving reflex
(E) causing gas embolism

Questions 627–630.

A 24-year-old welder is caught in a closed-space fire while repairing a gas tank. He suffers a 70 percent circumferential, full-thickness burn. Examination of the naso- and oropharynx reveals singed nasal hair and carbonaceous sputum. Laryngoscopy and bronchoscopy reveal significant airway erythema and swelling. The patient is electively intubated. Over the next several hours he requires massive volume resuscitation concordant with his severe thermal injury. Increasing oxygen requirements and progressive increase in the peak airway pressure (P_{peak}) to 60 cm H_2O are noted.

627. The appropriate initial diagnostic procedures should include all the following EXCEPT

(A) assessment of the peak-to-plateau gradient
(B) empirical trial of a bronchodilator
(C) empirical trial of a diuretic
(D) passage of a suction catheter through the endotracheal tube
(E) chest x-ray

628. The patient is treated with bronchodilators and has a good response. However, over the ensuing 24 hours he once again is noted to have worsening oxygenation and increasing airway pressures: P_{peak} = 65 cm H_2O, plateau airway pressure (P_{static}) = 52 cm H_2O, intrinsic PEEP ($PEEP_i$) = 0 cm H_2O. A chest x-ray reveals four-quadrant airspace filling. In this setting, the addition of appropriate levels of PEEP would be expected to

(A) leave the P_{peak} and P_{static} unchanged
(B) increase the P_{peak} without changing the P_{static}
(C) increase the P_{static} without changing the P_{peak}
(D) increase both the P_{peak} and the P_{static}
(E) decrease both the P_{static} and the P_{peak}

629. Once again the patient improves with the addition of PEEP, with stabilization of airway pressures and improvement in oxygenation. His pulmonary edema is treated with diuretics. Chest x-rays reveal partial resolution of the diffuse alveolar flooding. Five days after his injury, the patient is noted to develop higher airway pressures and hypotension. Oxygenation is preserved, but hypercarbia is noted. Physical examination reveals blood pressure 90/60, heart rate 110, and intact breath sounds bilaterally. Airway pressures are $P_{peak} = 65$ cm H_2O and $P_{static} = 57$ cm H_2O with tidal volume of 400 mL and PEEP set at 7.5 cm H_2O. There is no $PEEP_i$. The chest wall is remarkable for thick eschars and is tense to palpation. Which of the following is the appropriate therapy?

(A) Increase of tidal volume
(B) Bilateral full-thickness escharotomies
(C) Infusion of dopamine
(D) Antibiotic therapy
(E) Diuretic therapy

630. Two weeks after the initial injury, the patient is breathing spontaneously on CPAP of 5 cm H_2O with an FIO_2 of 0.4. Respiratory rate is 18, tidal volume 700 mL, heart rate is 84, and blood pressure is 110/65. The patient is afebrile and appears comfortable. ABG shows pH 7.35, $Paco_2$ 42 mm Hg, Pao_2 124 mm Hg, and Sao_2 99 percent. There is no air leak around the endotracheal tube when the cuff is let down. Which of the following statements is true?

(A) Weaning parameters are necessary before a decision about extubation can be made
(B) The patient has been intubated for 2 weeks and should be scheduled for a tracheostomy if he is not extubated in the next few days
(C) The patient is currently ready for a trial extubation
(D) Direct or fiber-optic laryngoscopy should be performed before extubation
(E) None of the above

DIRECTIONS: Each question below contains four suggested responses of which **one or more** is correct. Select

A	if	**1, 2, and 3**	are correct
B	if	**1 and 3**	are correct
C	if	**2 and 4**	are correct
D	if	**4**	is correct
E	if	**1, 2, 3, and 4**	are correct

Questions 631–632.

A 91-year-old victim of smoke inhalation was obtunded in the emergency room. After adequate volume resuscitation, the blood pressure was 140/70 mm Hg, the pulse was 110 beats per minute, and the respiratory rate was 34 breaths per minute. The room air blood gas was pH 7.27, Pa_{CO_2} 27 mm Hg, and Pa_{O_2} 105 mm Hg.

631. Possible diagnoses in this patient include

(1) hypoxic encephalopathy
(2) cyanide poisoning
(3) carbon monoxide poisoning
(4) aspiration pneumonitis

632. Given the diagnostic possibilities, appropriate initial management of this patient includes

(1) 100% oxygen
(2) corticosteroids
(3) CT of the head
(4) empirical hyperbaric oxygen

633. Complications of smoke inhalation include

(1) bronchospasm
(2) atelectasis
(3) pulmonary edema
(4) upper airway obstruction

634. A patient with a massive thoracic and abdominal burn and eschar formation required mechanical ventilation for smoke inhalation. Despite massive fluid challenge, the blood pressure was 85/56 mm Hg and the pulse was 120 beats per minute. Urine sodium was less than 10 mEq/L. Strategies to increase blood pressure should include

(1) more fluid
(2) dopamine
(3) escharotomy
(4) norepinephrine (Levophed)

635. Hematologic changes occurring after burns include

(1) underproduction anemia
(2) hemolytic anemia
(3) thrombocytopenia
(4) a hypercoagulable state

Questions 636–637.

A 62-year-old alcoholic was found unconscious on the floor of his heated apartment. His temperature was 29°C (84.2°F), blood pressure was 95/50 mm Hg, the pulse was 50 beats per minute, and the respiratory rate was 18 breaths per minute. The serum glucose was 290 mg/dL. Room air arterial blood gases measured at 37°C (98.6°F) were pH 7.20, Pa_{CO_2} 49 mm Hg, and Pa_{O_2} 80 mm Hg.

636. Drugs appropriately given at this time include

(1) bicarbonate
(2) atropine
(3) insulin
(4) oxygen

637. Possible causes of this patient's low body temperature include

(1) exposure
(2) Wernicke's encephalopathy
(3) alcohol
(4) sepsis

638. A 22-year-old man is brought to the operating room for elective hernia repair. On presentation he is awake with a temperature of 36.3°C (97.3°F), heart rate of 84, blood pressure of 124/66, and respiratory rate of 18. His abdomen is diffusely tender. He is taken to the operating room for an appendectomy. Anesthesia is induced with 500 mg of thiopental and 100 mg of succinylcholine and is maintained with isoflurane and nitrous oxide. Over the next 20 minutes, while the patient's abdomen is being prepped with betadine, the patient's heart rate is noted to increase to 140 (sinus tachycardia), respiratory rate increases to 40, and temperature increases to 39.8°C (103.6°F). An arterial blood gas during spontaneous ventilation with an F_{IO_2} of 40 percent shows pH 7.22, Pa_{CO_2} 28 mm Hg, and Pa_{O_2} 140 mm Hg. Appropriate initial steps include

(1) discontinuation of isoflurane and ventilation with 100% oxygen separate from the anesthesia machine
(2) initial attention to cooling measures with cooling blankets and cold intravenous saline
(3) dantrolene therapy (2.5 mg/kg IV) given immediately with the help of assistants to mix the solution
(4) proceeding with surgery *only after* dantrolene therapy has been completed

639. A 42-year-old man was admitted to the psychiatric unit for hallucinations. He had no previous medical history, was not taking any medication, and had no history of illicit drug abuse. He was started on daily chlorpromazine (Thorazine) on the day of admission. One week later he had developed fevers, marked rigidity, and tachycardia. Medications you would consider giving at this time include

(1) dantrolene
(2) corticosteroids
(3) bromocriptine
(4) haloperidol

640. True statements concerning decompression sickness and gas bubble embolism associated with ascent from diving with compressed gas include

(1) patients with "the chokes"—chest pain, cough and shortness of breath—will develop their symptoms immediately upon ascent
(2) pulmonary vascular rupture and arterial gas embolism can occur after a rapid ascent from shallow water
(3) hyperbaric oxygen or recompression is of value only in the first 12 hours
(4) experimental evidence clearly indicates that the formation of gas bubbles causes decompression sickness

641. Which of the following statements are true regarding the diagnosis of burn wound infection?

(1) The diagnosis of a burn wound infection is made by histologic examination of a full-thickness biopsy specimen at an interface between viable and nonviable tissue. The presence of bacterial invasion of viable tissue indicates true infection
(2) Surface cultures taken in nonpurulent areas after wound exudate has been removed identify only colonization and are of no use clinically
(3) *Staphylococcus aureus* is the most common organism involved in wound infection in the first week after a burn
(4) Surface cultures are useful in diagnosing wound infection in purulent-appearing areas only

642. Which of the following are true regarding the treatment of a 60 percent full-thickness burn with inhalational injury in the postresuscitation phase (days 2 to 6)?

(1) Early parenteral alimentation should be instituted until full enteral alimentation is possible
(2) Early antibiotic therapy for purulent tracheobronchitis is indicated
(3) Controlled surgical excisions should begin as soon as possible to avoid having extensive burns still in place with a high risk for subsequent infection
(4) Central venous access should be obtained early in anticipation of ongoing aggressive intravenous fluid administration with a frequent need to monitor central filling pressures

643. A 72-year-old man is admitted to the emergency room after being found in a burning building. He is obtunded. Arterial blood gases demonstrate a pH of 7.15, a Pa_{CO_2} of 30 mm Hg, and a Pa_{O_2} of 125 mm Hg on a 100% face mask. Pulse oximetry reveals a saturation of 98 percent. True statements include

(1) the metabolic acidosis probably is due to carbon monoxide or cyanide intoxication
(2) the patient's altered mental status may be due to head trauma or intoxication
(3) the pulse oximetry saturation is unreliable in this case
(4) given the patient's high Pa_{O_2}, a reduction in F_{IO_2} is appropriate

DIRECTIONS: Each group of questions below consists of four lettered headings followed by a set of numbered items. For each numbered item select

A   if the item is associated with   (A) **only**
B   if the item is associated with   (B) **only**
C   if the item is associated with   **both** (A) and (B)
D   if the item is associated with   **neither** (A) nor (B)

Each lettered heading may be used **once, more than once, or not at all.**

Questions 644–647.

(A) Postburn hypermetabolic state
(B) Postburn sepsis
(C) Both
(D) Neither

644. Fever

645. Lactic acidosis

646. Increased carbon dioxide production

647. Increased cardiac output

Questions 648–650.

(A) Neuroleptic malignant syndrome
(B) Malignant hyperthermia
(C) Both
(D) Neither

648. Muscle contracture caused by a central rather than a muscular abnormality

649. Genetic predisposition

650. Effective treatment with dantrolene

Questions 651–652.

(A) Rhabdomyolysis
(B) Severe electrolyte disturbance
(C) Both
(D) Neither

651. A 21-year-old man dove into shallow water at an inland lake and hit his head on the bottom. He was pulled from the water and was cyanotic. Immediate CPR was performed, and he was brought to the hospital. He was in respiratory failure and required mechanical ventilation. Cervical spine injury and skull injury were not apparent. Conditions that may present early in the patient's course include

652. A 50-year-old diver completed 6 hours of work at 30 feet depth. Twelve hours later he developed joint aches in both lower extremities. He is also at risk to develop

BURNS AND
ENVIRONMENTAL INJURY

ANSWERS

623. **The answer is C.** *(Chapter 11)* In patients with large burns, early intubation is indicated when intraoral or airway edema occurs. This is best accomplished with a large tube because thick secretions may develop as a result of lung injury. Nasal airways are best avoided because the tube used is often small and the tip of the airway may not be sufficiently below the vocal cords when massive edema develops. Once massive edema develops, it is very dangerous to change the tube.

624. **The answer is E.** *(Chapters 51, 94, 95)* *Staphylococcus aureus* is the most common early wound infection. β-hemolytic streptococcal infection also occurs early but is found in less than 5 percent of burn patients. Gram-negative infection occurs more commonly after the first week. Enterococcus and *Candida albicans* are being seen with increased frequency.

625. **The answer is C.** *(Chapter 104)* Erythema multiforme (EM) occurs primarily in young adults. EM minor is a mild, often recurring form of illness that sometimes is associated with herpesvirus infection. EM major is more likely to lead to critical illness and consists of the sudden onset of inflammatory bullous skin lesions and mucosal erosions. Mycoplasma is a well-established cause, as are many drugs, most notably the sulfonamides, phenylbutazone, phenytoin, and the penicillins. Sarcoidosis often results in erythema nodosum—tender erythematous subcutaneous nodules that usually are localized to the pretibial area.

626. **The answer is C.** *(Chapter 108)* The usual cause of cessation of a dive and return to the surface after a breath-hold is hypercapnia. When divers hyperventilate before a dive, respiratory drive is diminished and alveolar hypoxia with dysfunction of the central nervous system may occur before a diver reaches the surface. The result is drowning.

627. **The answer is C.** *(Chapter 32)* In acute airway injury, the increasing airway pressures probably are due to bronchospasm rather than pulmonary edema, although the latter should not be excluded. This differential diagnostic question would be served by additional data, in particular by evaluation of the peak-to-plateau gradient. An increased resistive pressure drop, which is characterized by the difference between peak airway pressure (P_{peak}) and plateau pressure (P_{static}), strongly suggests bronchoconstriction. Evaluation of other possible causes of airway obstruction, such as plugging of the endotracheal tube, also should be pursued. A chest x-ray would help confirm the presence of pulmonary edema if in fact the rising airway pressures were due to decreased compliance rather than to increasing resistance. In addition, it would help exclude the development of other causes of increased P_{static}, such as atelectasis, pneumothorax, and chest wall restriction from circumferential thoracic burns. Administration of diuretics without first confirming a diagnosis of pulmonary edema in a patient in whom intravascular volume depletion is likely would be injudicious. Furthermore, since the likely explanation of the increased airway pressures is airway obstruction, dynamic hyperinflation and intrinsic PEEP ($PEEP_i$) may be present. Administering a diuretic in this setting might reduce venous return and blood pressure to dangerous levels.

628. **The answer is D.** *(Chapter 33)* The addition of PEEP in patients with pulmonary edema results in the reexpansion of previously flooded lung units. This reexpansion results in improved compliance, which causes Pstatic to increase, though often to a lesser extent than the amount of PEEP added. Since PEEP does not have an impact on airway resistance, there should be no effect on the peak-to-plateau gradient.

629. **The answer is B.** *(Chapter 36)* This patient has a noncompliant respiratory system. Potential causes may involve the lung parenchyma (e.g., pulmonary fibrosis), the pleural space (e.g., pneumothorax), and the chest wall (e.g., kyphoscoliosis). In a burn patient with a circumferential burn of the chest wall, the eschar may limit excursion of the chest wall. Optimally, esophageal manometry would demonstrate this physiology with an increased esophageal pressure (approximating pleural pressure) and a low transpulmonary pressure. Escharotomy allows the expansion of the chest wall, decreasing intrathoracic pressure and increasing venous return. This increase in venous return should correct the hypotension.

630. **The answer is D.** *(Chapter 39)* Patients suffering from inhalational burn injuries are at high risk for significant upper airway injury with associated edema. In evaluating such patients for extubation, upper airway edema must be assumed to be present until disproved. Letting the cuff of the endotracheal tube down and listening for an air leak constitute an important first step. If no air leak is present, visualization of the glottic opening and larynx is helpful in making a decision regarding extubation. Formal weaning parameters correlate poorly with extubation success. Although tracheostomy may ultimately be necessary in this patient, at 12 days' duration of intubation it is not imminent, especially with a low-pressure, high-volume cuffed endotracheal tube.

631. **The answer is A (1, 2, 3).** *(Chapter 94)* Persistent metabolic acidosis in fire victims suggests carbon monoxide or cyanide poisoning. Arterial Pa_{O_2} may be normal. Despite normal arterial Pa_{O_2}, tissue hypoxia occurs because carbon monoxide displaces oxygen from hemoglobin, shifts the oxygen hemoglobin dissociation curve to the left, and causes cellular dysfunction of Fe^{2+}-containing enzymes. Although aspiration pneumonitis is a concern in anyone with an abnormal mental status, the normal alveolar-arterial Pa_{O_2} gradient in this patient argues against significant aspiration.

632. **The answer is B (1, 3).** *(Chapters 94, 95, 96)* Despite a normal Pa_{O_2}, FI_{O_2} of 1.0 is desirable in patients with suspected carbon monoxide poisoning to shorten the elimination half-time of CO from about 5 to 1.5 hours. This is best delivered through an endotracheal tube with a properly inflated cuff to avoid entrainment of room air. In patients with proven CO toxicity, hyperbaric oxygen is useful to decrease elimination half-time to 30 minutes. This therapy is often logistically difficult and should not be used empirically. CT of the head should be done in all obtunded patients who may have fallen during a fire. There is no role for empiric corticosteroids in this setting.

633. **The answer is E (all).** *(Chapters 94, 95, 96)* All the listed conditions are well-recognized complications of smoke inhalation. Bronchodilators and PEEP are useful therapies in many of these patients to treat bronchospasm and atelectasis, respectively, and large endotracheal tubes are indicated to allow for adequate suctioning of mucopurulent material.

634. **The answer is B (1, 3).** *(Chapters 94, 95, 96)* This patient should be considered hypovolemic (hypotensive with a narrow pulse pressure and low urine sodium) until proved otherwise by measurement of central pressures and should be given more fluid. Hypovolemia is common in burn patients because of tissue edema and often requires massive fluid resuscitation. Patients with edematous and scarred chest walls generate high airway pressures during mechanical ventilation that increase pleural pressure and decrease venous return to the right atrium to lower cardiac output and blood pressure. Lowering airway pressure with escharotomy provides an "intrinsic" volume challenge and may result in hemodynamic improvement. Vasoactive mediations should not be part of the initial management until volume resuscitation has been accomplished.

635. **The answer is E (all).** *(Chapters 94, 95, 96)* Hematologic changes after major burns include hemolysis, increased red cell fragility, decreased red cell hematopoiesis, thrombocytopenia, and leukocytosis. A hypercoagulable state can be seen initially in moderate burn injuries. A coagulopathic state resulting from depletion of clotting factors can be seen in massive burns.

636. **The answer is D (4).** *(Chapter 106)* Arterial blood gases that are not corrected for low body temperature will show falsely elevated Pa_{O_2} and Pa_{CO_2} and falsely decreased pH. In this case, corrected blood gases showed pH 7.31, Pa_{CO_2} 33 mm Hg, and Pa_{O_2} 55 mm Hg. Failure to correct for low body temperature may result in the unnecessary administration of bicarbonate, which can later result in a metabolic alkalosis once body temperature is normal. It is not uncommon for serum glucose to be high in hypothermic patients because hypothermia inhibits the release of insulin from the pancreas and decreases peripheral utilization of glucose. Hyperglycemia generally goes away with warming, and treatment with insulin runs the risk of hypoglycemia once body temperature is normal. Atropine is generally ineffective on the hypothermic heart and should be avoided unless absolutely necessary.

637. **The answer is E (all).** *(Chapter 106)* Causes of hypothermia are legion, including exposure (even in apartments heated to 21.1°C (70°F)), sepsis, drug ingestions (most commonly alcohol, barbiturates, and phenothiazines), metabolic irregularities (hypoglycemia, hypothyroidism, hypoadrenalism), and disorders of the central nervous system (cerebrovascular accident, trauma, Wernicke's encephalopathy).

638. **The answer is B (1, 3).** *(Chapter 107)* This patient is suffering from malignant hyperthermia (MH), which is characterized by features such as tachypnea, tachycardia, hyperthermia, metabolic acidosis, and hypermetabolic state. MH is a metabolic disorder of skeletal muscle that involves a loss of calcium control and a sudden rise in the myoplasmic concentration of ionized calcium. This leads to a large increase in oxygen consumption and carbon dioxide production, with lactic acidosis and muscle cell membrane damage. Inhaled anesthetic agents such as isoflurane and depolarizing neuromuscular blockers such as succinylcholine are classic triggering agents. Initial treatment of MH includes immediate discontinuation of all triggering agents and ventilation with 100% oxygen. Dantrolene is effective in treating MH and should be given as soon as possible. It is a skeletal muscle relaxant that prevents calcium release from the sarcoplasmic reticulum. Cooling measures are usually minimally effective and should not supplant the administration of dantrolene. MH is a life-threatening pharmacologic syndrome with associated complications such as disseminated intravascular coagulation and renal failure. Therefore, surgery should not proceed and the patient should be monitored closely in the ICU for at least 24 to 48 hours.

639. **The answer is B (1, 3).** *(Chapter 107)* This patient has neuroleptic malignant syndrome from the use of chlorpromazine. Manifestations include rigidity, fevers, and tachycardia in most patients. Therapy consists of discontinuing all neuroleptic and anticholinergic drugs, administering dantrolene or bromocriptine, and supportive care.

640. **The answer is C (2, 4).** *(Chapter 108)* Symptoms of "the chokes" can develop minutes to hours after ascent as gas bubbles enter the pulmonary circulation. When one is diving with compressed gas, a rapid ascent from a shallow dive can cause alveolar expansion and rupture, with the potential for arterial gas embolism. Hyperbaric oxygen within 24 to 48 hours is still the therapy of choice for gas embolism.

641. **The answer is B (1, 3).** *(Chapter 95)* The diagnosis of burn wound infection can be difficult. All burn wounds are colonized on the nonviable surface. Infection indicates

invasion of underlying viable tissue. The most reliable technique for diagnosing wound infection is full-thickness biopsy at an interface between viable and nonviable tissue, looking for histologic evidence of microbial tissue invasion. Identification of surface organisms is useful in the assessment of the effectiveness of topical antimicrobial agents. Surface cultures, even in purulent areas, do not reliably diagnose wound infection. *Staphylococcus aureus* commonly infects burn wounds in the first week.

642. **The answer is A (1, 2, 3).** *(Chapter 95)* Peak hypermetabolic state usually is seen at days 5 to 7 after a burn. Early alimentation (enteral and/or parenteral) is essential to allow wound healing in such a catabolic environment. Patients with inhalational injury often develop diffuse bronchopneumonia without chest x-ray evidence of consolidation. Antibiotic therapy for bacterial tracheobronchitis should be initiated, since such infections often progress rapidly if left untreated. Surgical procedures often are performed in the first week, since morbidity from early wound excision and closure is much lower than is the case later in the patient's hospital course. Central venous access should be avoided if possible because of the risk of line sepsis.

643. **The answer is A (1, 2, 3).** *(Chapter 99)* This patient is suffering from carbon monoxide intoxication with altered mental status and metabolic acidosis. The metabolic acidosis probably is due to inadequate tissue oxygen delivery from increased carboxyhemoglobin levels. Cyanide toxicity also may be present in a patient with smoke inhalation from a burning building. Unfortunately, both oxyhemoglobin and carboxyhemoglobin absorb light in the two wavelengths (660 nm and 940 nm) used by commercially available pulse oximeters. In fact, oximeters tend to read the sum of percentages of carboxyhemoglobin and oxyhemoglobin. The presence of carboxyhemoglobin is detected only by co-oximetry. Therefore, in this patient, carboxyhemoglobinemia would have to be excluded while other causes of metabolic acidosis were pursued. Certainly, cyanide intoxication may complicate smoke inhalation and should be evaluated. If carboxyhemoglobinemia was found, maximal oxygenation would be indicated, even to the point of intubation and hyperbaric oxygen therapy. Finally, while carboxyhemoglobinemia probably explains this patient's altered mental status, other causes, such as head trauma, or other intoxicants should be considered.

644–647. **The answers are 644-C, 645-B, 646-C, 647-C.** *(Chapters 94, 95)* Sepsis looks very much like the postburn hypermetabolic state. Both cause fever, leukocytosis, increased cardiac output, and increased oxygen consumption and carbon dioxide production. Impaired tissue oxygenation causing lactic acidosis and hypotension are not seen with hypermetabolism alone.

648–650. **The answers are 648-A, 649-B, 650-C.** *(Chapter 107)* Malignant hyperthermia (MH) and neuroleptic malignant syndrome (NMS) are life-threatening syndromes that share clinical and laboratory features such as hyperthermia, muscle rigidity, tachycardia, tachypnea, rhabdomyolysis, and hyperkalemia. MH is classically induced by inhalation anesthetics or depolarizing muscle relaxants, has a definite genetic predisposition, and is caused by a muscular abnormality. NMS is caused by neuroleptic agents and probably results from a central abnormality. A definite genetic predisposition has not been demonstrated. Early administration of dantrolene has reduced the mortality and morbidity significantly in both MH and NMS.

651–652. **The answers are 651-A, 652-D.** *(Chapter 108)* Near-drowning victims can develop rhabdomyolysis, but this is less common than ATN as far as renal complications are concerned. Human near-drowning victims rarely aspirate enough fluid to cause significant electrolyte disturbances. The 50-year-old diver demonstrates early symptoms of type 1 decompression sickness ("the bends"). He would not be expected to be at risk for either rhabdomyolysis or a severe electrolyte disturbance.

SPECIAL ANESTHESIOLOGIC AND SURGICAL MANAGEMENT IN THE PERIOPERATIVE AND PERIPARTUM PERIODS

QUESTIONS

DIRECTIONS: Each question below contains four or five suggested responses. Select the **one best** response to each question.

653. All the following criteria should be considered relative contraindications to lung resection EXCEPT

(A) diffusing capacity of carbon monoxide less than 60 percent of predicted
(B) mean pulmonary artery pressures in excess of 40 mm Hg with balloon occlusion of the pulmonary artery of the lung that will be resected
(C) resting hypercapnia
(D) predicted postoperative FEV_1 of 0.75 L in a 5-foot-tall woman
(E) metastatic cancer

654. Two days after repair of a ruptured abdominal aortic aneurysm, a 60-year-old man is noted to have fever and bloody diarrhea. Lactic acidosis and an increase in the white blood cell count to 20,000/mm³ are reported. True statements include which of the following?

(A) This is most likely a complication of antibiotic therapy
(B) This is a usual presentation of an infection of an aortic graft
(C) Surgery is not part of the management of this complication
(D) This complication is more common in emergency repair of an aortic aneurysm than it is in elective reconstruction
(E) This complication has no impact on mortality in patients with this condition

655. A 40-year-old man with a history of intravenous heroin abuse sustained a gunshot wound to the left hemithorax that required resection of the left lower lobe. Despite treatment with 20 mg of intravenous morphine in the first 2 hours postoperatively, he complained of severe chest pain. Arterial blood gases on 6 L/min of oxygen delivered by nasal cannula were pH 7.23, Pa_{CO_2} 57 mm Hg, and Pa_{O_2} 61 mm Hg. Respiratory rate was 20 breaths per minute. What would you administer next?

(A) More morphine
(B) Propofol, 1 to 3 mg/kg per hour
(C) Thoracic epidural blockade
(D) Intrathecal blockade
(E) Naloxone

656. Efforts to reduce closing volume and thus postoperative atelectasis include all the following EXCEPT

(A) reduction of pulmonary edema
(B) upright position
(C) cessation of smoking
(D) perioperative chest physiotherapy
(E) bronchodilators in patients with airways obstruction

657. A 64-year-old man with chronic obstructive pulmonary disease of the pure emphysematous type is two days postop from an open cholecystectomy. Over the past 24 hours he has noted progressive shortness of breath. An initial blood gas reveals pH 7.25, Pa_{CO_2} 70 mm Hg, and Pa_{O_2} 49 mm Hg. His respiratory rate then rises to 40 breaths per minute. He can speak only one word at a time and appears somnolent. The attending physician decides that mechanical ventilation is required. Considerations regarding the optimal ventilation of this patient would include all the following EXCEPT

(A) oxygen by face mask is contraindicated since it may suppress the patient's hypoxic drive to breathe and worsen ventilatory failure

(B) noninvasive mask ventilation should be instituted for acute-on-chronic ventilatory failure

(C) the patient should be ventilated in such a way that he supplies as much of the work of breathing as possible from the initiation of ventilation in order to avoid loss of respiratory muscle tone

(D) the pulmonary mechanical problem from the patient's pure emphysematous component of disease may not be reflected in a measurable resistive load on the ventilator

(E) correction of metabolic abnormalities may produce an increase in respiratory muscle strength

658. What is the usual physiologic response of a conscious patient in severe respiratory distress who is intubated without sedation?

(A) Tachycardia and bronchospasm followed by hypotension

(B) Tachycardia and hypertension followed by bronchospasm

(C) Tachycardia and hypertension followed by hypotension

(D) Bradycardia and hypotension followed by hypertension

(E) Bradycardia and bronchospasm followed by hypotension

Questions 659–661.

A 45-year-old woman with a 20-pack-year smoking history undergoes cholecystectomy for acute cholecystitis. The patient was extubated immediately postoperatively but several hours later was noted to become progressively more tachypneic. Physical examination reveals an obese woman with a distended abdomen who is lying flat and is in moderate respiratory distress, using accessory muscles. Vital signs are stable except for a respiratory rate of 34 breaths per minute with labored breathing and a tachycardia of 115 beats per minute. Chest examination revealed bibasilar crackles, cardiac examination showed II/VI systolic ejection murmur (SEM) but no S_3 or jugular venous distention, and abdominal examination a distended abdomen and a moderately to severely tender right upper quadrant (RUQ) in the area of her operation. There was no peripheral edema. Arterial blood gas revealed pH 7.48, Pa_{CO_2} 30 mm Hg, and Pa_{O_2} 50 mm Hg.

659. The most likely etiology of this patient's hypoxemia is

(A) pulmonary edema

(B) pulmonary embolism

(C) atelectasis

(D) pleural effusion

660. The pathophysiologic explanation underlying this patient's hypoxemia is

(A) shunting through an atrial septal defect

(B) alveolar flooding

(C) decreased functional residual capacity

(D) decreased total lung capacity

661. Which of the following therapies would be most useful in this patient's management?

(A) Vigorous diuresis

(B) Heparin

(C) Analgesia

(D) Thoracentesis

DIRECTIONS: Each question below contains four suggested responses of which **one or more** is correct. Select

A	if	**1, 2, and 3**	are correct
B	if	**1 and 3**	are correct
C	if	**2 and 4**	are correct
D	if	**4**	is correct
E	if	**1, 2, 3, and 4**	are correct

662. The risk of an intraoperative or postoperative morbid cardiac event

(1) is high in a patient who has frequent premature ventricular beats with no underlying cardiac disease

(2) can be predicted by a preoperative Holter monitor that indicates signs of ischemia

(3) is independent of ventricular function and is determined more by the risk of infarction

(4) may be predicted by a dipyridamole thallium scan in those with a moderate risk of coronary artery disease

663. Correct statements regarding epidural anesthesia include

(1) sympathetic blockade occurs with more dilute solutions

(2) accidental intrathecal injection can cause cardiovascular collapse

(3) the catheter should be placed at the spinal level approximating the center of the desired analgesic band

(4) it is often safer than general anesthesia for patients with severe cardiac or pulmonary disease

664. A 55-year-old man was admitted with a 50 percent full-thickness burn. His course in the ICU was notable for intermittent fever, hypotension, and on day 14 tenderness in the right upper quadrant. A diagnosis of acalculous cholecystitis was entertained. Which of the following tests would be helpful in making this diagnosis?

(1) Percutaneous bile aspiration for culture

(2) Ultrasound of the right upper quadrant

(3) Liver function tests

(4) Abdominal CT

665. Proposed mechanisms of improved pulmonary function after epidural blockade for thoracic surgery include

(1) relief from pain

(2) reduction of phrenophrenic inhibitory afferents

(3) relaxation of abdominal muscle tone

(4) improved diaphragmatic contractility

666. With regard to infections of vascular grafts, true statements include

(1) most infections of aortic grafts occur in the groin area

(2) infections of aortic grafts occur in less than 10 percent of cases

(3) *Staphylococcus epidermidis* is a common pathogen

(4) gram-negative organisms are rarely involved in infections of grafts

667. Correct statements regarding general principles of vascular surgery include

(1) there is a greater than 50 percent prevalence of coronary artery disease in the population under evaluation for vascular reconstruction

(2) most cases of graft thrombosis are due to technical error

(3) after vascular surgery, bleeding that requires surgical repair is uncommon

(4) in the immediate period after peripheral reconstruction, absent distal pulses and Doppler signals in the feet are poor signs

668. True statements regarding cardiac surgery include

(1) postoperative neurologic deficits may be more common in patients with diffuse atherosclerotic disease

(2) postoperative thrombocytopenia and coagulopathies often are seen in cases requiring longer than 4 hours of cardiopulmonary bypass

(3) prebypass ischemia is associated with an increased incidence of perioperative myocardial infarction

(4) desmopressin is effective in reducing bleeding after surgery

Questions 669–670.

669.   An 18-year-old woman (G_1P_0) presents at 31 weeks of gestation with complaints of headache, blurry vision, and abdominal pain. She has received no prenatal care to this point. On physical exam she is mildly lethargic but oriented to person, place, and time. Temperature is 37.0°C (98.6°F), blood pressure is 168/110, heart rate is 106, and respiratory rate is 26. Abdominal exam shows diffuse tenderness, most prominent in the right upper quadrant. She has peripheral edema in both the upper and the lower extremities. Lab findings include hemoglobin 8.8 g/dL, platelet count 36,000/mm³, AST 185 U/L, and ALT 168 U/L. Urine protein is 3+ by dipstick. Appropriate initial management steps include

(1)   aggressive control of blood pressure
(2)   avoidance of epidural anesthesia
(3)   delivery of the fetus
(4)   magnesium sulfate infusion

670.   Appropriate first-line pharmacologic management of this patient's hypertension includes

(1)   hydralazine
(2)   trimethaphan
(3)   nitroglycerin
(4)   captopril

671.   A 25-year-old woman with a previously normal pregnancy presents with premature labor at 30 weeks of gestation. Despite intravenous ritodrine therapy, labor progressed and the baby was delivered. Immediately after delivery the woman complained of dyspnea and was noted to have a respiratory rate of 40, a pulse of 145, and a blood pressure of 60/45. Lung examination revealed bilateral crackles. The most likely diagnoses include

(1)   pulmonary edema resulting from tocolytic therapy
(2)   amniotic fluid embolism
(3)   eclampsia
(4)   venous air embolism

672.   A 46-year-old man was admitted to the hospital for right leg cellulitis after a puncture wound of the right foot. He was otherwise healthy and was not taking any medications. He had no known drug allergies. His admitting doctors prescribed intravenous nafcillin. Shortly after his first dose, he noted severe shortness of breath and anxiety. Upon arrival, his doctors noted him to have a temperature of 38.1°C (100.6°F), a respiratory rate of 35, a heart rate of 125, and blood pressure of 70/40. His skin was notable for a diffuse erythematous rash. Appropriate interventions at this point include

(1)   maintenance of the airway and administration of 100% oxygen
(2)   epinephrine 0.1 mg IVP
(3)   immediate discontinuation of nafcillin
(4)   calcium chloride 200 mg IVP

DIRECTIONS: Each group of questions below consists of lettered headings followed by a set of numbered items. For each numbered item select the **one** lettered heading with which it is **most** closely associated. Each lettered heading may be used **once, more than once, or not at all.**

Questions 673–677.

For each side effect listed, select the drug with which it is most likely to be associated

(A) Vecuronium
(B) Pancuronium
(C) Atracurium
(D) Succinylcholine

673. Tachycardia

674. Hyperkalemia

675. Histamine release with bolus administration

676. Increased intracranial pressure

677. Malignant hyperthermia

Questions 678–681.

Match the descriptions below with the appropriate agent.

(A) Pancuronium
(B) Ketamine
(C) Morphine
(D) Succinylcholine
(E) None of the above

678. A depolarizing muscle relaxant that may cause hyperkalemia, bradycardia, and decreased intracranial pressure

679. A nondepolarizing muscle relaxant that may cause tachycardia

680. An intravenous anesthetic that may cause hypertension, tachycardia, bronchodilation, hallucinations, and dysphoria

681. An analgesic that may cause hypotension, respiratory depression, and bronchodilation

DIRECTIONS: Each group of questions below consists of four lettered headings followed by a set of numbered items. For each numbered item select

A   if the item is associated with   (A) **only**
B   if the item is associated with   (B) **only**
C   if the item is associated with   **both** (A) and (B)
D   if the item is associated with   **neither** (A) nor (B)

Each lettered heading may be used **once, more than once, or not at all.**

Questions 682–683.

   (A)   Regional anesthesia as opposed to general anesthesia
   (B)   Bedside spirometry and aggressive postoperative pulmonary care
   (C)   Both
   (D)   Neither

682.   A 65-year-old man who was a 15-pack-year smoker with a history of inferior wall myocardial infarction (MI) 15 years ago is to undergo a transurethral prostatectomy. He quit smoking after his MI 15 years ago and has no cardiac or pulmonary complaints. You find no cardiac or pulmonary abnormalities on physical examination. To offer clear benefit in reducing complications postoperatively, your suggestions should include

683.   A 59-year-old woman has a diagnosis of chronic obstructive pulmonary disease (COPD). Spirometry 4 years ago revealed an FEV_1 of 1.2 L. She continues to smoke and has dyspnea on exertion at two blocks and one flight of stairs. She also has been diagnosed with angina, which is well controlled with medication. She has not experienced chest pain in the last 3 weeks. To clearly minimize her perioperative complications, you would suggest

Questions 684–685.

   (A)   Sepsis
   (B)   Pregnancy
   (C)   Both
   (D)   Neither

684.   Increased cardiac output

685.   Increased systemic vascular resistance

SPECIAL ANESTHESIOLOGIC AND SURGICAL MANAGEMENT IN THE PERIOPERATIVE AND PERIPARTUM PERIODS

ANSWERS

653. The answer is D. *(Chapter 84)* While as a general guideline a predicted postoperative FEV$_1$ of 0.8 L is useful, it must be considered within the context of a given patient. If a man 74 inches tall had a predicted postoperative FEV$_1$ of 0.75 L, such a volume probably would not be adequate to support any exertion and perhaps not even spontaneous ventilation. The same FEV$_1$ in a small woman might be adequate to allow completion of minimal to moderate activities. The other criteria listed are highly predictive of postoperative respiratory (hypercapnia) or cardiac (DL$_{CO}$, PA pressure) failure.

654. The answer is D. *(Chapter 83)* Intestinal ischemia is a common complication after repair of an aortic aneurysm and is more common in the setting of repair of a ruptured aortic aneurysm. This complication increases the associated mortality. Bowel resection or revascularization may be required.

655. The answer is C. *(Chapters 10, 83)* Epidural local anesthetics can provide complete relief of pain and improve postoperative respiratory function. Selective spinal anesthesia with intrathecal injection tends to be more profound but is associated with a higher incidence of side effects. In critically ill patients, an epidural catheter is preferred. This permits repeated injections, administration of smaller incremental doses or continuous infusion, and maintenance of analgesia for prolonged periods. The use of morphine or propofol could cause respiratory depression, and naloxone might be expected to increase pain and agitation.

656. The answer is B. *(Chapters 30, 83)* Efforts to maintain airway patency and thus reduce closing volume will avoid atelectasis. These efforts include steps to reduce airway edema (reducing pulmonary edema), steps to decrease airway secretions (cessation of smoking and perioperative chest physiotherapy), and steps to decrease airway smooth muscle tone (bronchodilators). Upright position, while important in preventing postoperative atelectasis, does this by increasing functional residual capacity.

657. The answer is C. *(Chapters 30, 34, 83)* This patient most likely has respiratory failure from respiratory muscle fatigue. Postoperative pain may be contributing by causing shallow, ineffective breaths ("splinting"). This may cause hypoxemia (atelectasis) and hypercarbia (increased dead space fraction). Noninvasive ventilation is a reasonable intervention for ventilatory failure in this patient and may permit recovery from respiratory muscle fatigue without intubation. Hypoxemia should be corrected without concern about suppression of drive to breathe in this unstable patient, since it may cause significant complications (myocardial ischemia, dysrhythmias, hypoxic pulmonary vasoconstriction and right heart failure). At the outset of ventilation 24 to 48 hours of rest is necessary to restore muscle strength in most instances. The patient's obstructive lung disease will predispose him to air trapping and intrinsic PEEP. The emphysematous component of COPD results in expiratory airflow obstruction owing to dynamic airway collapse. This may not be reflected by large increases in inspiratory resistance as measured by the proximal airway pressure on the ventilator.

658. The answer is C. *(Chapter 10)* If the patient is not already maximally stressed by preexisting hypoxemia and hypercarbia, the initial response to intubation is hypertension and tachycardia. This is secondary to the sensitivity of the larynx and tongue to the pressure induced by laryngoscopy. Once the endotracheal tube is secured and mechanical ventilation is instituted, hypotension may ensue. Hypotheses to explain this hypotension include hypovolemia, the shift to positive-pressure ventilation, a sudden decrease of catecholamines as a result of diminished respiratory distress, and histamine release induced by direct laryngoscopy.

659–661. The answers are 659-C, 660-C, 661-C. *(Chapter 30)* This is a classic example of acute perioperative respiratory failure occurring secondary to atelectasis of dependent lung units. The underlying pathophysiology is a functional residual capacity (FRC) that is less than the patient's closing volume. Thus, factors that increase closing volume (age, history of smoking, overhydration) or decrease FRC (supine position, obesity, upper abdominal surgery, ascites, peritonitis) will cause atelectasis and resulting hypoxemia. Appropriate therapy includes placing the patient in an upright posture with regular turning to alter the dependent lung region, efforts to minimize elevations of abdominal pressure such as analgesia and muscle relaxants, and PEEP, which increases FRC.

662. The answer is C (2, 4). *(Chapter 84)* Preoperative Holter monitoring and dipyridamole-thallium (in at-risk groups) have been reported to be predictive of perioperative morbid cardiac events. Ventricular function has been found to be very important in assessing operative risk and may be more important than the presence of coronary artery disease. Dysrhythmias in patients with no underlying heart disease have not been found to signify perioperative risk.

663. The answer is A (1, 2, 3). *(Chapter 84)* With epidural anesthesia, neural blockade of sympathetic, sensory, and motor functions occurs at progressively increasing concentrations. Accidental intrathecal injection can result in central nervous system toxicity or cardiovascular collapse. Therefore, after checking for the presence of cerebrospinal fluid and blood, a test dose should be administered. The catheter should be placed at the spinal level approximating the center of the desired analgesic band (e.g., T4–6 after thoracotomy). Central neural blockade with epidural or spinal anesthesia is not safer in high-risk patients. Sympathetic blockade can lead to significant hemodynamic changes in patients with cardiac disease. Motor blockade of accessory muscles (abdominal muscles, intercostal muscles) leads to significant interference of respiratory function in patients with limited pulmonary reserve.

664. The answer is C (2, 4). *(Chapter 85)* Acalculous cholecystitis is a disease of chronic ICU patients and occurs in 0.5 to 1.5 percent of patients in the ICU for more than 1 week. These patients often do not have prior biliary tract disease but usually have suffered severe trauma or gastrointestinal dysfunction. It is insidious in onset, presenting with fever, tenderness of the right upper quadrant, septic hemodynamics, or multiple system organ failure. The most helpful tests are ultrasound and CT, which may show pericholecystic fluid, intramural gas, or a sloughed mucosal membrane. Percutaneous bile aspiration for culture is not helpful, as it has high false-positive and false-negative rates. Liver function tests are often abnormal, but not in a diagnostic manner.

665. The answer is A (1, 2, 3). *(Chapters 10, 83)* Thoracic epidural anesthesia decreases diaphragmatic dysfunction. Proposed mechanisms include relaxation of abdominal muscle tone, which may benefit diaphragmatic mechanics and decrease phrenophrenic inhibitory afferents. In addition, relief of pain allows for a deeper breath. There is no evidence that epidural anesthesia improves diaphragmatic contractility.

666. The answer is A (1, 2, 3). *(Chapters 83, 85)* Infections of aortic grafts are not common, and most occur in the groin. *Staphylococcus epidermidis, S. aureus,* and gram-negative organisms are the most likely pathogens.

667. The answer is A (1, 2, 3). *(Chapters 24, 83)* Given atherosclerotic disease as a cause of most obstructions that require revascularization, it is not surprising to find a high incidence of coronary artery disease in this population. Poor pulses and absent Doppler signals are common in the immediate postoperative period, when hypothermia is still present. This vasoconstriction often is relieved once normothermia is achieved. Graft thrombosis usually is ascribed to technical difficulties. Major bleeding, defined as that requiring surgical repair, is unusual after vascular procedures.

668. The answer is E (all). *(Chapters 24, 83)* Postoperative neurologic dysfunction appears to be caused by cerebral atheroemboli that possibly are related to aortic cannulation. Therefore, those with atherosclerotic disease of the aorta are at increased risk. Long periods of cardiopulmonary bypass are associated with increased platelet destruction and consumption coagulopathies. As bypass time reaches 4 hours, the risk increases substantially. Prebypass ischemia is associated with a threefold increase in the incidence of perioperative myocardial infarction. The use of desmopressin has been advocated to decrease bleeding after cardiac surgery. This effect is thought to be due to the ability of desmopressin to induce release of factor VIII and improve platelet function.

669. The answer is E (all). *(Chapter 102)* This primagravida woman is presenting with severe preeclampsia (hypertension with SBP > 160, proteinuria, and generalized edema) and HELLP syndrome (*h*emolysis, *e*levated *l*iver enzymes, *l*ow *p*latelets with RUQ tenderness). With headache and blurred vision, this patient is at high risk for progressing to eclampsia (seizures) and should be started on a magnesium sulfate infusion. With this degree of advanced disease, preparation for immediate delivery should be made. Aggressive control of blood pressure is an important component of this patient's management. Epidural anesthesia, when carefully titrated, is well tolerated in preeclampsia. Sympathetic blockade often will decrease blood pressure, and so epidural administration of a local anesthetic must be done cautiously; however, this patient's thrombocytopenia prohibits central neuraxis blockade because of the risk of epidural hematoma.

670. The answer is A (1, 2, 3). *(Chapter 102)* Hydralazine has been used extensively in pregnancy for hypertension, with an excellent record of efficacy and safety. Its vasodilating properties increase uteroplacental and renal blood flow. Trimethaphan is a ganglion-blocking agent which may be useful when cerebral edema and increased intracranial pressure are a concern because it does not cause vasodilatation of cerebral vasculature. Nitroglycerin has been used safely without compromising uteroplacental blood flow. Captopril (an ACE inhibitor) is not appropriate because it is available only in an oral form and therefore is not easily titratable. In addition, it is classified under FDA pregnancy risk category D, with known teratogenic effects.

671. The answer is C (2, 4). *(Chapter 102)* The differential diagnosis of acute pulmonary edema occurring postpartum includes tocolytic therapy, amniotic fluid embolism, eclampsia, venous air embolism, ARDS from sepsis or aspiration, and a postpartum cardiomyopathy. Amniotic fluid embolism presents as severe dyspnea during labor or soon after delivery. It is associated with circulatory collapse and pulmonary edema. Venous air embolism, while rare, presents with dyspnea, tachypnea, and tachycardia during or immediately after labor and then is followed by sudden hypotension. Tocolytic therapy is the most common cause of pulmonary edema in pregnancy, usually occurring *before* delivery. Most women have dyspnea, tachypnea, and tachycardia, which respond readily to oxygen and diuretics; circulatory collapse is rare. Eclampsia is characterized by seizures and usually is preceded by a preeclamptic phase, which consists of hypertension, proteinuria, and generalized edema.

672.   The answer is A (1, 2, 3). *(Chapter 103)*   This patient has an acute anaphylactic re-action to nafcillin. Clinical manifestations include dizziness, pruritus, tachypnea, edema of the face and upper airway, laryngeal stridor, cough, wheezing, chest tightness, and hypotension. Life-threatening reactions may include laryngeal edema, bronchospasm, and vascular collapse. Mediators such as histamine and leukotrienes induce vasodilation and translocation of fluid from capillaries, resulting in fluid loss from intravascular spaces and decreased systemic vascular resistance. Therapy is directed at maintaining the airway and oxygenation with supplemental oxygen (and intubation if necessary), ex-panding intravascular volume with fluids, and giving epinephrine to reverse hypotension and bronchospasm. Secondary treatment consists of the administration of antihistamines, aminophylline, and corticosteroids as necessary. Calcium may worsen anaphylaxis, as the release of mediators is a calcium-dependent process.

673–677.   The answers are 673-B, 674-D, 675-C, 676-D, 677-D. *(Chapter 10)*   Pancuro-nium increases heart rate, which may be dangerous in patients with ischemic heart dis-ease or arrhythmias. Atracurium, when given as a bolus, can result in the release of histamine with resulting hypotension. Cis-atracurium does not release histamine. Cis-atracurium and atracurium are the preferred agents in patients with severe renal fail-ure because they are metabolized by the Hofmann reaction (nonenzymatic degradation at body temperature and pH) and ester hydrolysis. The only clinically available depolar-izing agent is succinylcholine. Adverse effects from this drug include hyperkalemia, increased intraocular and intracranial pressures, and malignant hyperthermia. All nonde-polarizing neuromuscular blocking agents have been associated with prolonged paralysis when used in the ICU setting.

678–681.   The answers are 678-E, 679-A, 680-B, 681-E. *(Chapter 10)*   Succinylcholine is a short-acting depolarizing muscle relaxant. Side effects include cardiac arrhythmias (bradycardia, tachycardia, and ventricular premature beats), increased intracranial pres-sure, increased intraocular pressure, hyperkalemia, muscle fasciculations and pain, in-creased salivation, and increased intragastric pressure. Pretreatment with a subparalyzing dose of a nondepolarizing muscle relaxant such as *d*-tubocurarine attenuates but does not abolish the fasciculation and muscle pain as well as the rise in intragastric, intracranial, and intraocular pressures. The effectiveness of precurarization in preventing hyperkalemia is questionable. Atropine will prevent or treat the bradycardia and increased salivation.

   Pancuronium is a long-acting nondepolarizing muscle relaxant. Sinus tachycardia with or without hypertension is a common side effect. It causes little histamine release.

   Ketamine produces a dissociative mental state characterized by catalepsy, sedation, amnesia, and analgesia. Patients under ketamine anesthesia usually retain the laryngeal reflex and can maintain a patent upper airway without assistance. A rise in blood pres-sure of 20 to 40 mm Hg and an increase in heart rate of 30 to 40 beats per minute are usual, and so ketamine is contraindicated in hypertensive patients and those with ischemic heart disease. However, it is useful in patients who are hypovolemic. It is a potent bronchodilator and thus is useful in asthmatic patients. Emergence from ketamine anesthesia frequently is associated with hallucinations and dysphoria.

   Morphine is a narcotic analgesic that does not depress myocardial contractility but may cause arteriolar and venous dilatation. It may cause bronchial constriction by histamine release, though this is rare. Morphine depresses respiration and can cause nausea, vomiting, constipation, urinary retention, pupillary constriction, hyperreflexia, and convulsions.

682–683.   The answers are 682-A, 683-B. *(Chapter 84)*   Regional anesthesia has been found to reduce cardiac risk in ophthalmologic surgery and transurethral prostatectomy but not in other conditions yet. The patient has no signs of pulmonary disease and only a remote history of smoking. Therefore, pulmonary care will not predictably alter his risk of pulmonary complications.

   Spirometry has not been proved to be a good predictive test of pulmonary complica-tions, but it does help alert the clinician to the degree of pulmonary impairment. Aggressive pulmonary care in patients with pulmonary impairment has been of proven benefit in reducing complications and hospital stay even if preoperative measures that delay surgery are added.

684–685.   The answers are 684-C, 685-D.   *(Chapters 41, 42, 102)*   Sepsis is associated with a rise in cardiac output and a fall in systemic vascular resistance. The normal hemodynamic changes in pregnancy include an increase in cardiac output from a rise in both heart rate and stroke volume and a decrease in systemic vascular resistance mediated by the increased synthesis of prostacyclin and progesterone found in pregnancy. The diagnosis of sepsis in a febrile gravid patient can be confounded by the normal hemodynamic changes of pregnancy. Because of this, clinicians must be aware of situations that increase the risk of sepsis in a pregnant patient.

OVERDOSE AND POISONING

QUESTIONS

DIRECTIONS: Each question below contains four or five suggested responses. Select the **one best** response to each question.

686. Which of the following is the preferred benzodiazepine in patients with severe hepatic dysfunction?

(A) Oxazepam (Serax)
(B) Diazepam (Valium)
(C) Chlordiazepoxide (Librium)
(D) Flurazepam (Dalmane)
(E) Clorazepate (Tranxene)

687. Which of the following statements regarding opioid intoxication is true?

(A) Meperidine-induced seizures may be reversed with naloxone
(B) The triad of coma, respiratory depression, and mydriatic pupils suggests opioid intoxication
(C) A partial response to naloxone rules out the possibility of mixed agonist-antagonist opioids
(D) In extreme cases of opioid overdose, urine alkalinization, forced diuresis, and hemodialysis may be considered
(E) While unpleasant, acute narcotic withdrawal is seldom life-threatening in adult patients

688. The major cause of death from organophosphate poisoning is

(A) respiratory failure
(B) cardiac arrhythmias
(C) intractable seizures
(D) acute renal failure
(E) liver failure

689. A 24-year-old woman attempted suicide by ingesting an unknown substance. Which of the following signs would be most suggestive of organophosphate poisoning?

(A) Bronchorrhea
(B) Salivation
(C) Miosis
(D) Muscle fasciculations
(E) Involuntary urination

690. All the following statements regarding flumazenil, a benzodiazepine receptor antagonist, are true EXCEPT

(A) it can reverse both the respiratory depressant and sedative effects of some benzodiazepines
(B) it can be given only parenterally
(C) it may reduce the need for procedures such as CT of the head
(D) it may cause tachycardia, hypertension, and arrhythmias in patients who respond
(E) it may unmask the adverse effects of other drugs in a mixed overdose

691. A 28-year-old man arrives at a U.S. customs office in Chicago and is noted to be confused and to have generalized tremor of his hands. He vomits onto the customs officer and passes out. He is now admitted to your ICU. His blood pressure is 200/110 mm Hg, heart rate is 120 beats per minute, and temperature is 36.7°C (98.1°F). His cardiopulmonary examination is otherwise unremarkable. His neurologic examination is remarkable for confusion, mydriasis, and tremors. You should now

(A) perform a gastric lavage after intubation
(B) administer naloxone
(C) perform CT of the head
(D) administer physostigmine intravenously

692. A 16-year-old boy is admitted to the intensive care unit for close monitoring after a bite from a black widow spider. Potential complications include all the following EXCEPT

(A) hemolytic anemia
(B) hypertension
(C) respiratory insufficiency
(D) hypotension
(E) cardiac arrhythmias

Questions 693–695.

A 28-year-old farmer with a history of asthma was in his usual state of excellent health until 2 hours before admission, when he noted the onset of a nonproductive cough, weakness, and mild dyspnea on exertion. His symptoms began approximately 5 hours after working in a recently filled grain silo. He denied detecting any distinctive odors while working in the silo. Physical examination was notable for a respiratory rate of 24 breaths per minute, unlabored, and mild end-expiratory wheezing. His chest x-ray was notable for mild hyperinflation and peribronchial cuffing. Room air arterial blood gas measurements revealed pH 7.38, Pa_{CO_2} 30 mm Hg, and Pa_{O_2} 75 mm Hg.

693. While in the emergency room, the patient received inhaled β agonists and a theophylline infusion. Within minutes of treatment, he developed worsening shortness of breath, nausea, headache, and light-headedness. Physical examination was notable for slight lethargy and moderate respiratory distress with the use of accessory muscles. Blood pressure was 105/60, heart rate 118, respiratory rate 36, and temperature 40.2°C (104.4°F). Lung examination revealed mild to moderate expiratory wheezing and crackles over the lower two-thirds of the lung fields bilaterally. Cardiac examination was notable for a II/VI systolic ejection murmur. Extremities were warm, with good capillary refill. White blood cell count was 19,300 with 6 percent band forms. Room air arterial blood gas showed pH 7.20, Pa_{CO_2} 28 mm Hg, and Pa_{O_2} 40 mm Hg. Chest x-ray is shown below. The most likely etiology of this patient's symptoms is

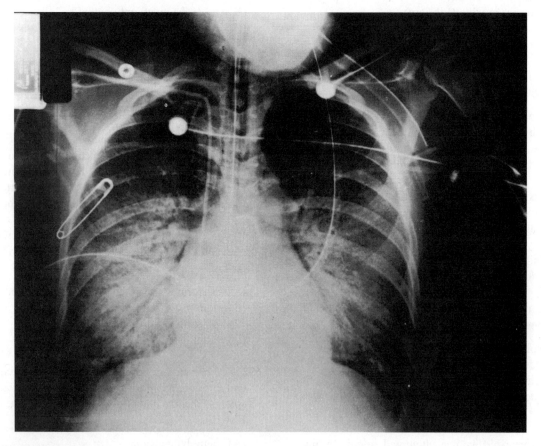

(A) allergic drug reaction
(B) nitrogen dioxide exposure
(C) acute myocarditis with cardiogenic pulmonary edema
(D) extrinsic allergic alveolitis
(E) bacterial bronchopneumonia

694. The most appropriate initial management would be to

(A) admit the patient to the hospital
(B) treat the bronchospasm and discharge arranging for follow-up in several days
(C) order a ventilation-perfusion scan
(D) administer heparin

695. The patient remained hypoxemic despite the application of a 100% nonrebreather face mask. He was intubated and required sedation because of an inability to coordinate with the ventilator. After several hours on an FIo$_2$ of 0.6 and PEEP of 5, the arterial blood gas showed pH 7.23, Paco$_2$ 35 mm Hg, and Pao$_2$ 75 mm Hg. Vital signs and the remainder of the physical examination remained unchanged. Blood chemistries were notable for an anion gap acidosis and normal creatinine and glucose. Optimal management of this patient's metabolic acidosis might include

(A) administration of dobutamine
(B) administration of methylene blue
(C) administration of bicarbonate
(D) administration of antibiotics
(E) increasing minute volume

Questions 696–697.

An 18-year-old woman arrives in the intensive care unit 20 minutes after ingesting an unknown amount of concentrated alkali. She is complaining of "burning in my mouth," a severe retrosternal "ache," difficulty swallowing, and dizziness. She denies vomiting, hematemesis, or difficulty breathing. Physical examination is notable for blood pressure of 89/72 mm Hg, heart rate of 135 beats per minute, respiratory rate of 26 breaths per minute (unlabored), and temperature of 37°C (98.6°F). Her skin is cool and clammy, and her oropharyngeal mucosa is severely inflamed and burned.

696. Appropriate initial management might include

(A) gastric lavage
(B) neutralization with a weak acid
(C) activated charcoal
(D) washout with milk mixed with egg white

697. Six hours after initial therapy in the emergency room, chest x-rays are taken (shown below). Of the following, the diagnosis most consistent with this clinical scenario is

(A) subdiaphragmatic abscess
(B) trauma
(C) esophageal perforation
(D) pancreatitis

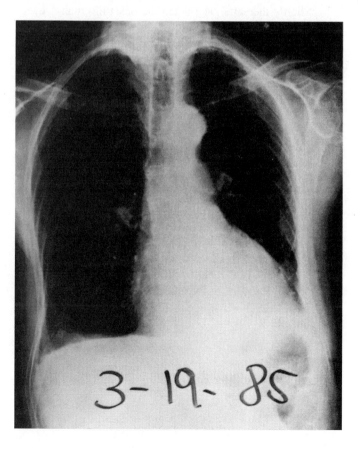
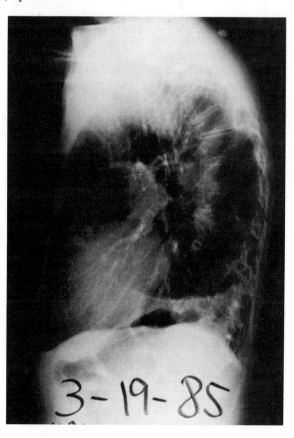

DIRECTIONS: Each question below contains four suggested responses of which **one or more** is correct. Select

A	if	**1, 2, and 3**	are correct
B	if	**1 and 3**	are correct
C	if	**2 and 4**	are correct
D	if	**4**	is correct
E	if	**1, 2, 3, and 4**	are correct

698. In a suicidal gesture, a 24-year-old black man ingested an unknown quantity of isoniazid (INH). The patient's mother states that she and her son have a "blood abnormality" and that she has a list of medications and foods they must avoid. The man is alert and in no acute distress. His vital signs reveal a regular heart rate of 120 beats per minute and a respiratory rate of 28 breaths per minute, unlabored. His mucous membranes and skin are pale, gray, and cyanotic. Accompanying findings might include

(1) elevated reticulocyte count
(2) chocolate-brown-colored blood
(3) decreased oxyhemoglobin saturation
(4) normal arterial Pa_{O_2}

Questions 699–701.

A 35-year-old, 100-kg man is brought to the emergency room 15 hours after he has swallowed approximately 1.5 g of amitriptyline. He is now admitted to the ICU.

699. His management should include

(1) activated charcoal
(2) ECG monitoring
(3) maintenance of serum pH 7.45 to 7.55
(4) forced diuresis

700. Cardiac arrhythmias associated with cyclic antidepressant overdose include

(1) torsade de pointes
(2) ventricular fibrillation
(3) bradycardia and asystole
(4) multifocal atrial tachycardia

701. His symptoms can include

(1) miosis
(2) urinary retention
(3) diarrhea
(4) hyperthermia

702. True statements about cocaine intoxication include

(1) it is the leading cause of illicit-drug-related emergency department visits
(2) benzodiazepines should be used for cocaine-related agitation and seizures
(3) it is the second leading cause of drug-related deaths
(4) cocaine-related fatalities generally occur within 4 hours of drug ingestion

703. Potential complications of inhalations of toxic gas include

(1) upper airway obstruction
(2) lactic acidosis without hypoxemia
(3) pneumonia
(4) bronchiolitis obliterans

704. While cleaning her bathroom, a 28-year-old woman with an unremarkable past medical history mixed a chlorine bleach (Clorox) with her toilet-bowl cleaner. Shortly thereafter, she noted the onset of "runny" eyes, "burning" throat, a nonproductive cough, a "choking sensation," and minimal wheezing. Physical examination was notable only for oropharyngeal erythema and mild, intermittent end-expiratory wheezing. A list of the potential complications of this patient's illness includes

(1) upper airway obstruction
(2) bronchospasm
(3) pulmonary edema
(4) atelectasis

705. A 35-year-old man is brought to the emergency room in a coma after being rescued from a fire. On examination he was noted to be unresponsive. His face and oral mucosa were charred. His pulse was 45, and his blood pressure was 85/50. Arterial blood gas on room air revealed pH 6.95, Pa_{CO_2} 35 mm Hg, and Pa_{O_2} 75 mm Hg with a carboxyhemoglobin level of 25 percent. His lactate level was 8 mg/dL. Appropriate measures include

(1) oxygen
(2) thiosulfate
(3) hydroxocobalamin
(4) sodium nitrite

Questions 706–707.

A 73-year-old man who has severe osteoarthritis presents with disorientation. Room air arterial blood gases show pH 7.35, Pa_{CO_2} 29 mm Hg, and Pa_{O_2} 90 mm Hg.

706.   Possible diagnoses include

(1)   urosepsis
(2)   carbon monoxide poisoning
(3)   salicylate toxicity
(4)   central nervous system infection

707.   Two hours later, the patient is more lethargic. Arterial blood gases show pH 7.25, Pa_{CO_2} 36 mm Hg, and Pa_{O_2} 65 mm Hg. The salicylate level is 50 mg/dL. Appropriate interventions at this time include

(1)   intravenous bicarbonate
(2)   acetazolamide to alkalinize the urine
(3)   intubation and mechanical ventilation
(4)   syrup of ipecac

708.   Clinical findings in patients with salicylate toxicity include

(1)   hyperpyrexia
(2)   oliguria
(3)   cerebral edema
(4)   wide QRS complex

709.   A 13-year-old girl presents 9 hours after ingesting an unknown amount of medications, including acetaminophen. Further therapy should include

(1)   administration of *N*-acetylcysteine immediately
(2)   administration of activated charcoal
(3)   determination of acetaminophen level
(4)   administration of cimetidine

710.   True statements about phencyclidine (PCP) overdose include which of the following?

(1)   Assays to confirm ingestion are not available
(2)   Haloperidol and droperidol are the tranquilizers of choice
(3)   Activated charcoal plays no role in the management of these patients and only carries a potential for harm
(4)   Nystagmus is a helpful finding and suggests this ingestion

Questions 711–712.

A 25-year-old asthmatic was admitted to the ICU with mental confusion and agitation. Earlier that day he was at a picnic and was seen tasting different plants, including jimson weed. On admission to the ICU his blood pressure is 165/95 mm Hg, respirations are 15 per minute and unlabored, and ECG demonstrates a sinus tachycardia at a rate of 125 beats per minute. Physical examination reveals flushed extremities, mydriasis, and dry mucous membranes. He remains quite agitated.

711.   Therapeutic interventions should include

(1)   chlorpromazine (Thorazine)
(2)   naloxone
(3)   β blockers
(4)   benzodiazepines

712.   After 1 hour the patient suddenly has a grand mal seizure of 30 seconds' duration and becomes unresponsive. Interventions at this time should include

(1)   administer 2 mg physostigmine intravenously over at least 2 minutes
(2)   place a central line
(3)   continue to observe the patient with no further intervention unless the seizure recurs
(4)   intubate the patient

713.   A 25-year-old man is admitted to the ICU after a rattlesnake bite in his left forearm. On examination, his forearm is swollen and his fingers are slightly cyanotic. He complains of severe pain and numbness in his left hand and fingers. His management now should include

(1)   elevation of the left arm
(2)   mannitol, 2 g/kg intravenously over 30 minutes
(3)   antivenin (Crotalidae) polyvalent, 10 to 15 vials intravenously over 60 minutes
(4)   emergent fasciotomy

714.   In snake bites, antivenin (Crotalidae) polyvalent is indicated if

(1)   there is a worsening platelet and hemoglobin count
(2)   compartment syndrome develops
(3)   hypotension develops
(4)   there is development of systemic signs

715. Which of the following are clinical manifestations of methanol ingestion?

(1) Severe anion gap acidosis
(2) Osmolar gap
(3) Visual difficulties
(4) Acute tubular necrosis

716. Complications of organophosphate poisoning that should be anticipated include

(1) hypoglycemia
(2) complete heart block
(3) torsade de pointes
(4) respiratory muscle weakness

717. Measures recommended in the treatment of organophosphate poisoning include

(1) washing of skin with mild alkaline soap and water
(2) administration of aminophylline
(3) administration of obidoxime or pralidoxime
(4) administration of scopolamine

718. A 42-year-old man was admitted 6 hours after ingesting 40 mL of a 20% concentrate of paraquat. The patient complained of burning in his mouth and throat, substernal chest discomfort, dysphagia, odynophagia, crampy abdominal pain, nausea, vomiting, and mild dyspnea on exertion. Physical examination was notable for a respiratory rate of 20, erythema of both arms, conjunctivitis, oral ulcers, and a lung examination that demonstrated bibasilar crackles. Laboratory data showed potassium 3.0, BUN 45, creatinine 3.1, and arterial blood gas values of pH 7.30, Pa_{O_2} 55 mm Hg, and Pa_{CO_2} 32 mm Hg. Chest x-ray showed bibasilar infiltrates. Appropriate initial management would include

(1) activated charcoal
(2) oxygen
(3) hemoperfusion
(4) gastric lavage and ipecac

DIRECTIONS: The group of questions below consists of lettered headings followed by a set of numbered items. For each numbered item select the **one** lettered heading with which it is **most** closely associated. Each lettered heading may be used **once, more than once, or not at all.**

Questions 719–722.

Match the ethanol withdrawal syndromes with times of onset after the cessation of drinking.

(A) 6 to 8 hours
(B) 7 to 48 hours
(C) 24 to 72 hours
(D) 3 to 5 days

719. Common abstinence syndrome

720. Delirium tremens

721. Alcoholic ketoacidosis

722. Seizures

DIRECTIONS: Each group of questions below consists of four lettered headings followed by a set of numbered items. For each numbered item select

A	if the item is associated with	(A) **only**
B	if the item is associated with	(B) **only**
C	if the item is associated with	**both** (A) and (B)
D	if the item is associated with	**neither** (A) nor (B)

Each lettered heading may be used **once, more than once, or not at all.**

Questions 723–724.

    (A) Tachycardia
    (B) Pupillary dilation
    (C) Both
    (D) Neither

723. A 32-year-old man presents to the emergency room with a history of hallucinations. A friend states that the patient has been a consumer of amphetamines. Which of the above signs would be consistent with amphetamine ingestion?

724. A 30-year-old woman is reported to have ingested large quantities of belladonna for a gastrointestinal condition. She is experiencing visual hallucinations and does not have a prior history of psychiatric illness. The patient has dry, flushed skin. Which of the above signs would you expect?

Questions 725–727.

    (A) Cocaine toxicity
    (B) Opioid toxicity
    (C) Both
    (D) Neither

725. Myocardial infarction

726. Pulmonary edema

727. Hypotension

Questions 728–731.

Regarding adverse drug reactions

    (A) Drug fever
    (B) Anaphylactic or anaphylactoid reaction
    (C) Both
    (D) Neither

728. Amphotericin B

729. Penicillin G

730. Phenytoin

731. Vecuronium

Questions 732–733.

    (A) Phenobarbital overdose
    (B) Meprobamate overdose
    (C) Both
    (D) Neither

732. Urinary alkalinization is helpful

733. Activated charcoal is helpful

OVERDOSE AND POISONING

ANSWERS

686. The answer is A. *(Chapter 99)* Oxazepam and lorazepam (Ativan) are short-acting benzodiazepines that are metabolized in the liver by glucuronidation and have no active metabolites. In general, sedatives should be used with caution in patients with hepatic dysfunction.

687. The answer is E. *(Chapter 99)* Acute opioid withdrawal in adults usually is not life-threatening. The fear of inducing opioid withdrawal should not deter the use of antagonists in the treatment of opioid intoxication. The increased incidence of seizures associated with meperidine use can be attributed to accumulation of the active metabolite, normeperidine. Naloxone is ineffective in the prevention or treatment of normeperidine-related seizures. The triad of coma, respiratory depression, and *miotic* pupils suggests opioid intoxication. A partial response to the opioid antagonist naloxone should prompt the intensivist to consider mixed agonist-antagonist opioids, mixed ingestions with other CNS depressants, and the possibility of a coexistent medical or surgical condition. Urine alkalinization, forced diuresis, and hemodialysis are not indicated in the management of opioid intoxication.

688. The answer is A. *(Chapter 99)* Although all the listed conditions may result from organophosphate poisoning, respiratory failure, often from aspiration pneumonitis, is the leading cause of death.

689. The answer is D. *(Chapter 99)* Muscle fasciculations, which are rare in other intoxications, should always suggest organophosphate poisoning.

690. The answer is B. *(Chapter 99)* Flumazenil is a benzodiazepine antagonist that reverses both the respiratory depressant and the sedative effects of benzodiazepines. It can result in a "catecholamine rush" not unlike that seen with naloxone, causing hypertension, tachycardia, and arrhythmias. It may unmask the adverse effects of coingested drugs, and it may be given by both the oral and intravenous routes.

691. The answer is A. *(Chapter 99)* This drug smuggler panicked and swallowed a bag of cocaine, which burst in his stomach. Therapy at this point should include gastric lavage, activated charcoal, and cathartics. The patient has mydriasis rather than miosis, and naloxone is not indicated.

692. The answer is A. *(Chapter 99)* Hemolytic anemia is a potential life-threatening complication of violin or brown recluse spider bites. It is not seen with black widow bites. Respiratory insufficiency, cardiovascular instability manifested as both hypertension and hypotension, and cardiac arrhythmias may all occur in patients with black widow spider bites.

693. The answer is B. *(Chapter 99)* The chest x-ray is consistent with pulmonary edema, either cardiac or noncardiac. With the temporal relation of this patient's symptoms to his working in a grain silo, the most likely diagnosis is noncardiac pulmonary edema secondary to exposure to nitrogen dioxide.

694. The answer is A. *(Chapter 99)* This patient was working in a recently filled silo with the potential of exposure to nitrogen dioxide. Although nitrogen dioxide is a reddish-brown gas with a distinctive sweet odor, it may be trapped in pockets below the grain surface. Thus, even an alert worker may be unaware of the presence of this gas. The onset of respiratory symptoms is typically delayed for 3 to 30 hours, and chest x-rays may be initially normal. Particularly with the tachypnea, hypoxemia, and metabolic acidosis, significant exposure to nitrogen dioxide should be assumed in this patient, and he should be observed closely for at least 48 hours.

695. The answer is B. *(Chapter 99)* The patient has a significant anion gap metabolic acidosis with normal Pa_{O_2}, glucose, and creatinine values. The physical examination rules out cardiogenic shock, and there is no reason to suspect a toxin exposure or sepsis. The toxicity resulting from nitrogen dioxide exposure may be complicated by the systemic absorption of nitrates and nitrites, which might produce methemoglobinemia. Since methemoglobin is not useful for carrying oxygen and has an increased affinity for oxygen, decreased oxygen delivery and subsequent anaerobic metabolism and lactic acidosis result. This occurs in the presence of a normal Pa_{O_2}. Measured oxygen saturation is reduced; however, if the laboratory calculates oxygen saturation from Pa_{O_2} levels rather than directly measuring saturation, this finding will be missed. In this patient, one should measure methemoglobin level. A significant level is greater than 30 percent. The therapy of choice for methemoglobinemia is the administration of methylene blue.

696. The answer is D. *(Chapter 99)* The emergency treatment of corrosive ingestion consists of dilution and washout with fluids. The time element of dilution is more important than the choice of the fluid. Therefore, if water is readily available, it should be used, although milk mixed with egg white is a better choice since it dilutes and buffers as well. Fluid washout is effective if it is delivered immediately after ingestion (less than 2 minutes) and is of questionable value after 30 minutes. Induced emesis, gastric lavage, and activated charcoal administration are contraindicated, as is neutralization. Neutralization generates an exothermic reaction, with resultant tissue damage and possible gas emission.

697. The answer is C. *(Chapter 99)* The major complications of corrosive ingestions are esophageal, gastric, or small bowel perforation; gastrointestinal hemorrhage; and upper airway obstruction. With alkali, most of the damage occurs in the esophagus. In this setting, a left-sided pleural effusion should raise the possibility of esophageal perforation.

698. The answer is E (all). *(Chapter 99)* With the family history of a similar "blood abnormality" and a list of medications and foods to avoid, one needs to consider that this patient may have glucose 6-phosphate dehydrogenase (G6PD) deficiency. INH is one of the medications that can cause methemoglobinemia and hemolysis in this group of patients. Above a methemoglobin level of 15 percent, a gray cyanosis appears on the skin and mucous membranes. Above 30 percent, tachycardia and tachypnea occur. The diagnosis is confirmed by the chocolate-brown color of venous or arterial blood. Arterial blood gas analysis by a spectrophotometric method demonstrates an increased methemoglobin concentration, decreased oxyhemoglobin saturation, and a normal Pa_{O_2}.

699. The answer is A (1, 2, 3). *(Chapter 99)* General management principles in cyclic antidepressant overdose include early intravenous access, activated charcoal, monitoring of QRS duration, early intubation and mechanical ventilation, gastric lavage if the airway is protected, and maintenance of serum pH between 7.45 and 7.55. There is no role for diuresis or dialysis.

700. The answer is A (1, 2, 3). *(Chapter 99)* Cardiac arrhythmias in cyclic antidepressant overdose are supraventricular and ventricular tachycardias, torsade de pointes, ventricular fibrillation, advanced heart block, bradycardia, and asystole.

701. **The answer is C (2, 4).** *(Chapter 99)* Anticholinergic crisis in cyclic antidepressant overdose can present as mydriasis, blurred vision, urinary retention, dry mucous membranes, constipation, ileus, sinus tachycardia, hyperthermia or hypothermia, confusion, agitation, and hallucinations.

702. **The answer is A (1, 2, 3).** *(Chapter 99)* In the United States, cocaine is the number one cause of drug-related emergency department visits and the number two cause of drug-related deaths. Treatment of cocaine involves initial cardiopulmonary stabilization and close observation for potential complications. The use of benzodiazepines such as diazepam is indicated in the treatment of cocaine-related agitation, seizures, and hyperadrenergic states. A particular challenge in the management of cocaine intoxication is the fact that cocaine-related fatalities often do not occur in close temporal relationship to ingestion. Serious complications of cocaine intoxication, including death, may occur up to 24 hours after ingestion.

703. **The answer is E (all).** *(Chapter 99)* Inhaled toxins such as methane can cause asphyxia by replacing atmospheric oxygen. They also can cause tissue hypoxia and resulting lactic acidosis by interfering with tissue oxygen delivery or utilization. Cyanide and carbon monoxide can do this in the presence of a normal arterial Pa_{O_2}. Airborne chemicals can cause bronchospasm, mucous hypersecretion, and direct injury to airway epithelium, with the last resulting in loss of normal ciliary activity, loss of the normal barrier against microbial invasion, airway edema, and airway obstruction and atelectasis from luminal plugging with sloughed epithelial cells. These effects play a prominent role in the upper and lower airway obstruction and the high incidence of pulmonary infection that follow acute inhalation of toxic gas. Inhaled toxins also can cause injury to bronchiolar epithelium, alveolar lining cells, vascular endothelium, and airspace macrophages. The result may be noncardiac pulmonary edema and, in a small minority, bronchiolitis obliterans.

704. **The answer is E (all).** *(Chapter 99)* Clorox contains sodium hypochlorite, while toilet-bowl cleaners are slightly acidic. Mixing chlorine bleaches with weak acids (vinegar is another example) liberates chlorine gas. Acute effects of exposure to chlorine gas include lacrimation, conjunctival irritation, rhinorrhea, cough, headache, sore throat, chest pain, dyspnea, and nausea. Airway injury may result in bronchospasm, hoarseness, stridor, upper airway obstruction, and atelectasis. Severe exposures may progress to tracheobronchitis, noncardiac pulmonary edema, and respiratory failure. Corneal abrasions and cutaneous burns also result from direct exposure. Symptoms usually begin within minutes of exposure, and asymptomatic patients may be safely triaged at the exposure site without fear of delayed development of symptoms.

705. **The answer is A (1, 2, 3).** *(Chapter 99)* The patient has suffered from smoke inhalation as evidenced by his singed oral mucosa and elevated carbon monoxide level. Coma, bradycardia, and lactic acidosis occur in cyanide poisoning and should prompt a search for this entity, since as many as 30 percent of domestic fire victims suffering from smoke inhalation also have high levels of cyanides. A whole blood cyanide level should be measured, and treatment should be begun with oxygen, sodium thiosulfate, and hydroxocobalamin, which are safe and proven antidotes to cyanide poisoning. The induction of methemoglobinemia with sodium nitrite or amyl nitrite is contraindicated in cases of smoke inhalation because the desired methemoglobinemia, together with the observed carboxyhemoglobinemia, decreases the oxygen-carrying capacity.

706. **The answer is E (all).** *(Chapter 99)* The diagnostic possibilities are many in elderly patients with respiratory alkalosis and metabolic acidosis and include all those listed. A history of osteoarthritis especially raises the possibility of chronic salicylate toxicity.

707. **The answer is B (1, 3).** *(Chapter 99)* In patients with salicylate toxicity, acidemia must be avoided because it enhances tissue penetration by salicylates. Blood pH should be corrected to above 7.30 with sodium bicarbonate. Alkalinization of the urine (if possible to pH 8 to 8.5) enhances renal excretion. Hypokalemia must be aggressively treated to achieve urinary alkalinization. Carbonic anhydrase inhibitors should not be used to alkalinize the urine because they may result in metabolic acidosis. Early intubation and mechanical ventilation are indicated in patients who are tiring or have progressive acidemia from increased Pa_{CO_2} or lactic acidosis. Emesis should not be induced in obtunded patients.

708.   The answer is E (all).   *(Chapter 99)*   Clinical findings of salicylate poisoning are many, including neurologic abnormalities, acid-base disturbances, pulmonary edema, fever, hypotension, ECG abnormalities (such as wide QRS and first- and second-degree AV block), coagulation disorders, renal failure, cerebral edema, hypoglycemia, and GI bleeding.

709.   The answer is A (1, 2, 3).   *(Chapter 99)*   Acetaminophen intoxication often is clinically silent on presentation. Therapy with *N*-acetylcysteine is most effective when initiated within the first 8 hours; therefore, it should not be administered if the ingestion is fairly remote. An acetaminophen level should be measured to assess the need for further therapy. Activated charcoal will remove residual acetaminophen from the gut and should be administered. Coincident charcoal and *N*-acetylcysteine administration does not seem to reduce the efficacy of the *N*-acetylcysteine. Cimetidine has not been shown to diminish hepatotoxicity when administered with *N*-acetylcysteine.

710.   The answer is C (2, 4).   *(Chapter 99)*   PCP overdose can be confirmed by urine assays, and activated charcoal may be helpful in binding ingested drug. Horizontal, vertical, and rotary nystagmus may be present, with seizures, muscular rigidity, violent behavior, and analgesia also reported. Urinary acidification is controversial for enhancing drug elimination with PCP.

711.   The answer is C (2, 4).   *(Chapter 99)*   The patient is suffering from an anticholinergic crisis caused by jimson weed. The typical patient has been described as "mad as a hatter, hot as a hare, dry as a bone, red as a beet, and blind as a bat." Agitation is best treated by benzodiazepines. Neuroleptics have anticholinergic effects and should not be used. Any patient who presents with mental confusion and mydriasis should be given naloxone to uncover opiate toxicity.

712.   The answer is D (4).   *(Chapter 99)*   Patients with anticholinergic syndromes (ACS) can develop seizures. The cholinergic stimulation associated with physostigmine may cause bradyarrhythmias, asystole, and seizures. Its use should be restricted to patients with life-threatening ACS that is unresponsive to conservative therapies. Physostigmine is contraindicated in asthma, peripheral vascular disease, bowel obstruction, urinary obstruction, and gangrene. Intubation may prevent aspiration of gastric contents.

713.   The answer is A (1, 2, 3).   *(Chapter 99)*   Elevated compartment pressure in envenomation is caused by the action of the venom on the tissues. Consequently, the most effective treatment is to neutralize the venom, which in most cases reduces the compartment pressure. Intracompartmental pressure should be measured, and if elevated compartment pressure (> 30 mm Hg) persists over 1 hour, fasciotomy should be considered.

714.   The answer is E (all).   *(Chapter 99)*   Antivenin polyvalent is recommended in envenomations that show evidence of poisoning and progression. Progression is indicated by an increase in local pain, ecchymosis, and swelling; falling platelet counts; a falling hematocrit; prolongation of clotting times; mental status changes; or the development of unstable vital signs. In addition, antivenin is recommended for life-threatening poisoning and in compartment syndrome.

715.   The answer is A (1, 2, 3). *(Chapter 99)*   Methanol ingestion should be considered in any patient who presents with a severe metabolic acidosis characterized by significant anion and osmolar gaps. Visual disturbances are common findings in methanol ingestion that may progress to blindness if not treated promptly. Acute tubular necrosis is a relatively common finding in many ingestions, including ethylene glycol, but is rarely seen as a direct result of methanol toxicity.

716.   The answer is E (all). *(Chapter 99)*   The major cause of death in organophosphate poisoning is respiratory failure resulting from muscle weakness, depressed drive, bronchoconstriction, bronchorrhea, or aspiration pneumonia. Brady- and tachyarrhythmias are the second most common cause of death. Whenever the QT interval exceeds half the RR interval, the ICU staff should be ready to insert an emergency temporary pacemaker. Hypo- and hyperglycemia, pancreatitis, rhabdomyolysis, acute nonoliguric renal failure, liver dysfunction, delayed peripheral neuropathy, and regression psychosis are other potential complications.

717.   The answer is B (1, 3). *(Chapter 99)*   Organophosphate compounds are absorbed through the skin and are hydrolyzed in an alkaline pH. Thus, removal of clothes and washing of skin with mild alkaline soap and water are recommended in all such intoxications. Organophosphate compounds are well adsorbed by activated charcoal. Bronchospasm, bronchorrhea, and bradycardia are treated by parenteral administration of atropine. Scopolamine, a centrally acting anticholinergic drug, is not recommended because of its narrow toxic-to-therapeutic range. Benzodiazepines are recommended for the control of convulsions and agitation. Aminophylline probably should not be given since hypoxemia and ventricular arrhythmias are common. Oximes reactivate acetylcholinesterase and are useful in serious poisonings.

718.   The answer is B (1, 3). *(Chapter 99)*   The decision to induce emesis and perform lavage must take into account the benefits versus the risks of esophageal injury and perforation. In this patient, the long time since ingestion, the presence of spontaneous vomiting, and the presence of oral ulcers argue against the use of gastric lavage and ipecac. Activated charcoal effectively binds paraquat and should be used in all ingestions. Although the effectiveness of hemoperfusion has not been confirmed, it is theoretically most useful when started within 15 to 20 hours of ingestion in the presence of renal failure. Forced diuresis, hemodialysis, and peritoneal dialysis are not recommended. Supplemental oxygen potentiates paraquat-induced pulmonary fibrosis and should not be used unless Pa_{O_2} is less than 50 mm Hg.

719–722.   The answers are 719-A, 720-D, 721-C, 722-B. *(Chapter 99)*   The common abstinence syndrome, occurring at 6 to 8 hours, is the earliest withdrawal syndrome and often is present when the patient awakens. Seizures typically appear at 7 to 48 hours and are usually single rather than recurrent. Alcoholic ketoacidosis is seen slightly later at 24 to 72 hours. Delirium tremens is usually seen at 3 to 5 days but occasionally is seen as late as 14 days. Knowledge of this timing is useful in that it may aid in the differential diagnosis. For example, the presence of agitation, delirium, and tachycardia on admission the morning after the cessation of drinking is unlikely to be delirium tremens and should prompt a diagnostic evaluation.

723–724.   The answers are 723-C, 724-C. *(Chapter 99)*   Tachycardia and pupillary dilation are signs seen with ingestions that cause excess sympathomimetic activity or anticholinergic activity. The finding of dry skin and mucous membranes is a helpful sign in implicating an anticholinergic effect and would indicate that drugs with further anticholinergic activity, such as haloperidol and phenothiazines, would be best avoided in the management of agitation.

725–727. **The answers are 725-A, 726-C, 727-C.** *(Chapter 99)* Cocaine may induce myocardial infarction in patients with or without coronary artery disease. The pathogenesis of cocaine-induced infarction involves increased myocardial oxygen demand with decreased coronary artery perfusion. The role of coronary artery vasospasm has not been proved. Opioids have not been shown to substantially increase the risk of myocardial infarction and may in fact decrease the incidence of myocardial infarction in patients at risk by blunting sympathetic discharges associated with pain. Hypoxemia in patients with opioid toxicity is usually secondary to alveolar hypoventilation. An abnormal alveolar-arterial oxygen gradient in a patient with opioid toxicity should raise concerns about opioid-induced noncardiogenic pulmonary edema. Pulmonary complications of cocaine toxicity include alveolar hemorrhage, pulmonary infarct, hypersensitivity pneumonitis, BOOP, and acute pulmonary edema. Hypotension is a common complication of opioid use caused by peripheral vasodilation. Cocaine intoxication usually is associated with hypertension. The exception is seen in severe intoxication in which circulatory collapse is the major concern.

728–731. **The answers are 728-C, 729-C, 730-A, 731-B.** *(Chapters 40, 99, 102)* Adverse drug reactions contribute significantly to morbidity and mortality in a critically ill patient. Antibiotics are a common cause of adverse drug reactions, including fever and anaphylaxis. Amphotericin B and penicillin G may both cause fever and anaphylaxis in a given patient. High fevers may result from hypersensitivity to phenytoin. Neuromuscular blockers such as vecuronium have been implicated in the development of anaphylaxis. Febrile responses to vecuronium have not been widely reported.

732–733. **The answers are 732-A, 733-C.** *(Chapter 99)* The treatment of sedative hypnotic drug overdose is supportive. There are no antidotes for these drugs. As a result of decreased gastrointestinal motility and delayed gastric emptying, gut decontamination with lavage and activated charcoal may lessen toxicity. Forced alkaline diuresis aids in the elimination of longer-acting barbiturates (phenobarbital).

NOTES

NOTES

NOTES

NOTES

NOTES

NOTES

NOTES

NOTES

NOTES

ISBN 0-07-052294-4

90000

9 780070 522947